SYSTEMIC PATHOLOGY / THIRD EDITION

Volume 1   Nose, Throat and Ears

SYSTEMIC PATHOLOGY / THIRD EDITION

General Editor

W. St C. Symmers

MD(Belf), PhD(Birm), DSc(Lond), FRCP(Lond, Irel, Ed), FRCS(Eng), FACP(Hon), FRCPA(Hon), FRCPath, FFPathRCPI

Emeritus Professor of Pathology, University of London; Honorary Consulting Pathologist, Charing Cross Hospital, London, UK

System Editors

M. C. Anderson   **Gynaecological and Obstetrical Pathology**

T. J. Anderson and D. L. Page   **The Breasts**

B. Corrin   **The Lungs**

M. J. Davies, R. H. Anderson, W. B. Robertson and N. Woolf   **Cardiovascular System**

I. Friedmann   **Nose, Throat and Ears**

K. Henry   **Thymus, Lymph Nodes and Spleen**

B. C. Morson   **Alimentary Tract**

K. A. Porter   **Urinary System**

R. C. B. Pugh   **Male Reproductive System**

H. A. Sissons   **Bone, Joints and Soft Tissues**

D. Weedon   **Skin**

K. Weinbren   **Liver, Biliary Tract and Pancreas**

R. O. Weller   **Nervous System, Muscle and Eyes**

S. N. Wickramasinghe   **Blood and Bone Marrow**

E. D. Williams   **Endocrine System**

SYSTEMIC PATHOLOGY / THIRD EDITION

Volume 1

Nose, Throat and Ears

EDITED BY

I. Friedmann

MD(Prague), DSc(Lond), FRCS(Eng), LRCP(Lond), FRCPath, DCP(Lond)

Emeritus Professor of Pathology in the University of London; Honorary Consultant Histopathologist, Northwick Park Hospital, Harrow, Middlesex; Research Fellow, Imperial Cancer Research Fund, London, UK; Consultant in Electron Microscopy, House Ear Institute, University of Southern California, Los Angeles, California; Visiting Professor in Pathology, University of California, San Francisco and Los Angeles, California, and University of Colorado, Denver, Colorado, USA; formerly Director of the Department of Pathology and Bacteriology, Institute of Laryngology and Otology, and Consultant Pathologist, Royal National Throat, Nose and Ear Hospital, London, UK

CONTRIBUTORS

M. H. Bennett
MA(Cantab), MB BChir(Cantab), FRCPath
Consultant Pathologist, Mount Vernon Hospital, Northwood and Harefield Hospital, Harefield, UK

J. Piris
DPhil(Oxon), LMS(Spain), MRCPath
Senior Lecturer in Pathology, University of Edinburgh; Honorary Consultant Pathologist, Lothian Health Board, Edinburgh, UK

CHURCHILL LIVINGSTONE
EDINBURGH LONDON MELBOURNE AND NEW YORK 1986

CHURCHILL LIVINGSTONE
Medical Division of Longman Group Limited

Distributed in the United States of America by Churchill
Livingstone Inc., 1560 Broadway, New York, N.Y. 10036,
and by associated companies, branches and representatives
throughout the world.

First published 1986

ISBN 0 443 03097 9

British Library Cataloguing in Publication Data

Systemic pathology.—3rd ed.
  Vol. 1: Nose, throat and ear
  1. Pathology
  I. Friedmann, Imrich   II. Bennett, M.H.
  III. Piris, J.
  616.07   RB111

Library of Congress Cataloging in Publication Data

Main entry under title:

Nose, throat, and ear.

  (Systemic pathology; v. 1)
  Includes bibliographies and index.
  1. Nose—Diseases. 2. Throat—Diseases.
3. Ear—Diseases.   I. Friedmann, I (Imrich)
II. Bennett, M.H.   III. Piris, J.   IV. Series.
[DNLM: 1. Ear—anatomy & histology.   2. Larynx—
anatomy & histology.   3. Nose—anatomy & histology.
4. Pharynx—anatomy & histology
5. Otorhinolaryngologic Diseases.   QZ 4 S995 v.1]
RB111.S97 vol. 1 [RF47.5] 616.07 s [617′.51] 85-19488

Printed and bound in Great Britain by
Butler & Tanner Ltd, Frome and London

Foreword to the Third Edition of Systemic Pathology

I. Friedmann

The foreword to the First Edition was written by Sir Roy Cameron, a cellular pathologist I have greatly admired. It is my great honour and privilege to write the foreword for the Third Edition of *Systemic Pathology*.

The first two editions were well received. *Systemic Pathology* grew over 15 years from the two volumes of the first edition to the six volumes of the second edition. The Third Edition will comprise 15 volumes, reflecting the advances in pathology in recent years; the complete series will cover the core of histopathology in recent years, each volume dealing with a particular organ system. The fundamental concepts of the earlier editions have been preserved in the present edition.

Recent development of biology and pathology has been marked by the blending of various disciplines of research in the study of fundamental processes and in the re-investigation of vast morphological fields. With the introduction of electron microscopy and the perfection of immunological methods and techniques a new era of cytology has begun. A flood of new discoveries has been reported concerning the fine structure of the protoplasm (cytoplasm), which was called the physical basis of life by the great Czech anatomist Jan Evangelista Purkyně. The long-drawn-out controversy over the very existence of the cytoplasmic organelles, such as the mitochondria, the Golgi apparatus and the endoplasmic reticulum, has been settled and the existence and structure of these essential organelles are no longer in doubt. New important details have been added by the wide application of monoclonal antibodies. A spectacular variety of lymphocytes has been revealed and poses an intellectual challenge for classic diagnostic histopathologists.

There is the danger that we may be misled in matters of interpretation, and overwhelmed by rapid technical progress. As was said by Bernard of Chartres, who died circa 1130, we are like dwarfs on the shoulders of giants so that we can see more than they, not by virtue of our sharper eyesight but because we are raised up by their giant size.

These thoughts have taken me back to Payling Wright's invitation to me to contribute to *Systemic Pathology*. I have admired his teaching and his ideals, which, as Sir Roy pointed out, 'were such as to place him among the great teachers of the world, both past and present'. We have attempted to emulate his ideals.

January, 1986
Stanmore, Middlesex, UK

General Editor's Preface

William St Clair Symmers

In 1956, Professor G. Payling Wright, the Sir William Dunn Professor of Pathology in Guy's Hospital Medical School, London, was invited by his publishers, Longmans, to write a book on special pathology, the pathology of the body systems. They suggested that this should be in one volume, complementary to his text on general pathology, *An Introduction to Pathology* (Longmans published this now classic work in three editions, in 1950, 1954 and 1958). Professor Payling Wright agreed that there was a need for an up-to-date textbook of special pathology but pointed out that the work would be too much for one author to complete in a reasonably short time. By chance, earlier in 1956, another London publishing house, J. & A. Churchill, had asked if I would write a textbook of general and special pathology. Churchills' invitation came while the Edinburgh publishers, E. & S. Livingstone, were considering a suggestion that I had put to them that they might bring out a book on systemic pathology, to be written by a team of practising pathologists, each with special experience in the diseases of a particular system or organ. Livingstones were interested, but wanted the book to be by not more than two authors, and preferably by one. It is notable that at that time, only thirty years ago, three leading medical publishers in Britain still regarded a comprehensive textbook of pathology as within the professional and temporal competence of one author.

Having kept in touch with Professor Payling Wright since working in his department in 1946–1947, I called on him to ask what he thought of the practicability of a book, particularly a multi-author book, on systemic pathology. I did not know until that meeting that he had been asked by Longmans to write a book on the same subject. The outcome of that meeting was the publication, ten years later, of the first edition of *Systemic Pathology*, by 28 authors, in two volumes.

Professor Payling Wright died in 1964, the year after his retiral from the Chair at Guy's, and more than two years before *Systemic Pathology* appeared. *Systemic Pathology* may be less than the greatest of his memorials, for it was work that he shared with 27 colleagues and so is not as personally his as most of the others, but it is probably the one most widely known throughout the world.

The second edition began to appear in 1976, ten years after the first. By then, Longmans had absorbed both J. & A. Churchill and E. & S. Livingstone, combining the two houses to form the heart of the Medical Division of the Longman Group: the three publishers who had had their place in the earliest history of the book had become jointly responsible for its future. It had been intended that the second edition should consist of four volumes, to be published simultaneously: this was soon found to be unrealistic, and the edition appeared instead in six volumes, the last published in 1980.

In preparing the third edition, which starts publication with this volume, the publishers invited 19 specialists to become the editors, each an expert on the diseases of a particular system. The eight volumes that it was thought the edition might comprise have become 15, each dealing with only one system or part of one system. This will ensure that delay in completion of work on any system will not hold up the publication of systems that are ready to go to the printers. The volumes will appear in the order in which they reach the printers, and they will be numbered in the order of their publication. It is appropriate that Volume 1 is the volume edited by Professor Friedmann, whose contributions have been the first to be received in each edition.

The 19 editors were commissioned by the publishers to plan the presentation of the work and to nominate further contributors, and then to edit the manuscript and correct the proofs. The general editor's role is no more than advisory.

Whether this new edition of *Systemic Pathology* will reach the readers who have need of such a work will be determined as much by the cost of acquiring it as by its potential value as a text. The true worth of the edition will prove to be in the achievement of the 19 editors of the volumes and of the other contributors in conveying their knowledge and skills, and their understanding of pathology, to their readers. The publishers have put their experience and resources enthusiastically into the book, endeavouring always to meet the requirements of the editors and contributors.

I hope *Systemic Pathology* will continue to help pathologists and their clinical colleagues.

November, 1985
Northwood, Middlesex, UK

Preface

The last decades have witnessed an enhanced interest in the diseases of the head and neck. The specialist-pathologist has played an active role by drawing the attention of other pathologists to the problems of the ear, nose and throat and by acquainting the otorhinolaryngologist with the advances in pathology which have provided a sounder base for diagnosis and research in this region.

The chapters on the pathology of the nose, throat, nasopharynx, tonsils and ears were contained in several volumes of the second edition of Systemic Pathology. Now that both interest and subject matter have grown, it has been considered appropriate to present these chapters in a single separate volume.

The upper respiratory tract plays an important role, not only in localized but also in systemic diseases. Moreover, certain neoplasms, commoner in other organs, have been recognized more frequently in this region.

This volume presents the structure and function of the normal tissues; some malformations and, in detail, the histopathological features of common and less common inflammatory granulomatous and neoplastic diseases of the upper respiratory tract and the ear. It is intended for the postgraduate student of pathology and otolaryngology, for the general pathologist working in close co-operation with an active and progressive department of otolaryngology and for the ENT surgeon.

Most of the sites comprising the upper respiratory tract and ear are relatively inaccessible and biopsy materials are often obtained by curettage. The use of the operating microscope and micro-surgical techniques have proved valuable in obtaining representative specimens. The tissue samples received by the pathologist are often small and may have been subjected to artefactual traumatic distortion. Furthermore, the histological appearances may also be complicated by ulceration and secondary inflammatory reaction. Consequently, the pathologist should learn to recognize and make allowances for these changes. Some of the neoplasms of the larynx are difficult to diagnose in the biopsy specimen; consequently the original diagnosis has to be revised after a more detailed examination of the surgical specimen by means of special staining and histochemical methods and electron microscopy.

The diagnosis of tumours of the region involves nomenclature which is always a divisive factor. With some significant exceptions the WHO classification is followed, although, as pointed out by Leslie Sobin, 'the WHO classifications are not intended as just another attempt to reach nosological perfection, although that is one major goal'.

Many difficulties stand in the way of an unambiguous classification of various neoplasms. Electron microscopy and, more recently, sophisticated immunocytochemical methods have been applied to the identification of the so-called intermediate filaments of the cytoskeleton. These innovations have given a new impetus to histopathology but have stretched to the limit the available facilities of the laboratory.

The great advance in otology, however, has not been matched by an enhanced interest of the general pathologist in the apparently barren regions of the temporal bone. Otologists and audiologists have remained the forerunners of research into the diseases of the ear and in particular of deafness. Otitis media, known to Hippocrates, and its sequelae have been attracting renewed interest and the pathologist would be rewarded by a systematic study of this apparently trivial disease.

Close clinico-pathological cooperation at every phase of a disease is advocated; to rely on clinical experience alone may be a 'practical' approach but lacks objectivity. Equally to practise so-called 'objective' pathology without any reference to clinical information may limit the diagnostic awareness of the histopathologist.

Both granulomas and neoplasms often present as 'nasal, laryngeal and aural polyps' and distinction may only be established after histological examination, when various bacterial and mycotic granulomas, idiopathic granulomas and neoplasms may be revealed in clinically unsuspected cases. It is emphasized that all tissues removed must be submitted for histopathological examination. Semantic and terminological intricacies and controversies abound also in this field and the authors have adhered to descriptive terms based on characteristic morphological patterns whilst not ignoring alternative opinions.

Readers of the first two editions have become familiar with the excellent contributions of my late colleague Denis Osborn. His untimely and tragic death has been a great loss to ENT pathology. I have been able to include several of his figures and of the instructive tables he prepared for our chapters which, together with his other work, are a fitting tribute to his memory.

We have been very fortunate in gaining the co-operation of Dr M. H. Bennett, Consultant Pathologist at Mount Vernon Hospital, whose vast experience has contributed greatly to the quality and material of the chapter on the pathology of the nose and paranasal sinuses. The chapter on the pathology of the larynx has been extensively revised by Dr Juan Piris, Senior Lecturer in Pathology at the University of Edinburgh.

Our thanks are due to the staff of Churchill Livingstone, for their interest and patience, only surpassed by that of our wives. Our typists and 'word-processors', Mrs Joan Friedmann, Mrs Janet Gilbert, Mrs Val Pilbrow and Mr G. Reynolds have our grateful thanks, so well-merited.
1986   I.F.

Contents

PART ONE

I. Friedmann and M.H. Bennett

The nose and paranasal sinuses

1

Structure and function

ANATOMY AND HISTOLOGY

The nose and paranasal sinuses form a complex system of airways and cavities. The anatomy of the external nose has been described in detail recently,[1] and attention was drawn particularly to the variable relations between the upper and lower lateral nasal cartilages that determine the shape of the external nose, a matter of considerable importance in plastic surgery.

The anatomy of the maxillary sinus was defined by Nathaniel Highmore in 1651[2] and the sinus rightly bears his name (antrum of Highmore). He also described the anatomy of the frontal sinuses. The gross anatomical relationships of the paranasal sinuses are shown in Figures 1.1 and 1.2.

The nasal mucous membrane

The anterior half to two-thirds of the vestibular part of the lateral wall of the nose (the inner aspect of the ala) is lined by an extension of the epidermis; this is provided with sebaceous and sweat glands and carries a number of short hairs (the vibrissae). The posterior part of the vestibule is lined by non-keratinized, stratified squamous epithelium; this merges a little farther back with the respiratory tract type of epithelium that lines the rest of the nose except for the olfactory area. The nasal columella—the movable structure that separates the nostrils—is covered with skin, which merges through a narrow, non-keratinized zone of stratified squamous epithelium into the respiratory tract epithelium of the septum. As a result of metaplasia squamous epithelium may occur also on the anterior ends of the middle and inferior turbinates. The mucosal lining of the nasal cavity has been referred to as the Schnei-

3

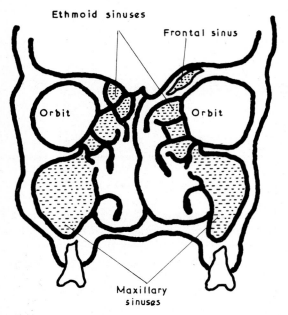

Fig. 1.1 Gross anatomical relations of the maxillary, ethmoidal and frontal sinuses.

cells and rests on a basal lamina. The ciliate cells bear a number of cilia projecting from their free surface (Fig. 1.3). It has been estimated that such cells in the trachea carry nearly 300 cilia. Fox et al[4] have studied the ultrastructure of the human nasal cilia. The internal structure of the axoneme of cilia has the classical 9+2 microtubular pattern.[5] The central microtubules are singlets, and the peripheral nine microtubules are doublets with a figure-of-eight appearance; there is one complete microtubule called subfibre A, and the other subfibre B shares a common wall with A. There are two short, diverging arms projecting from subfibre A (named dynein arms)[6] (Fig. 1.4a & b). Atypical or giant cilia are a variation of the normal structure, probably due to the precocious regeneration of the true cilia.[7, 8] Atypical cilia are usually multiple, two or more forming a complex enveloped by the bulging outer membrane of the cell. It seems likely that they would impede the regular rhythmic action of the mucociliary apparatus.

The immotile ciliary syndrome

Various syndromes are associated with defects and alterations in the classical ciliary structure. Kartagener's syndrome of sinusitis, bronchiectasis and situs inversus has been linked with the absence of dynein arms in the doublets of micro-

derian membrane. Schneider was the first to describe, in 1660, the nasal mucous membrane and disprove the theory that mucus was produced by the pituitary gland.[3]

The *respiratory epithelium* is pseudostratified columnar ciliate epithelium with secretory gobler

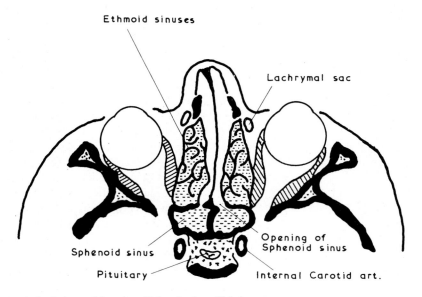

Fig. 1.2 Gross anatomical relations of the ethmoidal and sphenoidal sinuses.

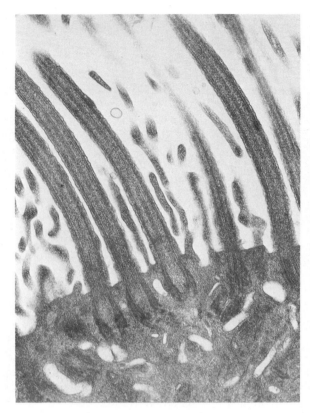

Fig. 1.3 Cilia in longitudinal section showing microtubules within the cilia terminating in basal bodies by which the cilia are anchored.

Electron micrograph   ×31 850

tubules of normal cilia, closely related to the immotility of respiratory cilia. The absence of the dynein arms may be accompanied by the transposition of the microtubules and the absence of radial spokes.[9] Since the cilia retain some motility but lack coordination, the immotile ciliary syndrome has been referred to by some authors as 'ciliary dyskinesis'.[9a]

Ciliary dyskinesis is a congenital defect which may be inherited as an autosomal recessive trait. It may be associated with neonatal respiratory distress, chronic and recurrent otitis media, chronic respiratory infections, bronchiectasis, chronic sinusitis, situs inversus, male sterility and some forms of hereditary deafness, e.g. Usher's syndrome. Reversible ciliary anomalies may be acquired during acute viral infections of the upper respiratory tract.

The nasal cilia in retinitis pigmentosa and congenital deafness (Usher's syndrome) have been shown to exhibit a high incidence of compound cilia with deviation from the $9+2$ pattern of microtubules and a relative absence of the dynein arms.[9c] Inflammation of the mucosa of the upper respiratory tract may result in loss of its cilia. Epithelium can be replaced through proliferation of the basal cells and subsequent differentiation and ciliogenesis, an important feature of the regenerating epithelium. Mucus is a necessary intermediary in the transport system and must be present if the cilia are to function properly. The failure of the ciliary system in such conditions as chronic bronchitis, sinusitis, asthma, mucoviscidosis and secretory otitis represents an inability of the mucosa to meet the transport demands under pathological conditions.

Varying numbers of goblet cells are scattered among the ciliate cells. The Golgi apparatus of the goblet cells produces a secretion formed mainly of mucopolysaccharide or mucoprotein; this is stored as granules, which are eventually discharged (Fig. 1.5).

Under inflammatory or toxic influences, the ciliate cells may undergo profound changes, although the cilia themselves may be retained under even quite extreme conditions. Goblet cells vary in number and it has been claimed that there are fewer in the paranasal mucosa. A study of the distribution of goblet cells in the developing human nose found no supporting evidence for the view that ciliate cells were capable of transmutation to goblet cells.[10] The modern view is that the goblet cells are derived from the basal cells of the respiratory type epithelium.

Under light microscopy with routine haematoxylin and eosin staining, goblet cells usually appear as unstained areas. Under the electron microscope, the cells are seen to contain numerous membrane-bound mucous granules, usually only moderately electron-dense but occasionally containing circumscribed denser material (Fig. 1.5). The free border exhibits microvilli which are often coated by mucopolysaccharides forming a glycocalyx.[8] Under the scanning electron microscope, craterlike spaces (Fig. 1.6) mark the sites of recent apocrine secretion of the goblet cells.[11]

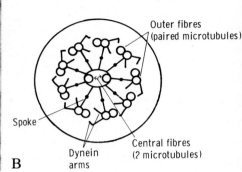

A   B

Fig. 1.4 Cross section of normal cilia showing the basic 9+2 pattern of the axoneme composed of 9 peripheral double microtubules which surround a central pair. There are two arms attached to one of each pair of outer microtubules which are referred to as 'dynein arms'.   A)   EM   ×53000

There are numerous *mucosal glands* lying deep in the lamina propria. These glands are mixed, comprising mucus-secreting cells and two types of serous secretory units. Random analysis of nasal secretions has revealed the presence of amylase-like activity. It has also been shown that tears and nasal secretion contain lysozyme (muramidase). On the periphery of both mucous and serous secretory units are located the myoepithelial cells. These are important since they have relevance to the pathogenesis of certain mucosal gland tumours. Electron microscopy reveals the myofilaments with their aggregation zones, resembling smooth muscle.

The *paranasal mucosa* is essentially similar to that of the nasal fossa, though there are slight differences. The columnar cells tend to be shorter, resulting in a somewhat thinner epithelium. Columnar cells bear cilia (Fig. 1.6) and there are large numbers of microvilli. The lamina propria also tends to be thinner and usually bears fewer mucosal glands. The lamina propria of the nasal and paranasal mucosa often contains a sprinkling of assorted inflammatory cells, including plasma cells, lymphocytes, macrophages and occasional polymorphonuclear leucocytes and eosinophils, even when the mucosa is apparently

healthy. Control of nasal secretion is believed to be under the influence of the parasympathetic system, fibres reaching the mucosa by way of the sphenopalatine ganglion. Vasoactive intestinal polypeptide (VIP) has been shown to be present in nerves in the nasal mucosa, in close association with seromucous glands and blood vessels. Its actions include stimulation of secretion and atropine-resistant vasodilation.[12]

The surface structure of the human nasal mucosa has been studied in detail by Boysen[13] who confirmed that squamous metaplasia of the nasal epithelium was a 'normal finding' and described five grades in the process of gradual metaplastic transformation that can be distinguished. It is interesting to note this author's reference to 'the transition' of the Grade III epithelium (mixed cuboidal/squamous) to metaplastic squamous epithelium (Grade IV). This may bear some relation to the papillomas of the nose described as of transitional type (see page 65).

The nasal lamina propria and the vascular system

The lamina propria of the mucosa of the respiratory passages of the nose is a vascular tissue that blends with the periosteum and perichondrium

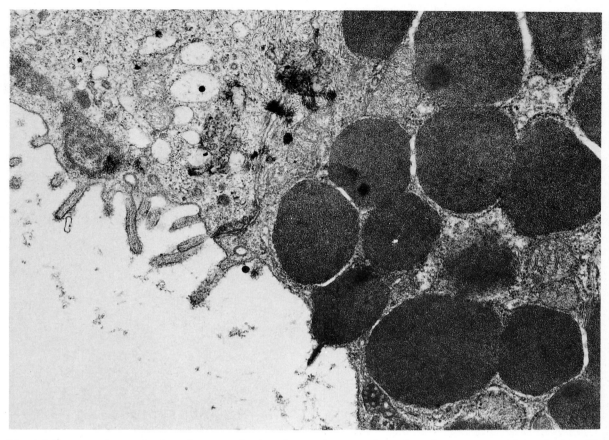

Fig. 1.5 Electron micrograph of nasal mucosa showing electron dense membrane bound secretory granules and microvilli coated with mucopolysaccharides forming a glycocalyx.

×·16 900

of the nasal skeleton. It contains much elastic tissue and abundant collagen enclosing the nasal mucous and seromucous glands. An interesting feature is the presence of complex blood vessels which are designated 'erectile tissue' (Fig. 1.7). This vascular component is found on the lateral walls and septum, concentrated posteriorly around the choanal orifices, and it may extend into the postnasal space. The vessels in this system contain a substantial amount of smooth muscle which, in contrast to the conventional pattern of ordinary arteries and veins, is oriented in a spiral fashion, thus giving rise to an irregular arrangement in cross section. The vessels develop in three strata, connected by arterial, venous and arteriovenous anastomoses. The plexuses are best developed in the mucoperiosteum of the middle and inferior conchae, and particularly the posterior part of the latter and the choanal region generally. They form an erectile tissue that can rapidly become so engorged with blood that it may partly or completely obliterate the nasal cavities.

The musculature of this tissue is controlled by the autonomic nervous system, and it also reacts to various pharmacologically-active agents, including some hormones.[12, 14] Its function is probably to bring about rapid changes in the local blood flow with consequent variation in the temperature of the inspired air. The structure of the nose is admirably adapted for the protection of the lower and more vulnerable parts of the respiratory tract. The arrangement of the septum and the turbinate bones ensures that the current

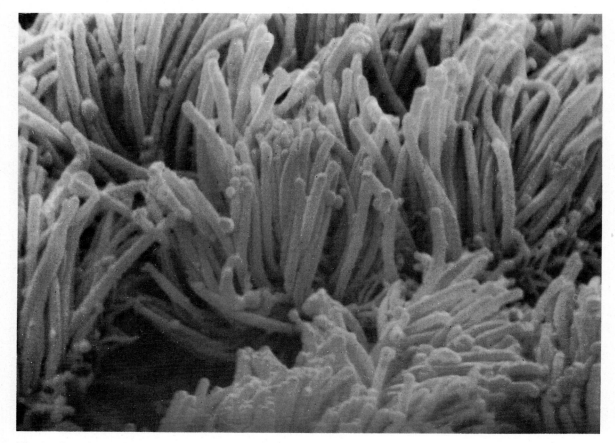

Fig. 1.6 Scanning electron micrograph of paranasal epithelium showing ciliated surface.
Provided by Mr R. Gray, Royal Free Hospital, London, UK

of inhaled air is directed against the mucous membrane, with the result that most of the finer particles, among them bacteria, become trapped in the surface mucus and later removed by ciliary action.

Not only does the nose serve as an effective filter, but it also warms and moistens the inhaled air, so that even with great variations in the temperature and humidity of the external atmosphere, the inspired air is nearly saturated with water vapour and raised to body heat before it passes the larynx. When this warming and humidification fails, as may happen in some forms of rhinitis, ciliary action and mucus secretion in the trachea and bronchi are adversely affected and a most effective means of protecting the lungs against infection is correspondingly handicapped.

Melanin-producing cells

Melanocytes have been readily demonstrated in the skin of the vestibule[15] but, in white races, melanocytes have not been demonstrated satisfactorily in the nasal fossa although they undoubtedly exist in the epithelial lining. Claims to have identified melanocytes in the nasal cavity on the basis of finding pigmented cells[16] have to be assessed in the light of the fact that melanocytes can inject their pigment into adjacent epithelial cells, hence pigmented cells are not necessarily melanocytes.

The human nasal mucous membrane in the menstrual cycle

The nasal mucous membrane is under hormonal control and various nasal symptoms have been ascribed to the effect of hormonal changes.[14] Dis-

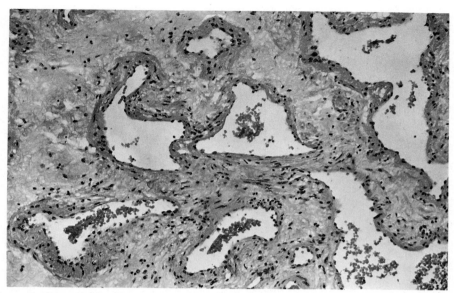

Fig. 1.7 Nasal erectile tissue showing the irregularity of the muscular wall of the vessels due to the spiral arrangement of the fibres.

Haematoxylin–eosin   × 135

turbances in hormonal balance may account for the rhinitis and sinusitis that sometimes occur at the menopause, and the hormonal changes accompanying pregnancy are probably the cause of the swelling of the nasal mucosa that is occasionally observed then. Some women are troubled by swelling of the nasal mucosa during the premenstrual phase of the menstrual cycle, with a tendency to epistaxis, the so-called 'vicarious nasal menstruation'. The erectile parts of the nasal lining may become swollen in some individuals, of either sex, during sexual excitement. The swelling may be accompanied by excessive secretion of watery mucus, and a comparable state may develop during emotional disturbances; the nasal obstruction that accompanies crying is a familiar example, the effects of the mucosal engorgement being then aggravated by the drainage of tears through the lacrimal ducts. It is clear that these responses must be mediated through the autonomic nerves. Bleeding from hereditary telangectasia increases ahead of, or during the menstrual flow.[17]

The ultrastructural and histochemical features of the normal nasal mucosa have been widely studied.[18, 19] The ultrastructural features of the human adult male and female respiratory nasal mucous membrane are alike, the female mucosa showing no cyclical change during the various phases of the menstrual cycle.[20] This suggests that the hormonal receptors of the nasal mucosa may be less sensitive to the physiological fluctuations of the levels of oestrogen and progesterone during the menstrual cycle than the hormonal receptors of the endometrial mucosa.

The mucous membrane of the normal human maxillary sinus

Light microscopy shows both similarities in the mucous membrane of the nose and paranasal sinuses and also some differences. The mucosa of the sinuses is thin and less specialized; the epithelium is lower and contains fewer goblet cells, a basal lamina is for the most part absent, the glands are fewer and smaller and the venous erectile plexus is absent.[21]

A study of the fine structure of the maxillary sinus mucosa[22] has shown it to be more delicate with fewer cilia than the nasal mucosa. The activity of the seromucinous glands and the exchange rate between tissue fluid and blood appeared to be diminished. These features would correlate with a lower resistance of the sinus mucosa to infection.

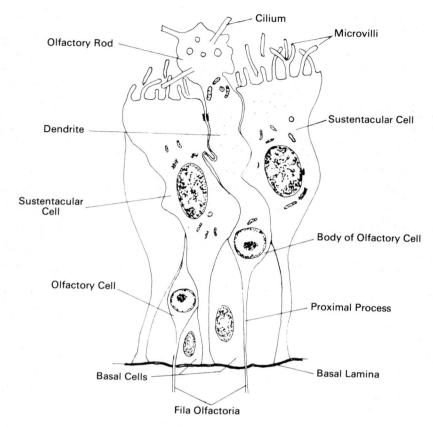

Fig. 1.8 Diagram: the cells of the olfactory mucosa.

The 'human compass'

The results of magnetometric and histological examination of various tissues from the human head have revealed that the bones of the region of the sphenoid and ethmoid sinuses contain a conspicuous band of ferric iron and are magnetic. It has been suggested that these form part of a magnetic sense organ (the 'human compass') as in mice and tuna fish.[23]

The olfactory area of the nose

The mucous membrane of the olfactory area has a highly specialized structure, in keeping with its function as the end-organ of one of the special senses. It includes not more than the upper one-third of the mucosa of the septum in the region opposite to the superior concha, the corresponding part of the very narrow roof of the nasal cavity, and the mucosa above and on the upper and medial aspects of the superior concha itself. It is slightly yellowish compared with the pinker colour of the respiratory mucosa.

The histological organization of the olfactory mucosa consists in the adult vertebrate of an epithelial layer, a basal lamina and the lamina propria which directly adheres to the underlying bony or cartilaginous tissue. The olfactory area is covered by a pseudostratified columnar epithelium which tends to be not only more extensive but thicker in lower animals than in man. There are three types of cell in the olfactory epithelium (Fig. 1.8) and three layers of nuclei can be recognized.[24] The nuclei of the supporting cells lie nearest to the epithelial surface, the nuclei of the middle layer are those of the olfactory receptor cells and the deepest layer is formed by the nuclei of the basal cells (Fig. 1.9). There is a fluid layer covering the epithelial surface in which the pro-

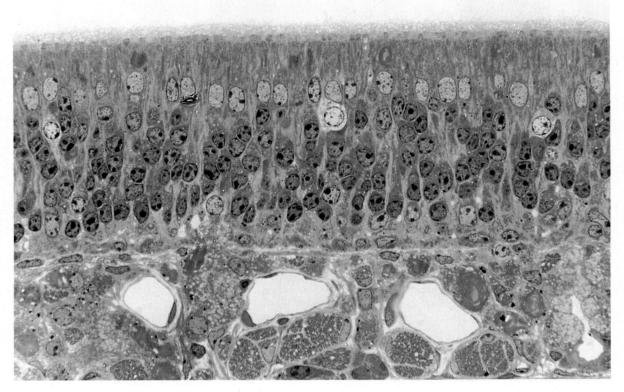

Fig. 1.9 Olfactory mucosa. The paler staining, more superficial nuclei belong to the supporting cells whilst the darker more rounded nuclei lie in the receptor cells. Note the duct of Bowman's gland (lower right).

Haematoxylin–eosin   × 1000

Provided by Dr P.P.C. Graziadei, Florida State University, Tallahassee, Florida, USA.

jections from the cells are embedded. Under the electron microscope these cells bear a large number of microvilli (Figs 1.8, 1.9) on their free surface, projecting into the fluid layer and forming a dense meshwork both in vertebrates and man.[24, 25] In addition to mitochondria and flattened profiles of rough endoplasmic reticulum, the supporting cells also contain yellowish-brown pigment which accounts for the gross appearance. The basal cells are roughly conical in shape and lie between the basal portions of the supporting cells. They may also envelop the proximal parts of the receptor cells and possibly function as Schwann cells.[24, 25]

The olfactory cells are essentially bipolar receptor neurons. The slender, flask-like cells contain rounded nuclei and are provided with distal and proximal processes. The distal process, known as the dendrite, passes towards the surface between the supporting cells. Under the electron microscope it can be seen to contain microtubules and mitochondria. When the dendrite reaches the surface it expands slightly to form the olfactory rod (Fig. 1.8). This contains a number of small vesicular structures; projecting from its surface are several cilia which lie in the fluid layer in association with the microvilli of the supporting cells. The olfactory cilia have a short proximal segment containing the 9 + 2 pattern of microtubules typical of kinocilia and a longer distal portion with two subfibres. Within the olfactory rod, the cilia terminate in basal bodies. The number and the length of cilia varies in different species.

Embryologically, olfactory receptors derive from neuroblasts differentiating directly from olfactory placodes. The central part of each placode invaginates, giving rise to an olfactory sac open anteriorly.

It may be noted that the olfactory organ is the only part of the body in which the cell bodies of neurons are at the surface, directly in contact with the external environment; this accounts for the frequency with which the sense of smell may be permanently impaired or destroyed by inflammatory disease of the nasal lining. The olfactory mucosa contains the tubuloacinar exocrine glands of Bowman, which are peculiar to this region; they lie deep to the basal lamina and their ducts traverse this and the olfactory epithelium to reach the surface. It is their function to bathe the surface with the thin fluid in which odoriferous substances are thought to become dissolved before their presence can effectively stimulate the processes of the sensory cells.

The practical importance of disturbances of these functions is indicated by the estimate that approximately 2 000 000 American adults have disorders of taste and smell and that a chemosensory problem can be the major presenting symptom in a large number of patients.[26]

The specialized receptor portion of the bipolar olfactory cell undergoes continuous renewal with a turnover time averaging 30 days, making the olfactory receptors rather vulnerable. Accidental blows to the head can shear these fine bundles, causing anosmia.

Radioactive labelling of the cells of the nasal cavity of hamsters treated with tritiated N-nitrosodiethylamine has been studied.[27] In the respiratory portion of the nose (nasal septum and conchae) most bound radioactivity was concentrated in the mucous cells of the respiratory epithelium and the secretory cells of submucous glands. In the olfactory epithelium only the sustentacular cells were labelled, and these only slightly so. It is of interest that the olfactory sensory cells were unlabelled. If these cells are the source of neurogenic tumours in this area, as is believed by many investigators, the above findings would indicate that factors other than metabolic activation may lead to their malignant transformation.

MALFORMATIONS

Malformations of the external nose range from slight deformity to bizarre anomalies. They are less frequent than congenital anomalies of the external ear. Least rare are involvement of the nose in defects of closure of the facial clefts (cleft lip), atresia of the anterior naris on one or both sides, and stenosis ('collapse') of the anterior parts of the nasal passages. The bridge of the nose is characteristically widened ('saddle nose') in association with hypertelorism (abnormally wide separation of the eyes), which may occur with or without other defects as a genetically-determined condition; some of these cases are instances of what has been called the 'first arch' syndrome, sometimes attributed to premature involution of the artery of the first branchial arch.

Internal malformations of the nose include involvement in cleft palate and unilateral or bilateral choanal stenosis or atresia.

Congenital malformations must be distinguished from deformities caused by acquired disease, including trauma, specific infections—particularly tuberculosis, leprosy and syphilis—and other destructive conditions, especially neoplasms, involving the nose or nasal sinuses.

Other congenital nasal lesions

Congenital nasal lesions are rare and include encephalocele, meningocele, glioma, dermoid and haemangioma. A review of the congenital nasal lesions seen in two children's hospitals in Liverpool over a 20-year period listed 67 nasal dermoids, 32 haemangiomas, 5 nasal gliomas and 2 encephaloceles.[28]

A nasal encephalocele may develop as a result of faulty closure of the anterior neuropore leading to protrusion of the intracranial contents into the nasal area. A nasal glioma may be considered a nasal encephalocele without connection with the subarachnoid space (see p. 87).

Faulty closure of the bones in the nasal area may result in dermal elements being trapped through the fronto-nasal suture line, thus explaining the origin of the 'complex' nasal dermoids.

The 'simple' nasal dermoid which accounts for 65% of all nasal dermoids may result from entrapment of dermal elements in the facial cleft, and consequent aberrant development of skin appendages.

REFERENCES

1. Dion MC, Jaffek BW, Tobin CE. Arch Otolaryngol 1978; 104: 145.
2. Highmore N. Corporis humani disquiritio anatomica. Haquae-comitis: S Broun, 1651.
3. Schneider CV. In: Pagel W. Virchows Arch (Pathol Anat) 1974; 363: 183.
4. Fox B, Bull TB, Arden GB. J Clin Pathol 1980; 33: 327.
5. Fawcett DV, Porter KR. J Morphol 1954; 94: 221.
6. Rungger-Brandle E, Gabbiani G. Am J Pathol 1983; 110: 361.
7. Kawabata I, Paparella M. Acta Otolaryngol (Stockh) 1969; 67: 511.
8. Friedmann I, Bird ES. Laryngoscope 1971; 81: 1852.
9. Sturgess JM, Chao J, Wong J et al. New Engl J Med 1979; 300: 53
9a. Mehlum DL, Parker GS, Bacher-Wetmore B. Laryngoscope 1983; 93: 573.
9b. Carson JL, Collier AM, Hu Sh H. New Engl J Med 1985; 312: 463
9c. Arden GB, Fox B. Nature 1979; 279: 534.
10. Poulsen J, Tos M. Acta Otolaryngol (Stockh) 1975; 80: 434.
11. Andrews PM. In: Hodges G, Hallowes RC, eds. Biomedical research applications of scanning electron microscopy. New York: Academic Press, 1979: 1.
12. Polak JM, Bloom SR. Exp Lung Res 1982; 3: 313.
13. Boysen M. Virchows Arch (Cell Pathol) 1982; 40: 279.
14. Polak JM, Bloom SR. In: Polak JM, Van Noorden S, eds. Immunocytochemistry. Bristol: PSG Wright, 1983: 197.
15. Szabo G. In: Gordon M, ed. Proceedings of the 4th Conference on Biology and Atypical Pigment Cell Growth. New York: Academic Press, 1959: 99.
16. Zak FG, Lawson W. Ann Otol Rhinol Laryngol 1974; 83: 515.
17. Harrison DFN. J Laryngol Otol 1957; 71: 597.
18. Toppozada HA, Gaafar HA. J Laryngol Otol 1973; 87: 639.
19. Mygind N, Winther B. Acta Otorhinolaryngol Belg 1979; 33: 591.
20. Toppozada HA, Michaels L, Toppozada M, El-Ghazzawi E, Talaat A, Elwany S. J Laryngol Otol 1981; 95: 1237.
21. Arey LB. Human histology. 4th ed. Philadelphia: WB Saunders, 1974.
22. Toppozada HA, Talaat MA. Acta Otolaryngol (Stockh) 1980; 89: 204.
23. Baker RR, Mather JG, Kennaugh JH. Nature 1983; 301: 78.
24. Graziadei PPC. In: Friedmann I, ed. Ultrastructure of sensory organs. Amsterdam: Elsevier, 1973.
25. Moran DT, Rowley JC III, Jafek BW, Lovel MA. J Neurocytol 1982; 11: 721.
26. Schiffman SS. N Engl J Med 1983; 308: 1275.
27. Reznik-Schuller HM. Cancer Letters 1982; 16: 109.
28. Bradley PJ, Singh SD. Clin Otolaryngol 1982; 7: 87.
29. Friedmann I, Osborn DA. Pathology of granulomas and neoplasms of the nose and paranasal sinuses. Edinburgh: Churchill Livingstone, 1982.

2

Inflammatory conditions of the nose

RHINITIS

Acute rhinitis

By far the commonest form of acute inflammation of the nasal passages is the common cold (see below), which is primarily a viral infection, familiar to everybody from personal experience. Acute rhinitis may also occur as a prodromal or symptomatic manifestation of the acute infectious fevers, particularly measles, and it may be the result of specific bacterial infections, such as diphtheria and, exceptionally, gonococcal infection. In some cases, acute rhinitis is caused by exposure to irritant chemical substances or is due to working in a dusty environment. Acute allergic rhinitis is a common clinical problem, particularly in hay fever.

In any of these conditions the disease may be confined to the nasal cavities, or it may also involve the nasal sinuses. Acute rhinitis, especially when due to infection, is very likely to be accompanied by acute nasopharyngitis as a natural consequence of the continuity of the nasal passages and nasopharynx. It must be stressed that the conventional distinction between these parts of the upper respiratory tract is a purely arbitrary topographical one, with no functional basis.

The common cold
The common cold (*acute coryza*) is of viral origin[1] the viral infection usually being followed within two or three days by secondary bacterial infection. The bacteria most frequently involved include *Streptococcus pneumoniae, Staphylococcus aureus* and *Streptococcus pyogenes* and, possibly, *Branhamella catarrhalis, Klebsiella pneumoniae* and *Haemophilus influenzae*, some of which are ordinarily part of the nasal and pharyngeal flora.

Immunity to the common cold is very transient, perhaps partly because of the occurrence of numerous immunologically-distinct strains of virus. The viruses have been isolated in tissue cultures and can be grown on the chorioallantoic membrane of eggs. The infection can be transmitted to human volunteers, although not to any animals. No means of immunization has been discovered, but *interferon* used prophylactically has been shown to protect volunteers from experimental rhinovirus infection.[2, 3] Although the disease usually runs a short course, it is the cause of a serious annual loss of productivity wherever it occurs, for it is very infectious. In most urban communities in temperate climates it is endemic throughout much of the year, and particularly frequent in cold, damp periods. Exposure to wet and cold predisposes to the infection, and local disease—such as deflection of the nasal septum sufficient to cause partial obstruction of one airway, or the presence of adenoids—is also a predisposing factor.

Except in very young or weak babies whose feeding and sleeping are interfered with by nasal obstruction, an uncomplicated common cold is a minor malady as far as the individual patient's health is concerned. The potential severity of the disease is, in fact, wholly determined by the effects of the secondary bacterial invaders, and these effects in their turn are largely determined by the potential pathogenicity of the bacteria themselves. In the average case the bacterial infection has no effect other than to convert the abundant, serous nasal discharge that characterizes the first two or three days of the viral infection into a scantier mucopurulent or sometimes purulent discharge, occasionally flecked with blood; this stage lasts only a further two or three days, recovery then following rapidly. If, however, the sinuses become involved during the stage of bacterial rhinitis the resulting infection may linger on for many weeks, and may pass into a chronic phase.

In some cases, especially in debilitated people, or at the extremes of age, the bacterial phase of the common cold leads to tracheobronchitis and bronchopneumonia.

Histopathology of acute rhinitis. The mucosal blood vessels are engorged and the mucosa in general is oedematous and rather sparsely infiltrated by neutrophils. There is considerable overactivity of the mucous and seromucous glands. With the development of the bacterial phase the number of neutrophils in the inflammatory exudate increases quickly, and these cells migrate through the surface epithelium in considerable numbers. There may be considerable loss of the ciliated cells of the surface epithelium, but this necrobiotic process is superficial and the cells regenerate rapidly once the infection subsides.

Nasal diphtheria

Diphtheria of the nose, in common with other forms of diphtheria, has become a rare disease in most parts of the world. It seems to have occurred mainly in childhood. The characteristic diphtheritic membrane forms mainly on the middle and inferior conchae or on the septum. In the great majority of cases the strain of *Corynebacterium diphtheriae* is of the mitis type. The patients are highly infective.

Toxaemia is strikingly uncommon in cases of nasal diphtheria, and the usual presenting manifestation is unilateral or bilateral nasal obstruction, sometimes with epistaxis, and often of several weeks' duration. The infection clears up without sequelae in almost all cases, although some patients become chronic nasal carriers of the organism. The ozaena type of chronic atrophic rhinitis may be the outcome of infection by a non-toxigenic strain of *Corynebacterium diphtheriae* (see ozaena).

Chronic rhinitis

Chronic hypertrophic rhinitis

Repeated attacks of acute rhinitis may be followed by chronic hypertrophic rhinitis. It is possible that unhealthy conditions of work, such as dusty or damp surroundings, or frequent exposure to nasal irritants are predisposing factors. Marked displacement of the septum, chronic sinusitis and adenoids are often accompanied by hypertrophic rhinitis.

Histopathology. The condition is characterized by hyperplasia of the mucosal glands and thickening of the mucous membrane, much of which is due to the persistent engorgement of the vascular plexuses. The engorgement is to some extent explained by rigid fibrous thickening of the walls of the vessels, with replacement of muscle fibres by collagen. The thickening is further increased by the considerable infiltration of the lamina propria by lymphocytes, often with the development of many well-formed lymphoid follicles with conspicuous Flemming centres. Plasma cells and macrophages also collect, but are less numerous. There is considerable thickening, and often hyalinization, of the basal lamina and there may be a general increase in the fibrous tissue throughout the mucosa.

Chronic atrophic rhinitis

Clinically, two varieties of chronic atrophic rhinitis are generally distinguished—a *simple atrophic rhinitis* and *ozaena* (atrophic rhinitis associated with foetor). In addition, a special clinical variety, *rhinitis sicca*, is sometimes described; rhinitis sicca has been regarded as an occupational disease of those who work in a hot, dry, dusty atmosphere—for example, in smelting works, steel mills, foundries, vulcanizing shops, glassworking shops, bakeries and stokeholes.

Ozaena. The characteristic fetor of ozaena comes from the presence of dry crusts formed from viscid secretion; these crusts collect in the meatuses under the conchae, and elsewhere in the nasal cavities, causing considerable obstruction of the airways. The patient is usually quite unable to detect the smell, and in fact the condition is almost always associated with complete anosmia. The disease is much commoner in women than in men and it often begins at about the time of puberty. It was formerly seen most frequently among the poor, in association with undernourishment and anaemia, and there seems to be no doubt that its incidence has fallen appreciably with the general rise in the standard of living. It remains predominantly a disease of town dwellers, and particularly of indoor workers. The causes of ozaena are obscure. The sex incidence suggests that there may be a hormonal factor; in

this context it may be significant that both the intensity of the smell and the amount of crusting may be markedly increased during menstruation. However, most authorities consider ozaena to be the result of infection. There are two main theories of infection—that the disease is the end-result of various non-specific forms of infective rhinitis, or that it is a specific infection. It was sometimes attributed to tuberculosis or syphilis. In some cases of ozaena, however, there is good evidence that the atrophic state is the outcome of inadequately-treated chronic suppurative rhinitis of the type that may be a sequel to the acute rhinitis of measles and scarlet fever, or that may accompany chronic suppurative sinusitis. Iron deficiency has been considered to be a cause of the disease. Iron therapy has been successful in many cases[4] except when there was irreversible atrophy of the mucosa.

Bacteriology. Many different types of bacteria have been isolated from cases of ozaena and supposedly identified as its immediate cause. They include organisms of three main types—klebsiellae, corynebacteria, and an ill-defined group of coccobacilli (of which the so-called *Coccobacillus fetidus* of Perez is the only one that has some claim to consideration). The klebsiellae include particularly *Klebsiella pneumoniae* subsp. *ozaenae*, the classic ozaena bacillus of Loewenberg and Abel, which can be isolated from between 70% and 100% of cases of the disease; it is noteworthy that *Klebsiella pneumoniae* subsp. *ozaenae* has only exceptionally been isolated in the absence of atrophic rhinitis. This organism is a serologically distinct species-serotype 4(D) of the capsulate, Gram-negative bacteria. Other klebsiellae, including *Klebsiella pneumoniae* (Friedländer's bacillus), have been isolated from cases of ozaena.

More recently, corynebacteria have been described as possible causes of ozaena: these include a non-toxigenic organism, *Corynebacterium belfantii*, which has been isolated in a high proportion of cases when selective culture media have been used. It is believed that *Corynebacterium belfantii* is, in fact, a non-toxigenic form of the mitis type of *Corynebacterium diphtheriae*: it can be converted in vitro into a toxigenic and lysogenic form by *phage beta*. It is known that toxigenic strains of *Corynebacterium diphtheriae* can be transformed to a non-toxigenic, non-lysogenic state by cultivation in broth containing anti-*phage-beta* antiserum, and it has been assumed that this might occur in vivo as a result of the natural production of antiphage antibodies in cases of infection by these organisms. It has been suggested, therefore, that ozaena is a late result of nasal diphtheria:[5] diphtheria might cause irreparable damage to the nasal mucosa, leading to atrophy, a reduction in blood supply and lessened resistance to infection; these conditions would favour persistence of the diphtheria bacilli, which in the course of time could become transformed into non-toxigenic variants, the continuing infection ultimately manifesting itself as ozaena.

Histopathology. There is marked atrophy of the mucous membrane throughout the nose and also of the bone of the conchae—when the characteristic dry, greenish, sickeningly fetid crusts are removed, the nasal cavities and the subchonchal meatuses appear strikingly roomier than in the normal nose. Microscopical examination shows changes that are sometimes considerably less remarkable than the clinical impression of severe atrophy leads one to expect. Usually, however, the surface epithelium is thinner than normal, with replacement of the ciliate columnar cells by simple columnar or cuboidal cells; there is a marked reduction in the proportion of goblet cells, or they may have disappeared completely. In many cases there is some squamous metaplasia, and this may be very widespread; keratinization does not occur, or, at most, is of very limited extent. The basal lamina may be thickened and hyaline, or it may be normal. The mucosal glands are atrophic and the lamina propria is often very thin and fibrous.

SINUSITIS

Acute sinusitis

Acute inflammation of the nasal sinuses is almost always the result of extension of infection from the nose itself. The common cold, influenza and the acute infectious fevers are the usual precipitating causes. Occasionally, acute sinusitis is the direct consequence of the entry of fluid into the nose, for instance while bathing or diving. The presence of an excess of fluid in a sinus may encourage bacterial growth, especially if the opening of the sinus does not allow its ready escape. Occasionally, infection may spread directly into the maxillary sinus (antrum of Highmore) from the roots of the teeth, especially the first and second molars. Again, infection may pass from one sinus to another as a result of the gravitation of infected secretion. Anomalies of the position and size of the openings between the sinuses and the nasal cavities may also predispose to infection, mainly by hindering free drainage.

Bacteriology of acute sinusitis
Most cases of acute sinusitis are due to infection by Gram-positive cocci: *Streptococcus pyogenes*, *Streptococcus pneumoniae* and sometimes *Staphylococcus aureus*. Rarer causes are *Klebsiella pneumoniae*, *Haemophilus influenzae* and *Escherichia coli*. In cases arising as a complication of dental sepsis, such organisms as *Treponema vincentii* and its associated fusiform bacteria may be present, contributing a characteristic fetor to the purulent exudate filling the maxillary sinus. It should be noted that anaerobic organisms may be associated with these infections, particularly maxillary sinusitis, taking the place of the aerobic pathogens as the local conditions alter during the progress of the inflammatory changes. In about one-quarter of our cases no organisms could be isolated.

If inflammatory oedema leads to persistent blockage of the ostium, the exudate accumulates within the sinus, and, if the infection is a pyogenic one, an acute empyema results with extensive destruction of the mucosal epithelium. If drainage is established at this stage the inflammatory changes will usually subside, but in a proportion of cases chronic suppurative sinusitis results, or even a chronic closed empyema.

Histopathology
The earliest change in the mucous membrane in a case of acute sinusitis is intense hyperaemia accompanied by moderate oedema, a slight infiltration by neutrophil leucocytes and active secretion by the goblet cells and mucosal glands.

Complete resolution is possible if the inflammatory reaction does not progress beyond this stage. In more severe cases there is an increasingly heavy accumulation of neutrophils, with the formation of seropurulent or mucopurulent exudate on the surface of the mucosa; at this stage there may be some erosion of the epithelial lining although recovery may still be accompanied by a virtually complete return to normal.

Chronic sinusitis

As the acute stages of sinusitis subside, the neutrophils in the exudate are replaced by a variably heavy accumulation of lymphocytes, often with a conspicuous admixture of plasma cells. Histiocytes and, in some cases, eosinophils may also be present. Fibroblastic proliferation leads to fibrosis, and there is eventually much mucosal atrophy. There may be widespread squamous metaplasia of the epithelium although the ciliate epithelium is often well preserved. Chronic sinusitis in children is usually associated with nasal polyps or a deviated nasal septum affecting drainage and causing retention of purulent secretion and consequent fibrotic and cystic changes in the mucosa.

The normal thickness of the mucosa of the maxillary sinuses is between 0.5 and 1.0 mm. In chronic sinusitis of children there is often radiological evidence of opacity, interpreted as thickening of the mucosa. Histological studies, however, showed no evidence of mucosal thickening but a layer of viscous secretion covering the antral mucosa was noted at operations on the sinus.[6] This protein-rich fluid resembles the secretion present in the so-called glue ear (see p. 265) and offers a reservoir for infection. The secretion may become inspissated, forming a mass imitating a tumour.[7]

Bacteriology of chronic sinusitis

Cultured specimens of the mucosa obtained during Caldwell–Luc operations for chronic maxillary sinusitis showed no obvious correlation between the bacteriological and clinicopathological findings, except that *Haemophilus influenzae* was isolated mainly from purulent sinuses.[8]

In one representative series of dental-related infections of the maxillary sinus[9] anaerobic streptococci were grown on culture in 76% and aerobic streptococci in 72%; other anaerobic organisms were also found (for example, *Bacteroides* sp. in 41%, *Actinomyces* or *Bifidobacter* in 40% and fusobacteria in 26%). *Staphylococcus aureus* was found in only 3% of the cases. Anaerobic organisms are a common cause of paranasal sinusitis.

Complications of sinusitis

Acute suppurative osteitis

In some cases of acute sinusitis the infection extends into the bony wall of the sinus, causing *acute suppurative osteitis*. This may lead, for instance, to an acute spreading osteomyelitis of the maxilla, but more usually the destruction of the bone is followed by spread of the infection directly into the adjacent tissues, with the formation of a subcutaneous abscess or the development of *orbital cellulitis* or of *intracranial suppuration*.

Intracranial complications

The intracranial complications of sinusitis include suppurative leptomeningitis, extradural or intracerebral abscesses and septic thrombosis of the cavernous venous sinus. In other cases these complications may develop without destruction of the bony wall of the sinus, presumably as a result of lymphatic spread or, possibly, of septic thrombosis of the blood vessels of the sinus mucosa. Infection of the orbit may, in its turn, be the immediate source of infection of intracranial structures, but by far the commonest source of intracranial complications is frontal sinusitis, with direct extension of the infection from the sinus into the meninges and brain. *Cavernous sinus thrombosis*, however, is almost always the result of sphenoidal sinusitis.

Orbital cellulitis

This is frequently associated with infection by *Staphylococcus aureus* and *Streptococcus pyogenes*. Less common causes of bacterial orbital cellulitis include *Pseudomonas aeruginosa* and *Escherichia coli*. A number of other bacteria have been related to more chronic or at least subacute infections of the sinuses or orbits and can invade the central nervous system. These bacteria include *Actinomyces israelii, Nocardia asteroides,*[10] *Nocardia madurae, Streptomyces griseus, Treponema pallidum, Mycobacterium tuberculosis, Mycobacterium leprae,* and atypical mycobacteria. Mucormycosis (see page 36) occurs most often in association with poorly-controlled diabetes mellitus, especially with ketoacidosis.[11]

Complications of chronic sinusitis

Any of the complications mentioned above may occur either in the course of acute sinusitis or as a result of chronic sinusitis. There are some other complications of chronic sinusitis that deserve to be noted. In some cases there is a well marked *polypoid hypertrophy* of the mucosa, which may become very considerably thickened: much of the thickening may be due to oedema, the accompanying cellular accumulation being largely confined to the zone immediately underlying the epithelium. This type of mucosal change may be the origin of some nasal polyps, particularly those that arise in the maxillary sinus (*antronasal polyps*) or in the ethmoidal air cells.

Mucocele results when mucus secretion accumulates in a sinus as a consequence of obstruction of its ostium. It is found most frequently in the anterior ethmoidal air cells or in the frontal sinuses, and, exceptionally, in the posterior ethmoidal air cells or the sphenoidal sinus: it also occurs in the maxillary sinus. The accumulation of mucus eventually leads to pressure atrophy of the bone around the sinus, and in the case of anterior ethmoidal and frontal mucoceles this gives rise to a painless swelling that may displace the contents of the orbit. Mucoceles develop very slowly. If they become infected they are transformed into abscesses (the so-called *pyoceles*): the consequences are then likely to be grave.

Chronic fibrosing osteitis is the sequel of low-grade inflammatory changes in the wall of chronically-infected sinuses. There may also be marked new bone formation amounting even to the development of cancellous osteomatoid masses that are sometimes misinterpreted as osteomas.

POLYPOSIS OF THE NOSE AND SINUSES

The existence of nasal polyps was noted over 100 years ago and, initially, there were differences of opinion as regards their nature. Many believed them to be neoplasms but others maintained that they represented the consequences of chronic infection and this latter view was ultimately established. Subsequently, they were recognized as projections of mucous membrane developing in association with chronic rhinitis and sinusitis but more especially with allergic disease of the upper respiratory tract.

In terms of material submitted for histopathology, nasal polyposis represented about 4% of patients registered with the Royal National Throat, Nose and Ear Hospital, London, over a period of 27 years.

Nasal polyps tend to occur most frequently in middle-aged males. In one year's material, 75% of polyps were removed from patients between 40 and 70 years of age and the male:female ratio was 3:1. Nevertheless, the age distribution is broadly based and polyps may be encountered in young patients. Clinical presentation is characterized by nasal obstruction, nasal discharge and sneezing. The lesions may appear at the anterior nares. They are often multiple and bilateral and may lead to visible broadening of the external nose.

Nasal polyps are, essentially, rounded projections of oedematous mucous membrane. They may develop in association with chronic hypertrophic rhinitis, chronic sinusitis and allergic diseases of the nose. They arise most commonly in the ethmoidal region, and particularly from the mucosa of the middle concha: the ethmoidal air cells may be filled by sessile polyps. Polyps that arise from the surface mucosa are likely to become pedunculated.

As seen clinically, polyps are smooth, shiny, movable swellings, usually bluish-grey in colour and occasionally traversed superficially by sparse, fine, ramifying blood vessels. Exceptionally, they are more vascular, appearing pink or red, and such polyps may be mistaken for swollen conchae, until probing reveals their mobility, uniform softness and lack of sensitivity. Nasal polyps may best be described in two categories, non-allergic and allergic. This grouping is adopted in the following account of their pathology.

Non-allergic polyps

Like the allergic polyps (see below), non-allergic nasal polyps consist of very oedematous fibrous tissue, the sparse fibres of which are often so widely separated by the accumulation of fluid that they are difficult to demonstrate. Reticulin staining reveals a characteristic alveolar pattern. A consistent feature is a hyaline condensation of the basal lamina, generally referred to as a thickening of that structure although in fact probably a product of the interstitial material in its vicinity.

The surface of the polyp is covered by well-ciliate epithelium of respiratory tract type, often showing goblet cell hyperplasia and only rarely becoming ulcerated. Squamous metaplasia is not unusual on the exposed surface of a polyp that has long presented at the nostril. There is a variable, but usually rather scanty lymphocytic infiltration of the tissue immediately under the epithelium; the lymphocytes may be accompanied by some plasma cells and neutrophils. In some instances plasma cells are exceptionally numerous and may even give rise to a suspicion of plasmacytoma.

Eosinophils are conspicuous in the cases in which there is an associated allergic state: these are the majority—their special histological features are described below under the heading Allergic polyps.

Antronasal polyps differ from the usual non-allergic nasal polyps in two respects—they arise in the maxillary sinus, and occur predominantly in children or young adults. They are solitary, as a rule, although one may be present on each side. The polyp grows through the ostium of the sinus into the middle meatus, extending forward toward the front of the nose, or more characteristically backward to present at the choana (hence the alternative names *choanal polyp* and *antrochoanal polyp*). Their pathological appearances are similar to those of ethmoidal polyps, except that they are liable to pseudocystic degeneration: a considerable amount of serous fluid may escape

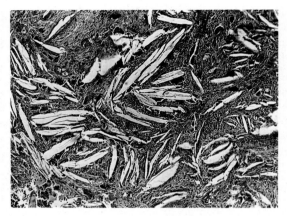

Fig. 2.1 Cholesterol granuloma of the maxillary sinus formed by chronic inflammatory granulation tissue with giant cells surrounding needle- or cigar-shaped spaces from which the cholesterol crystals have been dissolved during processing.

Haematoxylin–eosin   × 50

from these pseudocystic foci when they are ruptured during removal of the lesion or on probing it. Haemorrhage may occur into the degenerating tissue. In some cases *cholesterol granulomas* form (Fig. 2.1): these are quite similar to the familiar cholesterol granulomas of the middle ear. Similar polyps occasionally arise within the sphenoidal and ethmoidal sinuses.

Studies[12, 13] of the ultrastructure of the respiratory type epithelium covering nasal polyps have shown large numbers of goblet cells in the pseudostratified epithelium which ranges from 40–100 μm in thickness. Microvilli, with or without complex branching, are abundant near the edge of the free border of the ciliate cells, the cilia being closely packed in the central area (Fig. 2.2). Ultrastructural examination of the stroma of simple nasal polyps[14] has shown that there is an oedematous framework of fibroblasts with abundant interdigitating cytoplasmic processes, a plexus of inflamed blood vessels and a mixed infiltrate of active inflammatory cells. Solitary cilia were seen to arise from the stromal mesenchymal cells. No mycoplasma or viral inclusions were present. These features may have a relationship to the pathogenesis of nasal polyps.

An immunologically-induced liberation of vasoactive amines from mast cells results in increased capillary permeability and a consequent excess of intercellular fluid; the stromal cells

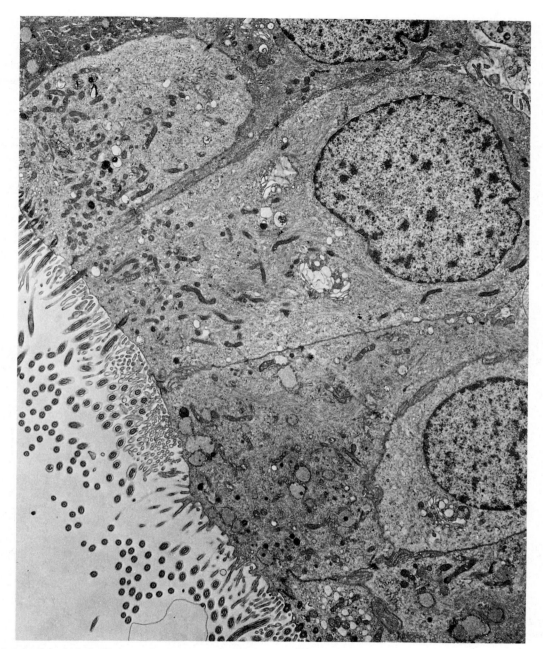

Fig. 2.2 Surface epithelium of a nasal polyp showing cilia and numerous microvilli.

Electron micrograph   × 6000

Provided by Dr R. A. Busuttil, Royal Infirmary, Glasgow, UK.

attempt to check this expansion by an increase in collagen synthesis. It has been shown that in vasomotor rhinitis the VIP immunoreactive nerves are greatly increased, forming thick bundles around blood vessels and seromucous glands. This may be a significant feature of the disease.[15]

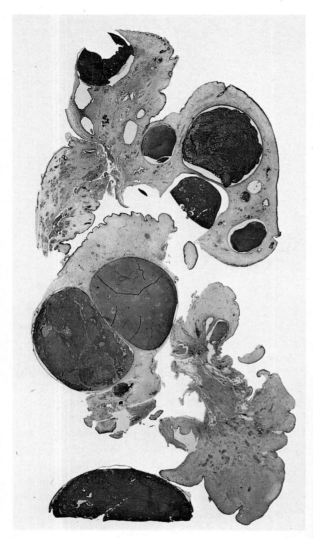

Fig. 2.3 Antronasal polyp showing cystic distension of sero-mucinous glands.

Haematoxylin–eosin   × 4

Allergic polyps

The essential feature in the pathogenesis of the allergic type of nasal polyp is the presence of oedema. The fluid has the characteristics of an inflammatory exudate, particularly a high content of protein. Its accumulation is the direct consequence of increased capillary permeability, mediated by vasodilator substances that have been liberated in the course of antigen–antibody reactions at cell surfaces. When such antigen-antibody reactions occur repeatedly, the oedema that thus results tends to become persistent: polyps form because the accumulation of fluid leads to progressive distension of the lamina propria of the mucosa and consequent protrusion of the epithelial covering, which may show patchy atrophy. Once polyps have developed in this manner, their histological appearances are often characteristic to the point of being pathognomonic. There is extensive replacement of the ciliate cells of the surface epithelium by large goblet cells. The mucous glands in the stroma become hyperplastic and distended and there is prominent hyalinization of the basal lamina. Cyst formation may result if the glands are obstructed by stretching or kinking or by the surrounding oedema. The cysts are filled with fluid that may be mucous or pro-

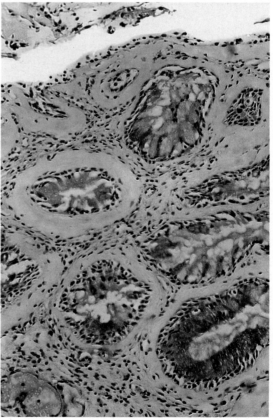

Fig. 2.4 Allergic type nasal polyp. There is intensive secretory activity of the mucous glands and hyaline thickening of their basal laminae.

Haematoxylin–eosin   × 190

teinaceous (Figs 2.3, 2.4). Infiltration of the stroma by eosinophils is characteristic: their number varies greatly, and whenever such an infiltrate is found in any biopsy specimen from this region its presence should raise the question of an allergic process. The distribution of the eosinophils may be uniformly diffuse, or confined to the subepithelial zone, or in scattered foci. A frequent feature is the presence of sharply-defined accumulations of eosinophils and plasma cells together with lymphocytes. Plasma cells and lymphocytes predominate in the lesions only in the presence of secondary infection. Their presence in smaller numbers does not necessarily indicate infection: it may indicate a reaction to an allergen, and the possibility that the antibodies are being produced locally.

Allergic polyps are often a part of the clinico-pathological picture of allergic rhinitis, particularly *vasomotor rhinitis*. The spectrum of conditions included under such diagnostic terms as allergic rhinitis, vasomotor rhinitis, allergic polyps and simple polyps is continuous: none of the varieties is an entity, for there is overlap in clinical picture and pathological findings between them all.

Aetiology of nasal polyps

The aetiology of benign mucous nasal polyps is not clear. Allergy and infection or a mixture of the two have been incriminated[16] but in a majority of patients with nasal polyps, skin tests to a wide range of allergens are negative. Passive transfer experiments have shown that nasal polyp fluid from allergic individuals with positive skin tests may contain a higher concentration of reagin than the serum,[17] and it has been postulated that this is indicative of primary local nasal allergy. But the role of allergy in nasal polyps of patients who are not obviously reaginic is not clear, and there are limits to the possibility of further study by tests using allergens. The essential prerequisite for the development of polyps is the occurrence of oedema. In so far as the formation of oedema is a particular feature of acute allergic reactions, this would explain why the majority of polyps are of allergic origin. Furthermore, the firmer attachment of the septal mucosa to underlying structures accounts for the lack of origin of

polyps from this location. In a study of the concentrations of various immunoglobulin components in both serum and polyp fluid,[18] it was noted that the IgE fraction, believed to be responsible for the reaginic activity, was present in the polyp fluid in higher concentration than could be accounted for by simple filtration, thus confirming local antibody production.

IgA constitutes about 80% of immunoglobulins in the secretions of the epithelial cells of mucous membranes. The mechanism by which IgA reaches the nasal mucosa is unclear. An ultra-structural study of the nasal mucosa[19] has shown that IgA produced by plasma cells is taken up by endocytosis in the epithelial cells where it can be demonstrated in the Golgi apparatus and in the secretory granules, thus eventually to reach the nasal secretion.

Differential diagnosis

It may be quite impossible to distinguish clinically between simple nasal polyps, polypoid lesions due to specific granulomatous diseases and polypoid neoplasms, including cancers. For this reason it is essential that all polyps removed from the nose and nasal sinuses should be fully examined histologically.

Abnormal connective tissue cells seen in the stroma of polyps are, as a rule, of no pathological significance. Two cases with pseudosarcomatous changes in antrochoanal polyps have been reported,[20] the authors warning against a mistaken diagnosis of malignancy in an otherwise benign lesion. Attention has also been drawn to the importance of recognizing that atypical mesenchymal cells in the stroma of simple nasal polyps do not indicate malignancy.[21, 22] Rarely ossification may occur in the stroma.[23]

GRANULOMATOUS DISEASES[23]

Granulomas of the nose and sinuses may be caused by specific or non-specific agents. Specific causes are largely infections which will be dealt with individually. Certain unknown agents produce characteristic clinical and histological patterns, such as sarcoidosis and the midfacial granuloma syndrome: these also merit separate

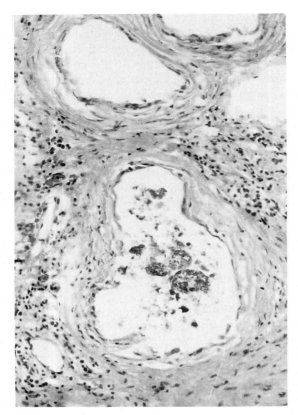

Fig. 2.5 'Myospherulosis'. Nasal biopsy showing distended spaces containing cluster of spherules.

Haematoxylin–eosin   × 180

consideration. One of the commonest non-specific granulomas is caused by reaction to foreign bodies but these are not commonly encountered in pathological material from the nose and sinuses. Two distinctive varieties of foreign-body-type granuloma encountered in the nasal and paranasal region, cholesterol granuloma and myospherulosis, will be described here. Eosinophilic granuloma is described on page 107.

Cholesterol granuloma of the sinuses

This lesion has become more commonly recognized[24, 25] though in former times there was confusion between cholesterol granuloma and 'cholesteatoma'. A proportion of cases reported under the latter name were clearly cholesterol granulomas.[26]

Cholesterol granulomas have been reported in the frontal and maxillary sinuses. The patients were almost invariably very young. Clinical presentation takes the form of nasal discharge, local discomfort and nasal obstruction, especially when the granuloma is found in an antrochoanal polyp.

Microscopically, the lesion is indistinguishable from that seen in the middle ear and elsewhere (see p. 274). Chronic inflammatory granulation tissue contains numerous foreign-body-type giant cells which surround and engulf the cholesterol crystals, the position of which is marked by empty needle-shaped spaces in paraffin-wax-embedded material (Fig. 2.1). Recent haemorrhage or iron pigment indicating previous haemorrhage is often seen.

As in all cholesterol granulomas, the basic cause is believed to be haemorrhage though the cause of this in the maxillary lesions cannot always be defined. However extraction of the upper

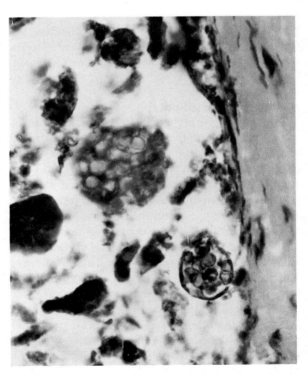

Fig. 2.6 'Myospherulosis'. Incidental finding in mucosa of maxillary sinus. There are clusters of spherules present closely packed within a delicate membrane. The spherules are, in fact, altered red blood cells.

Haematoxylin–eosin   × 760

molar teeth accounts for a proportion of cases. Removal of the granuloma is seldom followed by recurrence.

Myospherulosis of the nose and sinuses

Myospherulosis was first described in 1969 in six Africans with nodular swellings, often painful and apparently developing in relation to skeletal muscle.[27] A further five cases, also in Africans, were reported in which skeletal muscle was not always involved.[28] Histologically, the lesion consists of fibrous and inflammatory granulation tissue in which there are cyst-like spaces lined by flattened foam cells presumed to be histiocytes. Some of the spaces contain clusters of rounded bodies slightly larger than red blood corpuscles and surrounded by a thin refractile membrane (Figs 2.5, 2.6).

Involvement of the nose, paranasal sinuses and ear was reported in 1977 in a series of 16 patients in Missouri.[29] The ages ranged from 15 to 86 years and the sexes were equally divided. Over 50% involved the maxillary sinus with or without other cavities being affected. All cases had had operative procedures prior to the first histological identification of the lesion and about one-third had been operated upon for neoplasms of the region. Review of the initial biopsy was carried out in the majority of cases and revealed no evidence of 'myospherulosis'. A common feature in these cases was the use of gauze packing with petrolatum-based ointments and the author considered the possibility that the lesion represented an unusual reaction to this material. Subsequently the lesion was induced in experimental animals using petrolatum-based antibiotic ointments.[30]

The same lesion has been described in the maxillary sinus of an 8-year-old boy[31] in whom a previous biopsy had revealed fibromatosis. The biopsy site was packed with tetracycline ointment. A subsequent maxillectomy specimen showed, in addition to fibromatosis, the lesion of 'myospherulosis'. The author incubated red cells in test tubes internally coated with tetracycline ointment. After 5 days, smears showed appearances identical with the clumps of spherules in the lesions. The conclusion was that the spherules were red cells modified by the petrolatum-based ointment. Similar experiments[32] have confirmed this result with petrolatum and have also produced 'myospherules' in vitro with lanolin and emulsified human fat.

SPECIFIC GRANULOMAS

The chronic specific infections of the nose include a considerable variety of diseases, many of which are rare. Some of them have a special geographical distribution, for example, scleroma, leprosy and some of the fungal infections. In these days of greatly increased travel, however, cases of diseases that ordinarily would be regarded as exotic may be encountered anywhere in the world. Moreover, the relative frequency and importance of some of the hitherto less common nasal granulomas have been enhanced by the fall in the incidence of such formerly common diseases as tuberculosis and syphilis. It is important, however, to realize that, in spite of their much lower incidence nowadays, both tuberculosis and syphilis must still always be considered in the differential diagnosis of ulcerative granulomatous and neoplastic diseases of the nose.

Tuberculosis

There are two clinical forms of tuberculosis of the nose—lupus vulgaris and the so-called granulomatous tuberculosis of the nasal mucosa.

Lupus vulgaris

Lupus vulgaris is a slowly destructive tuberculous infection of the skin which may extend into the nasal vestibule. In drawing attention to the rare occurrence of lupus vulgaris in Britain, Warin & Wilson Jones have described five patients whose cutaneous tuberculosis of the nose presented with unusual clinicopathological features causing a delay in the accurate diagnosis.[33] A deep biopsy is required in the diagnosis of granulomatous disease affecting the nose and a full excision biopsy might be essential in arriving at the correct diagnosis of lupus vulgaris.

Granulomatous tuberculosis

The so-called granulomatous tuberculosis of the nose starts on the anterior part of the septum and

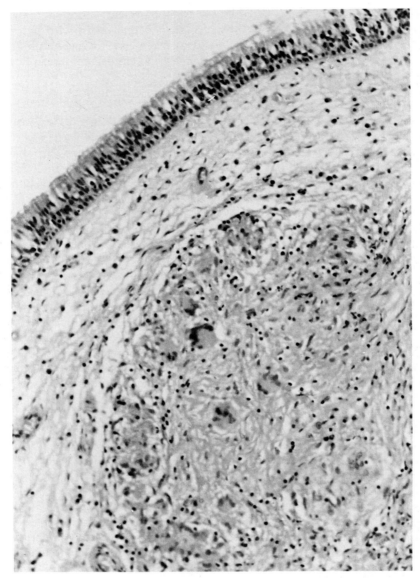

Fig. 2.7 Tuberculosis of the nose presenting as a nasal polyp. Note confluent tubercles underneath the respiratory epithelium. Haematoxylin–eosin   × 225

does not involve the skin. Early symptoms consist of nasal discharge with subsequent crusting, fetor and nasal obstruction; there may be epistaxis. The lesion is intranasal and commonly appears as a smooth lobulated mass, 5–10 mm in diameter, with an unbroken surface but may sometimes resemble granulations with a tendency to bleed. Although this lesion slowly breaks down it never involves the bony septum and there is no collapse of the bridge of the nose. If the vestibule and columella are affected, scarring and retraction follow the ulcerative process and result in the tip of the nose being drawn inward and downward towards the upper lip, with stenosis and even complete occlusion of the nostrils. Granulomatous tuberculosis is more common in

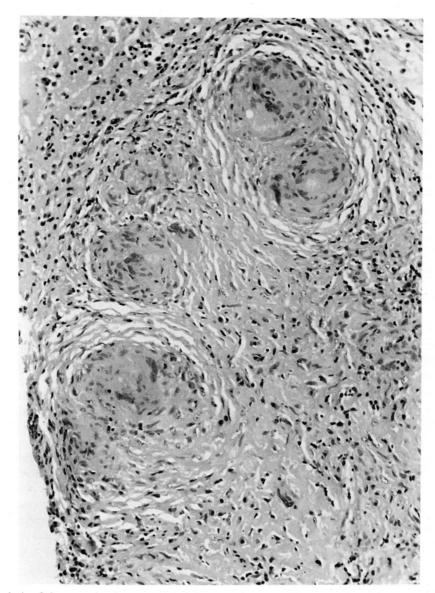

Fig. 2.8 Tuberculosis of the nose showing many scattered tubercles with Langhans-type giant cells in fibrotic granulation tissue.
Haematoxylin–eosin   × 225

the elderly, in whom it is particularly liable to be confused with malignant neoplasms.

Nasal tuberculosis may involve the lacrimal duct and spread along it to give rise to dacryocystitis and, occasionally, tuberculous ulceration in the region of the inner canthus of the eye.

Atrophic rhinitis is a frequent sequel, particularly when the conchae have been involved.

Occasionally, active pulmonary lesions are found but in many cases there is no evidence of such. It would appear that the relationship of nasal to pulmonary infection is an inconstant one, raising the question whether a tuberculous infection in the nasal region is primary or secondary. Failure to find tubercle bacilli in nasal material does not necessarily exclude tuberculous infection; antral washouts, sputum and urine should also be examined.

The *microscopical picture* is that of tuberculosis (Figs 2.7, 2.8). However caseation is uncommon, and secondary infection may obscure the picture of the tuberculous lesion. Acid fast bacilli may or may not be demonstrable. The diagnosis depends not only on the histological findings but, more important, on the isolation of the causal organism.[34]

Control of tuberculous infection generally has resulted in a marked reduction in the frequency of the disease. Nasal and paranasal involvement has shared in this trend. There has also been a shift towards an older age distribution. The declining incidence of infection with *Mycobacterium tuberculosis* has led to a relative increase in the importance of disease caused by other myobacteria.[35] These include *Mycobacterium kansasii*, *Mycobacterium avium*, *Mycobacterium xenopei* and *Mycobacterium scrofulaceum*. These organisms are capable of producing diseases which are clinically, radiologically and histopathologically identical with tuberculosis.

Mycobacterium balnei may cause nasal granulomas in those who have been exposed to infection in contaminated swimming pools.

Sarcoidosis

Boeck,[36] who in 1899 recognized the generalized nature of the disease, drew attention to its nasal manifestations. Reviews of sarcoidosis have emphasized upper respiratory involvement.[37-39] In a review of nasal involvement in sarcoidosis, published in 1976, 64 cases altogether were collected from the literature in English; 3 additional cases demonstrated that nasal lesions may be the presenting manifestation of sarcoidosis.[40]

Aetiology

The aetiology of this condition is still obscure and many of the theories have been examined by Scadding[39] but, 'whether the agent is primarily infective or chemical, this pattern of nasal involvement would be consistent with the concept of assault by some extraneous, probably airborne antigen'.[41] It has been suggested that atypical mycobacteria or some other organism might be involved. Homogenates from human sarcoid in-

oculated into footpads of mice or intraperitoneally or intravenously into mice produced local and disseminated epithelioid and giant-cell granulomas.[42] These experiments provide some evidence that transmissible agents are present in human sarcoid.

The demography of the disease suggests that it is not of genetic origin and, if contagious, it is of only low infectivity.[43] The adult North American Black living in rural areas of the South-eastern United States and Scandinavians appear to be most susceptible. Women are more prone to the disease. The clinical features suggest that the causative agent enters the body via the upper respiratory tract and later becomes blood-borne to affect any part of the body.

Histopathology

Sarcoid lesions of the nose are found principally on the septum and inferior turbinate. The histological picture is that of non-caseating histiocytic and giant-cell granulomas which tend to remain discrete even though they may be closely packed. Small foci of central necrosis are occasionally present. Reticulin staining shows the presence of a fibrillary pattern in the sarcoid granulomas but not in tuberculous nodules. Schaumann bodies are relatively infrequent in upper respiratory tract lesions. The microscopical picture is such that the diagnosis can be no more than suspected on histological grounds alone and will depend on other supporting evidence such as signs of generalized disease, raised serum calcium level, negative bacteriological investigations, negative tuberculin test and positive Kveim test.

Leprosy

Leprosy is the only bacterial disease included among the six selected for the World Health Organization's special programme for research and training in tropical diseases.[44] It is a complex and chronic inflammatory disease of man caused by the intracellular *Mycobacterium leprae*, displaying a wide clinical spectrum related to host ability to develop and sustain specific cell-mediated immunity.[45]

The nose is frequently involved in leprosy and granulomatous nodules, ulceration or perforation

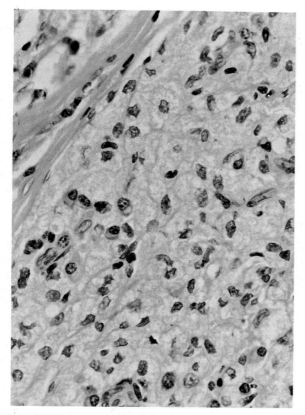

Fig. 2.9 Lepromatous leprosy of the nasal cavity showing clear 'lepra cells'.

Haematoxylin–eosin   × 480

may be found, particularly on the septum and the inferior conchae. The course of the disease is often marked by spontaneous remissions. Atrophic rhinitis develops as the granulomatous lesions heal. Nasal involvement is not uncommonly the first manifestation and it is important to bear this in mind when children who may have been exposed to the infection begin to have nose-bleeding.

The diagnosis is made by demonstrating the acid-fast but not alcohol-fast mycobacteria in scrapings or biopsy specimens from the mucosal lesions by a modification of the Ziehl–Neelsen method. Histological preparations are preferable to films of scrapings because they greatly facilitate recognition of the characteristic lepra cells (Fig. 2.9) with clustered intracytoplasmic masses

of the bacilli. Care must be taken not to mistake scleroma for leprosy, particularly in those parts of the world where both infections occur. Leprosy must also be distinguished from tuberculous rhinitis.

The nasal mucosa is affected in 95% of cases of early disease. The sites of election within the nasal cavity are the inferior concha (97% of cases) and the anterior part of the septum (85%).[46, 47] The posterior nasal structures are less frequently affected.

The nose clearly presents a favourable environment for the multiplication of *Mycobacterium leprae*. It is, therefore, important as a site of discharge of the bacilli from the body (with epidemiological implications). It may well be an important portal of entry of the bacilli also.[48] The nasal discharge is not merely mucoid material but is, in fact, an inflammatory exudate containing large numbers of macrophages, often loaded with the bacilli. The proportion of the organisms that survive in voided material has been found to be 100% up to 24 hours and 10% still surviving after nearly 2 days.[49] This would imply that susceptible individuals could be infected by inhalation, the bacilli invading the anterior part of the inferior concha at an early stage. Progressive destruction of nasal structures is not uncommon but there may be some degree of healing with fibrosis. Although therapy with dapsone and rifampicin has modified the course of the disease, it is not always curative. Rifampicin is rapidly bactericidal so that the public health risk presented by patients with lepromatous disease may be quickly reduced.

Syphilis
The nose is always involved in congenital syphilis and it may be affected at any stage in the course of the acquired disease.

Primary chancre
A primary chancre of the nose is usually the result of an accidental inoculation. It occurs in the vestibule or on the anterior part of the septum and it is associated with enlargement of the preauricular or submandibular lymph nodes on the same side.

Secondary stage

The nasal lesions of secondary syphilis are essentially of the same type as those in the mucous membrane of other orifices, particularly the mouth.[50]

Tertiary stage

Tertiary syphilis of the nose[51] may present as a gummatous mass with or without ulceration, or as perichondritis with necrosis of the cartilage, or as an atrophic rhinitis with ozaena. These lesions may appear at any time following the secondary stage, and their onset may even be recognizable before the symptoms of the latter have fully subsided. In most cases, however, they present in about the fifth year of the disease, although they may be delayed for up to 20 years or more. The sites most frequently affected are the septum, the inferior conchae, the floor of the nose and the alae. Involvement of the alae may take the form of indolent, brawny ulcerating granulation tissue and the appearances of the lesion may easily be mistaken for lupus vulgaris, malignant granuloma, rodent ulcer or squamous carcinoma. Perforation of the septum may occur in the anterior cartilaginous part, usually near the floor of the nose. If this is accompanied by destruction of the columella, the subsequent retraction of the tip of the nose produces a characteristic and peculiarly ugly deformity. Much more commonly the perforation is situated far back in the vomerine part of the septum. A posterior septal perforation is, in fact, usually due to syphilis; an anterior perforation, on the contrary, is rarely syphilitic, more usual causes being trauma, lupus vulgaris, the use of chromic acid as a cauterizing agent or industrial exposure to chromium or arsenical compounds.[52]

The inflammatory process in cases of tertiary syphilitic rhinitis may be very extensive. Syphilitic caries of the lateral nasal wall may lead to erosion of the maxillary sinus, or destruction of the lacrimal canal, or even invasion of the cranial cavity. It is important to note that the presence of necrotic bone in the nose should always raise the suspicion of syphilis.

Congenital syphilis

The nasal lesions of congenital syphilis may correspond in type to those of the secondary or tertiary stages of the acquired infection. Lesions of secondary type may be present at birth, but more often they first appear between 1 and 6 weeks afterwards, and they may be delayed until the third to the sixth month. The lesions are erythematous or mucous patches, and attention is usually drawn to them by the persistent catarrhal signs that are known as 'snuffles'. The discharge is often thick, yellow and blood-streaked: crusts form when it dries and increase the obstruction. It is the chronicity of the condition that distinguishes it from a simple coryza. The tertiary type of congenital lesions, which account for the characteristic nasal deformity, may follow immediately on the secondary symptoms: more often, however, they are delayed either to the age of 3 or 4 years or to the time of the second dentition, when the other later stigmas of the infection become apparent. Collapse of the bridge of the nose, perforation of the septum and of the hard palate, and ulceration of the vestibule or of the outer surface of the alae are the commonest manifestations.

Yaws (framboesia)

Caused by *Treponema pertenue*, yaws has a clinical and histological pattern somewhat similar to that of acquired syphilis. Transmission is believed to be by contagion or insect vectors. There is no congenital manifestation. The disease is indigenous in some tropical regions. Patients with the disease are seen occasionally in other parts of the world to which they have travelled. Tertiary lesions of yaws in the nose are hardly distinguishable from those of syphilis and in many cases the Wassermann reaction is positive.[53, 54]

Scleroma

Scleroma, or rhinoscleroma, is a chronic progressive granulomatous disease of long duration that begins in the nose and eventually extends into the nasopharynx and oropharynx, the larynx and sometimes the trachea and bronchi. It was first described by Hebra, in 1870: his term for it, rhinoscleroma, has been replaced by scleroma, which is more appropriate for a disease that is not necessarily confined to the nose.

Scleroma occurs at any age but its greatest fre-

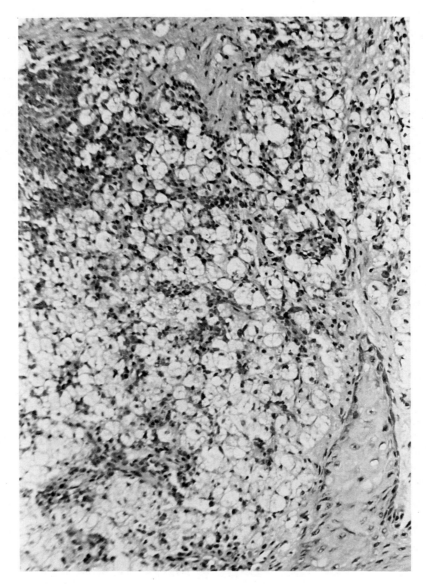

Fig. 2.10 Scleroma of the nose showing large numbers of clear Mikulicz cells.   Haematoxylin–eosin   × 308

quency is in the third decade. Both sexes are equally affected. People of any race may be affected. It has been endemic in Eastern Europe, including parts of Hungary, Slovakia, Poland and the Ukraine, in some countries on the Mediterranean (particularly in North Africa), in Pakistan and Indonesia and in parts of Central America and Central Africa. Strict epidemiological measures seem to have eradicated the disease from some countries, for example Slovakia.

Occasional cases are seen in other parts of the world. It has been observed in immigrant families in Britain. An indigenous case was recognized in County Fermanagh, in Northern Ireland, in 1940 and another in Edinburgh in 1942 (the Scottish patient was the wife of a Polish officer, who was free from evidence of the disease).[55]

Three clinical stages of the disease are recognized: 1) the catarrhal rhinitis stage; 2) the in-

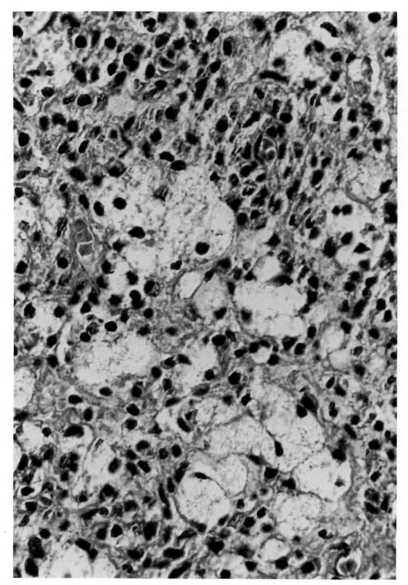

Fig. 2.11 Scleroma of the nose. There are groups of Mikulicz cells containing bacilli surrounded by plasma cells. Haematoxylin–eosin × 880

flammatory and proliferative granulomatous stage; and 3) the cicatricial, deformative stage.

The disease may result from the exposure of the members of an affected household to a common source of infection, aggravated by a poor standard of domestic hygiene. This does not imply that infection is necessarily conveyed by person to person contact.

Aetiology

There is general agreement that scleroma is due to infection by *Klebsiella pneumoniae* subsp. *rhinoscleromatis*, the organism described by von Frisch in 1882. This bacillus, which is serologially related to *K. pneumoniae* of serotype C, can always be found in the lesions of scleroma and specific antibodies are found in a considerable proportion of patients with the disease. Serolog ical investigations are, in fact, valuable in establishing the diagnosis of scleroma.[56] Further evidence that *K. pneumoniae* subsp. *rhinoscleromatis* is causally concerned has been provided by the successful treatment of the disease by various antibiotics to which this organism is sensitive, particularly streptomycin.

The disease has been reproduced in the skin of experimental mice[57, 58] by repeated inoculation of *K. pneumoniae* subsp. *rhinoscleromatis* mixed with hog gastric mucin. After many weeks typical lesions, including the classical Mikulicz cells, appeared in inoculated mice and the klebsiella was subsequently recovered from the lesion, thus fulfilling Koch's postulates. There seems to be little doubt now that the causal agent belongs to the *Klebsiella* group although there may be variants.[59] However the majority of strains of *Klebsiella* isolated from cases of scleroma appear to be antigenically and biochemically homogeneous.

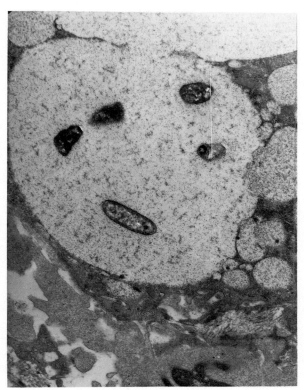

Fig. 2.12 Electron micrograph showing organisms in a cytoplasmic vesicle of a Mikulicz cell.   × 11 550

Scleroma is characterized by the growth of nodular masses of sclerotic, granulomatous tissue that has a strikingly cartilaginous consistency. Ulceration and foul discharge are typically present. The initial sites of involvement are usually the septum, the floor of the nose or a concha: the process then extends throughout the interior of the nasal cavities, although ordinarily sparing the superior meatus. The sinuses become involved, and the disease eventually spreads to the rest of the respiratory passages. In some cases the skin of the upper lip is involved.

Histopathology

Microscopically, the only specific feature of the inflammatory reaction is the presence of the intracellular *Klebsiella*. The mucosa is greatly thickened by an accumulation of plasma cells, lymphocytes and macrophages. The most characteristic aspect of the picture is the Mikulicz cell: this is a large macrophage with foamy-looking cytoplasm in which the bacilli are loosely clustered (Figs 2.10, 2.11, 2.12). The mucous capsule that the bacilli produce gives a positive periodic acid/Schiff reaction, and this is helpful in demonstrating their presence. An immunoperoxidase technique has now been developed for the identification of the organism in paraffin wax sections.[60]

The Mikulicz cells are to be found anywhere in the affected tissue, although most frequently in the subepithelial zone (Fig. 2.10). They may be so numerous as to be very readily seen, or many sections may have to be searched. There is often some degree of ulceration of the lesions, and secondary infection by other organisms may result in infiltration by neutrophils. Extensive fibrosis is found in the older lesions.

There are numerous Russell bodies in scleromatous lesions. The name Mott cell has been suggested for the type of plasma cell that is the origin of the Russell body. This cell is also known as the thesaurocyte because the cisternae of its endoplasmic reticulum are distended with stored globules of secretory matter. Coalescence of these globules results in the formation of the Russell body.[61, 62, 63] These bodies were described by Russell in 1890 in cells located at the margins of malignant tumours, and he misinterpreted them as an essential component of the neoplastic process.

There is frequently squamous metaplasia of the surface epithelium and pseudocarcinomatous hyperplasia may develop. The individual cellular components of the scleroma lesion are not in themselves specific features but, in combination, they produce a characteristic morphological pattern. Bacteriological confirmation of this diagnosis must always be sought.

There has been much speculation regarding the nature and origin of the Mikulicz cells. The generally accepted view is that they are derived from macrophages, a view which is supported particularly by ultrastructural studies.[64, 65, 66] Mikulicz cells contain mucopolysaccharide derived from the causal organisms. This material, which often lies within phagosomes, has been shown to have antigenic identity with the capsular substance and may protect the organism against antibodies or antibiotics. Under the electron microscope the Mikulicz cell is seen to contain numerous organisms, distended vesicular structures and a variable quantity of granular material (Fig. 2.12). This material resembles that seen surrounding the intracellular organism and also the organism in culture.[66] The inability of the cells to destroy or inactivate the phagocytosed microorganisms may be due to peculiar qualities of the bacteria, cellular deficiencies or impaired cellular immunity. It has been shown that serum from normal individuals and from patients with active or inactive rhinoscleroma kills *K. pneumoniae* subsp. *rhinoscleromatis* (this bactericidal effect is complement-dependent).[67]

MYCOSES

There is no mycosis that will not occasionally affect the nose and nasal sinuses. Some, like actinomycosis and nocardiosis, are very rare in these parts of the upper respiratory tract; others are relatively frequent, and some seem even to have a predisposition to occur here. Those that occur with special frequency include candidosis, zygomycoses, aspergillosis and rhinosporidiosis, all of which will be dealt with below. Paracocci-diodomycosis (South American blastomycosis)

also has a particular tendency to involve the nose, spreading from the mouth. Cryptococcosis, histoplasmosis, blastomycosis (North American blastomycosis), coccidioidomycosis, chromomycosis, and sporotrichosis are occasional causes of cutaneous or mucocutaneous ulceration of the nose. The specific nature of such lesions can be established only by identifying the fungus in histological sections[68] or, preferably, by culture. The cutaneous lesions of some of these infections are often difficult to distinguish clinically from ulcerated basal cell carcinomas.

It is noteworthy that examples of nasal involvement in all the fungal infections named above, including those that are not indigenous, have been seen in Britain since the first edition of this book appeared in 1966. This reflects again the importance of considering rare and exotic diseases in an increasingly international environment.

Fungal infections of the upper respiratory tract have been increasing in frequency and variety. These increases in part result from the great volume of international travel, which brings hitherto exotic mycoses to the attention of doctors, and in part to the occurrence of so called opportunistic mycoses as a consequence of steroid and antibiotic therapy and of the use of powerful cytotoxic drugs. Many common saprophytic organisms that under normal conditions have little or no pathogenic capacity may produce disease in debilitated or otherwise immunologically compromised patients. Such disease may escape diagnosis before autopsy; however, biopsy, culture and occasionally serological tests[69] may assist in establishing the diagnosis clinically.

MYCOSES CAUSED BY TRUE FUNGI

Candidosis

It is generally said that candidosis is the commonest fungal infection of the nose. In most cases the organism is *Candida albicans* and the nasal involvement accompanies superficial mucosal candidosis of the mouth and throat (thrush). Nasal thrush is much less frequent than oral thrush.

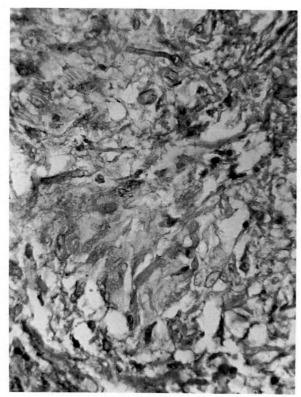

Fig. 2.13 Candidosis of the frontal sinus showing pseudohyphae lying in granulation tissue.

Haematoxylin–eosin   × 550

Candida granuloma
Granuloma formation is very seldom the result of infection by species of candida and examples in the nose are particularly rare. The diagnosis demands isolation of the fungus in pure culture as well as its identification in the granulomatous tissue (Fig. 2.13). In this context it is important to note that other fungi that may cause granulomas in the respiratory tract may be overgrown by candida.

Histologically, the candida granuloma resembles a straightforward tuberculoid lesion with multinucleate giant cells and foci of suppurative or caseous necrosis. The fungal elements are present both within the giant cells and free in the tissues, especially in the microabscesses. Differentiation from granulomas caused for instance, by species of aspergillus, is often impossible by conventional histological means, for the appearances

of the fungi in the sections are not always distinctive. In one case, that of a Sikh, candida infection of a frontal sinus was not recognized until a second biopsy following the failure of anti-tuberculous treatment showed the presence of the fungus in some of the giant cells in a necrotic granuloma;[70] (the granuloma had been misinterpreted as tuberculosis when the original biopsy was examined).

Zygomycosis (phycosmycosis)— entomophthoramycosis and mucormycosis
There are two clinically, aetiologically and mycologically distinct forms of zygomycosis of the nose and sinuses. Fungi of the order Entomophthorales cause very chronic infections that develop without recognized predisposing causes. In contrast, fungi of the order Mucorales cause rather rapidly progressive infections, originating in the sinuses, in patients whose resistance is lowered by other diseases or their treatment. Both forms of zygomycosis are important and will be considered in more detail.

Entomophthoramycosis[71]
There are two distinct clinicopathological forms of entomophthoramycosis; entomophthoramycosis due to infection by *Basidiobolus ranarum*,[72] which is a chronic granulomatous disease of the subcutaneous tissue, and entomophthoramycosis due to infection by species of conidiobolus (usually *Conidiobolus coronatus*)[73] which is the condition described below.

This mycosis was first described in 1961, as a nasal granuloma of horses in Texas, in the United States of America,[74] and in 1965 as the cause of a comparable condition in a boy in the West Indies.[75] The disease had been defined clinically in Nigeria in 1963 and was mycologically confirmed there in 1967;[73] most of the published cases have been from West Africa. It has been recognized in Brazil[76] and probably in India[77] and Malaysia.[78] It seems thus to be a disease of hot climates. Most of the patients have been young adults, men predominating, but children and old people may also be affected. The source and method of infection are unknown. The earliest lesions are commonly on the inferior concha on one side, the infection spreading

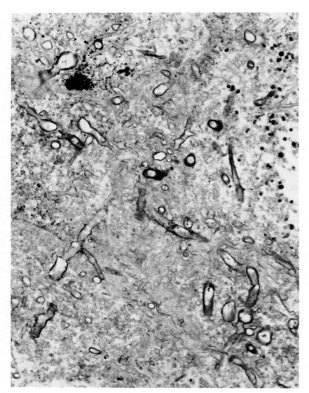

Fig. 2.14 Entomophthoramycosis showing the clear, sharply outlined hyphae surrounded by a broad eosinophilic deposit (from a pulmonary granuloma in a case of nasal infection by *Conidiobolus coronatus*).

Haematoxylin–eosin   × 340

Provided by Dr W. St C. Symmers.

This material contains lipid substances and is autofluorescent; ultrastructural examination has revealed nuclear and cytoplasmic debris derived from the cellular infiltrate. Some of the amorphous material is probably an antigen–antibody complex similar to that in the Arthus type hypersensitivity reaction.[79] Microabscesses and pseudotubercles may be present; the fungus is usually said not to penetrate the blood vessels.

Mucormycosis

Infection by species of *Rhizopus*, *Absidia*, *Mucor* or other zygomycetes is the cause of a rapidly fatal infection that originates in the sinuses and spreads to the orbit and brain. These fungi are ubiquitous saprophytic moulds that seem incapable of causing disease unless the patient's resistance to their invasion is broken by the effects on the body's defences of other diseases or of drugs and other therapeutic procedures: the mycoses that they cause are, in fact, classic examples of so called 'opportunistic' infection. The fungi belong to the order Mucorales and the infections they cause are given the name mucormycosis. Usually the portal of infection is the maxillary sinus or the ethmoid air cells;[80-84] usually one side only is affected. The nasal cavity is frequently involved.[80, 81, 85, 86] Involvement of the sphenoid sinus has been reported on several occasions.[83, 84, 86] A frontal sinus has been affected more rarely.[87]

In most cases the infection is a complication of some severe metabolic disorder characterized by persistant acidosis, particularly uncontrolled diabetes mellitus.[11, 84, 86] The association of severe diabetes mellitus, orbital cellulitis with ophthalmoplegia, and signs of meningoencephalitis makes up a syndrome that is diagnostic of *rhinocerebral mucormycosis*.[88, 89a] Clinical evidence of the underlying sinus involvement is rarely apparent. In the absence of effective antifungal treatment the disease is inevitably fatal. *Cunninghamella* has been recognized as a new cause of rhinocerebral mucormycosis. The organism is a zygomycete in the order *Mucorates*.[89b]

Histopathology. Microscopy shows granulation tissue with haemorrhage and necrosis. There is infiltration by polymorphonuclear leucocytes,

widely to involve the rest of the nasal passages, the sinuses, the orbits and the subcutaneous tissue of the face, but the infection is usually confined to these regions. Pain is unusual and secondary infection rare. Little is known about the outcome; it is doubtful whether the infection regresses spontaneously, as is sometimes the case in the very similar condition of the subcutaneous tissues referred to above.[72] Extension to the lungs has been noted in a fatal case.[78]

Histopathology.[78] The cellular infiltrate consists of eosinophils, with histiocytes, lymphocytes and plasma cells. Giant cells of foreign-body type are also present. The characteristically non-septate hyphae are commonly surrounded by a zone of eosinophilic granular material, with or without a peripheral palisade of histiocytes (Fig. 2.14).

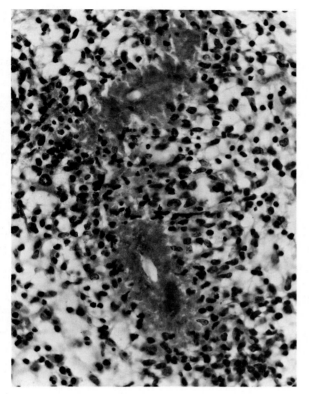

Fig. 2.15 Field in renal infarct in a case of naso-orbital zygomycosis caused by a species of *Mucor*. The variable width of the non-septate hyphae is characteristic.

Haematoxylin–eosin   × 215

Provided by Dr W. St C. Symmers.

histiocytes foam cells and multinucleated giant cells which may be of the Langhans type.[90] Non-septate fungal hyphae are found in the inflammatory tissue (Fig. 2.15), sometimes within the giant cells. A particular characteristic of mucormycosis is involvement of blood vessels. The mycelium of the fungi responsible penetrates the wall of vessels, including arteries: this induces intravascular thrombosis with consequent local infarction and necrosis. The fungus colonizes the thrombus and the dead tissue: it is readily recognized by its very broad, ribbon-like non-septate hyphae, which range from 3–35 μm in diameter.

Aspergillosis

Aspergillosis presents in two main forms in the nasal region. As so often, the facts have been unnecessarily confused by abuse of terminology. For instance, the granulomatous disease that results from invasion of the mucosa of the sinuses by an aspergillus has been described as an aspergilloma. This term in the context of bronchopulmonary disease is used exclusively to denote the common intracavitary fungal ball colony, a condition that is only exceptionally accompanied by fungal invasion of the tissues. It would be in the interests of everybody if this misuse of conventionally accepted terminology ended.

Aspergillus is an opportunistic fungus which can give rise to a variety of forms of infection—pulmonary, cutaneous and cerebral infection and systemic dissemination are recognized and are often superimposed on some other debilitating disease; the predisposition may be aggravated by therapy. A fatal case of meningoencephalitis due to *Aspergillus* following treatment of pulmonary tuberculosis with anti-tuberculous drugs and a steroid compound has been reported.[91] Immuno-suppressants may allow formerly saprophytic aspergillus to reach blood vessels which they penetrate, resulting in a septicaemia. *Aspergillus fumigatus* has been injected intravenously into rats which developed a cerebral infection,[92] whilst experimental intracranial aspergillosis has been produced by an intranasal route coupled with intensive cortisone administration.[93]

Aspergillosis is the most common fungal infection in the maxillary sinus.[94] Paranasal infections by *Aspergillus* are usually primary, not a complication of other diseases. The species most frequently involved in human paranasal infections are *Aspergillus fumigatus* and *Aspergillus flavus*. Of six such cases investigated at the Mycological Reference Laboratory in London two were caused by *Aspergillus fumigatus*, two by *Aspergillus flavus*, one by *Aspergillus glaucus* and one by *Aspergillus niger*.[95]

Aspergillus fungal ball (aspergilloma)

A ball colony of *Aspergillus*, usually—as in the lungs—*Aspergillus fumigatus*, is a rare finding in a nasal sinus. In most cases it occurs in a maxillary sinus or frontal sinus, particularly the former. The colony lies free wtihin the lumen of the sinus, and in some cases its mobility can be demonstrated radiologically. A characteristic histological feature is the onion-skin-like structure of the fungal ball.[96] Although the fungal ball predisposes to secondary infection by pyogenic bacteria and may therefore be associated with erosion or ulceration of the lining of the sinus, it is rare for the tissues to be invaded by the fungus. Nevertheless, as in the case of the pulmonary aspergilloma, if the patient's resistance is lowered by other disease or by drugs such as corticosteroids and cytotoxic agents, the fungus may invade the blood stream and establish a fatal septicaemia.

Aspergillus granuloma

This is the condition that has been mistermed 'aspergilloma' (see above). It is a granulomatous infection, usually confined to one of the sinuses but occasionally more widespread. It is particularly frequent in hot, dry climates; many of the reported cases occurred in the Sudan. The fungus most frequently identified as its cause has been *Aspergillus flavus*.[95-98]

Histopathology. The lesion consists of nonspecific granulation tissue containing microabscesses and multinucleated giant cells (Fig. 2.16), there may also be areas of necrosis. The fungus is abundant and consists of septate hyphae, which are often surprisingly hard to see in sections stained with haematoxylin and eosin. The hyphae give a positive periodic-acid/Schiff reaction. The hexamine-silver method (Grocott's methenamine-silver stain) is the most satisfactory of the special fungal stains for showing the organism in the granulomas (Fig. 2.17): its use should be a regular practice in the investigation of all granulomas of the nasal region.[68] The hyphae may be found lying in microabscesses or within the giant cells (Fig. 2.18). Sometimes they penetrate the wall of blood vessels and induce thrombosis; this tendency is not as marked as in mucormycosis. As the lesion progresses, fibrosis develops and areas may become almost completely sclerotic.

Rhinocerebral aspergillosis

Although very rare in comparison with the two varieties of nasal aspergillosis described above, this form of infection is important because of its high mortality. It is comparable in aetiology and

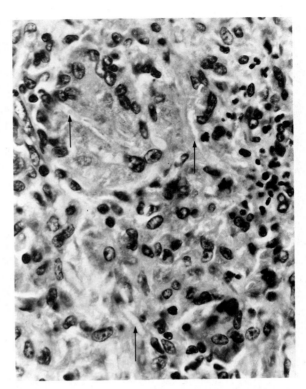

Fig. 2.16 Orbital aspergillosis from a case of naso-orbitocerebral infection. Hyphae (arrowed) appear unstained and are seen lying in multinucleated giant cells.
Haematoxylin–eosin   × 630
Provided by Dr W. St C. Symmers.

course to the opportunistic form of rhinozygomycosis (see above), occurring as a complication usually of persistent severe metabolic disturbances, such as uncontrolled diabetes mellitus. The infection spreads from the sinus to the orbit and thence to the meninges and brain. It tends to be less rapidly progressive than zygomycosis, perhaps because the aspergilli have less affinity for the blood vessels, tending to spread through the tissue spaces. As in the case of the aspergillus granuloma, this type of aspergillosis is usually caused by *Aspergillus flavus*. Invasive aspergillosis is difficult to diagnose. Blood cultures and serologic tests are usually negative.

Aspergillosis may also develop in the sphenoidal sinus. In this situation the infection may spread into the cranial cavity and usually is fatal. Surgical cure has been recorded in one case.[99]

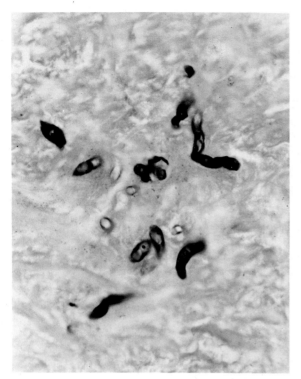

Fig. 2.17 Orbital aspergillosis showing fragments of hyphae.
Grocott's methenamine-silver stain   × 500
Provided by Dr W. St C. Symmers.

Fulminant aspergillosis
Fulminant aspergillosis of the nose and paranasal
sinuses is a new clinical entity occurring in individuals with depressed immunological responses.[91] It is marked by a rapid malignant
course, requiring early recognition and radical
surgery and chemotherapy. Its manifestations
include rapidly progressive gangrenous muco-
periostitis, advancing to destruction of the nasal
cavity and the paranasal sinuses within a few
days. The recent emergence of this form of aspergillosis appears to be directly related to the increased intensity of chemotherapy and immuno-
suppression in the treatment of cancer.

Oxalosis in aspergillus infection
The association of oxalate crystal deposition and
Aspergillus infection has been reported on a number of occasions. The presence of oxalate crystals
in specimens from the respiratory tract and in

pleural fluid may have diagnostic significance.
While oxalate deposition is more frequently associated with *Aspergillus niger* infections, mild
oxalosis has also been reported in association
with *Aspergillus fumigatus*. The production of oxalate by *Aspergillus niger* has been studied biochemically. The organism apparently possesses
the enzymes of the tricarboxylic acid cycle and
degrades oxaloacetate to oxalate by this route.[100]

Chromomycosis

Chromomycotic granuloma of the skin of the
nose is a rarity. Its usual cause is *Fonsecaea
(Phialophora) pedrosoi* or *Phialophora verrucosa*.
These organisms have been responsible for chromomycosis of the nasal septum of which only two
cases are on record.[101, 102] The fungus appears in
the tissues as dark brown bodies about 10 μm in
diameter in microabscesses or in multinucleate
giant cells.

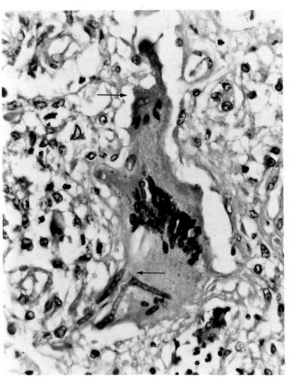

Fig. 2.18 Orbital aspergillosis showing hyphae (arrowed)
lying within a multinucleated giant cell.
Periodic-acid/Schiff reaction   × 400
Provided by Dr W. St C. Symmers.

Rhinosporidiosis

Rhinosporidiosis is a chronic infection caused by *Rhinosporidium seeberi*, an endosporulating organism that is nowadays generally classified among the fungi, although it has not yet been isolated in culture or transmitted successfully to animals. The morphology and life cycle have been widely studied and electron microscopy has provided further details.[103-106] The consistent presence of the parasite in its various forms is irrefutable evidence in favour of the cause of the lesion but animal inoculation has completely failed to reproduce the disease nor has the organism been grown on artificial media. Seeber, who first described the disease, believed the organism to be a protozoon, noting its resemblance to the coccidia.[107] Nothing is known about its occurrence outside infected tissues. The disease also occurs in some animals, particularly horses. Neither the route nor the source of infection has been discovered. The mode of transmission has not been finally settled. The condition occurs naturally in a variety of animals including horses, mules, cattle, goats, dogs, wild ducks and geese and the parrot *Psittacus ondulatus*.[108] It is of interest to note that the distribution of animal infections in India corresponds closely with the distribution of the human disease in the same country.

Rhinosporidiosis is seen most frequently in Sri Lanka and in parts of India and of Central and South America. It is rare elsewhere. It has been recognized exceptionally in patients who have never been out of Europe. Similarly, nasal rhinosporidiosis was recognized in a 73-year-old man who had lived all his life in the United States of America. His lesions were removed surgically and he remained free of disease 4 years later.[109] Occasional cases of the disease are met with in Britain in visitors or immigrants from parts of the world where the disease is endemic.

The lesions are vascular polypoid masses that develop on the nasal mucosa and occasionally in the conjunctiva or on the skin. They may be multiple.[110, 111, 112] Obstruction of the airway may occur and predisposes to bacterial infection. Occasionally, rhinosporidial infections develop at a distance from the initial site of the infection in the nose, the characteristic polypoid masses growing from the mucosa of the trachea or bronchi.

Histopathology

The microscopical appearances are distinctive for the spherical sporangia, which range from about 50–350 μm in diameter, are unmistakable. The sporangium has a thick structureless wall and contains innumerable spores that when mature are about the size of a red blood cell (Fig. 2.19). The tissue reaction is a nondescript chronic inflammation. Lymphocytes and plasma cells predominate rather than macrophages and giant cells, although these may be conspicuous in some specimens.

Outcome

There being no effective medicinal treatment, excision of the diseased areas is the only expedient. Even radical procedures may not prevent recurrence. Cases with widespread dissemination have been reported.[113, 114]

Rarer mycoses caused by true fungi

Alternaria species and *Curvularia* species are among the ubiquitous, saprophytic fungi which occasionally cause infection if resistance is lowered by diabetes or by diseases or treatment that interfere with immunity. An infection of the nasal septum by fungi of both of these genera occurred in a neutropenic patient.[115] There was histological evidence of invasion of the tissue. The patient recovered without the use of antifungal agents following surgical excision of the nasal septum.

MYCOSES CAUSED BY ACTINOMYCETES

Actinomycetes are considered to be bacteria. Others suggest that they form a separate group of organisms between the fungi and the bacteria.

Actinomycosis

Although the head and neck are the site of over 50% of cases of actinomycosis, involvement of the nose and sinuses is exceptional.

The usual site of infection is the maxillary sinus,[116-119] the condition developing over a period of weeks or months. Swelling of the cheek,

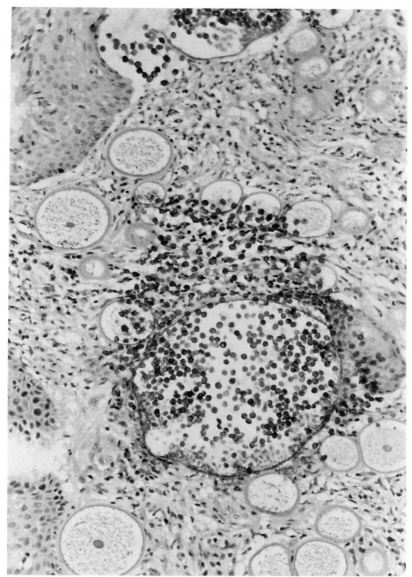

Fig. 2.19 Rhinosporidiosis showing detail of a large ruptured sporangium containing numerous spores. The smaller cysts are trophic forms of the organism.
Haematoxylin–eosin   × 225

with facial pain, is the usual presenting manifestation. Irrigation of the sinus may produce foul pus containing the causal organism, often in the form of so called 'sulphur granules' which are its colonies.

The cause of the disease in almost all cases is *Actinomyces israelii*; other species are seldom involved, the least rare being *Actinomyces bovis*. Infection of the maxillary and ethmoid sinuses has been reported following dental extraction. It would appear that the organism must have been present as a saprophyte in the mouth prior to the dental operation.[120] An infection of the maxillary sinus of a housewife living in an agricultural area, caused by *Actinomyces bovis*, could have been caused by direct inhalation of the organism.[119]

Nocardiosis

It has been suggested that the aerobic varieties of *Actinomyces* should be called *Nocardia*. Nocard, in 1888,[121] first recognized the condition and its causative organism in cattle in Guadeloupe. Eppinger[122] reported the first human case, a cerebral abscess. The two human strains are *Nocardia asteroides* and *Nocardia brasiliensis*. Some members of this group are non-acid-fast, but others such as *asteroides* are acid-fast, and rod forms may simulate *Mycobacterium tuberculosis*. Strongly acid-fast strains occur[123] but most strains are decolourized by 5% aqueous sulphuric acid.

Nocardia infection of the nose[124] and sinuses[125] is even rarer than actinomycosis. In one case,[124] that of an 80-year-old woman, biopsies from the nose revealed tuberculoid tissue. Fite's modification of the Ziehl–Neelsen stain revealed acid-fast bacilli: cultures for *Mycobacterium tuberculosis* were negative but an aerobic actinomycete (*Nocardia*) was isolated.

OTHER UNUSUAL INFECTIONS AND INFESTATIONS

Leishmaniasis[126]

Both Old World and New World cutaneous leishmaniasis may involve the nose. The lesions of the former, which is due to *Leishmania tropica*, seldom extend to the mucous membrane. In contrast, the nose is the commonest site of the mucocutaneous form of New World leishmaniasis, which is caused by *Leishmania brasiliensis*.

Mucocutaneous leishmaniasis

Involvement of the skin and mucous membrane at body orifices is a characteristic feature of the form of New World cutaneous leishmaniasis that is known as *espundia*. Espundia occurs in Central and South America, particularly in the Amazon basin and in the northern parts of the basin of the River Paraguay and the Gran Chaco. The reservoirs of infection are various rodents, particularly forest rats, and the vectors are sandflies of the genus *Lutzomyia*.

The initial lesion of infection with *Leishmania brasiliensis* is a cutaneous sore, usually on a foot or leg. This is quite comparable to the Old World leishmanial ulcer caused by *Leishmania tropica*. Mucocutaneous lesions develop in a proportion of cases that ranges from about 1% in parts of Central America to over 20% in parts of Brazil and considerably higher in some endemic areas of Paraguay. They may appear within a few months of the development of the initial sore, or the interval may be many years. The nose and upper lip are by far the most frequent site of mucocutaneous involvement. The occurrence of these lesions at a distance from the primary sore is conventionally attributed to 'metastasis'. There is doubt about the means of such metastatic spread: rather than being haematogenous it may well be effected merely by digital transfer of the organisms from the initial lesion to the nose or other mucocutaneous site, with their implantation through 'picking' and the resulting damage to the mucosa by the contaminated finger nail. While the sore at the site of the primary inoculation usually heals within a matter of months, or at most a couple of years, leaving a distinctive scar, the mucocutaneous lesions tend to be chronic and may not heal without treatment.

The affected mucocutaneous tissues are thickened by oedema, inflammatory cellular infiltrate and fibrosis. Within the nose the lesions may resemble polyps.[127] Superficial ulceration and secondary bacterial infection contribute to the picture. Gross distortion and destruction of the tissues eventually result. The so called 'tapir nose' is characteristic, although like many classic features of disease it is seldom seen in its typical form: it results from involvement and collapse of the anterior part of the cartilaginous septum, with loss of the columella and the lower parts of the alae.

The leishmaniae are usually easily found in the lesions in the earlier stages of the infection (Fig. 2.20). Later, they are fewer: at this stage the earlier diffuse scattering of the infected macrophages throughout the lesion may give way to a strikingly tuberculoid picture. This change in the character of the lesion and the parallel fall in the number of recognizable parasites suggest that a change has taken place in the patient's state of immunity.

New World leishmaniasis, like Old World

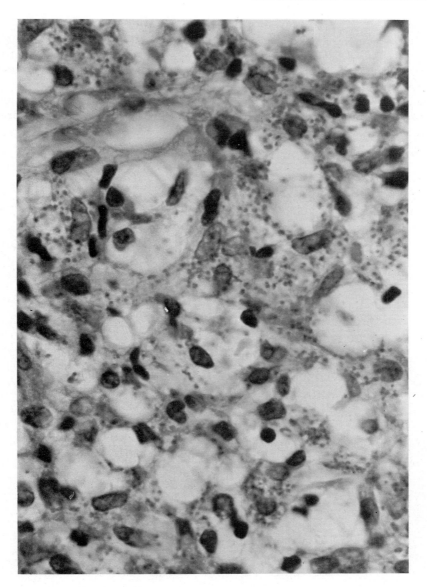

Fig. 2.20 Leishmaniasis of the nose. The parasites are mostly intracellular.
Haematoxylin–eosin   × 1250
Provided by Professor S. Haim, Haifa, Israel.

leishmaniasis included among the 'six diseases' of WHO,[128] is seen from time to time in practice in countries like Britain where neither occurs naturally.[129] The importance of knowing the patient's geographical history is clear, assuming the doctor to be sufficiently familiar with geographical medicine. It is worth noting again that care is needed to avoid mistaking *Histoplasma capsulatum* for a leishmania, or a leishmania for the histoplasma.[130] Both are intracellular parasites of the macrophages, and their similarity of size can cause them to be confused (see Fig. 7.5). The leishmaniae do not give a positive periodic-acid/Schiff reaction and are not shown by the hexamine-silver (methenamine-silver) method of staining fungi.

Viral granuloma

A patient who had recently received a cadaver kidney transplant developed fatal herpes simplex infection. The infection manifested itself as a progressive, ulcerating, destructive granuloma of the nose, complicating herpes of the upper lip.[131] Herpetic and other viral infections have become more frequent in consequence of the increased use of immunosuppressive therapy.

Hydatid disease

A 34-year-old Egyptian woman presented with a slowly growing swelling of the left side of her face. A cystic lesion removed from the maxillary sinus at operation proved to be a hydatid cyst. This appears to be the first case of hydatid disease of a paranasal sinus in the literature.[132]

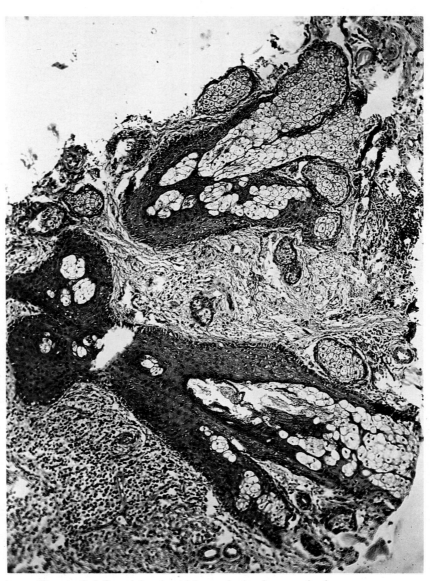

Fig. 2.21 Rhinophyma. Chronically inflamed dermis with hyperplastic sebaceous glands. Haematoxylin–eosin   × 75

RHINOPHYMA

Rhinophyma is preceded by a rosacea type of dermatitis, with transient episodes of erythema and vasodilation: indeed, it is now generally believed to be an outcome of rosacea. Its development is slow, taking anything from 5 to 20 years. Papules and pustules appear in crops, and repeated recurrence over the years leads to the characteristic picture. Hypertrophy of the tissues of the nose produces lobulate, dull red or purplish masses, ranging from 3 mm to several centimetres in diameter. When the condition is advanced the nose may be greatly enlarged, and the changes may affect other parts of the face that are liable to rosacea, such as the cheeks and forehead.

Histopathology

The essential microscopical features are hyperkeratosis of the epidermis, and hypertrophy and hyperplasia of the sebaceous glands. The follicles are distended by large accumulations of keratin and abscesses may develop within them. There is overgrowth of the connective tissue of the affected parts, and dilatation of the blood vessels. Lymphocytes and sometimes plasma cells and macrophages accumulate round the follicles and, particularly, the adjacent blood vessels (Fig. 2.21).

The incidence of rhinophyma is decreasing, perhaps because of earlier and more effective treatment of rosacea. There is no evidence that excessive consumption of alcohol plays any part in its causation, and this formerly popular theory has been abandoned by most dermatologists. The small metazoan parasite *Demodex folliculorum* is often present in large numbers in the follicles but it has no pathogenic significance.

REFERENCES

1. Tyrrell DAJ, Bynoe ML. Br Med J 1961; i: 393.
2. Scott GM, Wallace J, Greiner J, Phillpotts RJ, Gauci CL, Tyrrell DAJ. Lancet 1982; ii: 186.
3. Editorial. Lancet 1982; ii: 369.
4. Barnat I. Br Med J 1968; iii: 315.
5. Henriksen SD, Gunderson WB. Acta Pathol Microbiol Scand 1959; 47: 380.
6. Bailey QR. J Laryngol Otol 1981; 95: 55.
7. Wenig BL, Sciubba JJ, Zielinski BZ, Stegnjajic A, Abramson AL. Laryngoscope 1983; 93: 621.
8. Karma P, Jokipii L, Spila P, Luotenen J, Jokipii AM. Arch Otolaryngol (Stockh) 1979; 105: 386.
9. Sabiston CB, Grigsby WR, Segerstrom N. J Oral Surg 1976; 41: 430.
10. Katz P, Fauci AS. JAMA 1977; 238: 2397.
11. Blitzer A, Lawson W, Meyers BR, Biller HF. Laryngoscope 1980; 90: 635.
12. Busuttil A, More IAR, McSeveney D. J Anat 1977; 124: 445.
13. Busuttil A, More IAR, McSeveney D. Arch Otolaryngol 1978; 104: 260.
14. Busuttil A, More IAR, McSeveney D. Arch Otolaryngol 1976; 102: 589.
15. Kurian SS, Blank MA, Sheppard MN et al. IRCS Medical Science 1983; Respiratory System 11: 425.
16. Samter M. Arch Otolaryngol 1961; 73: 334.
17. Berdal P. Acta Otolaryngol (Stockh) 1954; 44 (Suppl 115): 1.
18. Donovan R, Johansson SGO, Bennich H, Soothill JF. Int Arch Allergy Appl Immunol 1970; 37: 154.
19. Crifo S, Russo M. Acta Otolaryngol (Stockh) 1980; 89: 214.
20. Smith CJ, Echevarria R, McLelland CA. Arch Otolaryngol 1974; 99: 228.
21. Klenoff BH, Goodman ML. J Laryngol Otol 1977; 91: 751.
22. Kindblom LG, Angervall L. Acta Path Microbiol Scand (A) 1984; 92: 65.
23. Friedmann I, Osborn DA. Pathology of granulomas and neoplasms of the nose and paranasal sinuses. Edinburgh: Churchill Livingstone, 1982: 34.
24. Graham J, Michaels L. Clin Otolaryngol 1978; 3: 155.
25. Hellquist H, Lundgren J, Olofsson J. ORL 1984; 46: 153.
26. Osborn DA, Wallace M. J Laryngol Otol 1967; 81: 1021.
27. McClatchie S, Warambo MW, Bremmer AD. Am J Clin Pathol 1969; 51: 699.
28. Hutt MSR, Fernandes BJJ, Templeton AC. Trans R Soc Trop Med Hyg 1971; 65: 182.
29. Kyriakos M. Am J Clin Pathol 1977; 67: 118.
30. De Schryver-Kecskmeti K, Kyriakos M. Am J Pathol 1978; 87: 33.
31. Rosai J. Am J Clin Pathol 1978; 69: 475.
32. Wheeler TM, McGavran MH. Am J Clin Pathol 1980; 73: 685.
33. Warin AP, Wilson Jones E. Clin Exp Dermatol 1977; 2: 235.
34. Waldman SR, Levine HL, Sebek B, Parker W, Tucker HM. Laryngoscope 1981; 91: 11.
35. Marks J. Tubercle 1969; 50: 78.
36. Boeck C. J Cut Genit Urin Dis 1899; 17: 543.
37. Robinson B, Pound AW. Med J Aust 1950; 2: 568.
38. Lindsay JR, Perlman HB. Ann Otol Rhinol Laryngol 1951; 60: 549.
39. Scadding JG. Sarcoidosis. London: Eyre & Spottiswoode, 1967.
40. Gordon WN, Cohn AM, Greenberg SD, Komorn RN. Arch Otolaryngol 1976; 102: 11.
41. James GD. Chest 1973; 64: 675.
42. Mitchell DN, Rees RJW, Goswami KKA. Lancet 1976; ii: 761.
43. Wright RE, Clairmont AA, Per-Lee JH, Butz WC. Laryngoscope 1974; 84: 2058.
44. Waters MF. Br Med J 1982; 282: 1320.

45. Ridley DS, Jopling WH. Int J Lepr 1962; 33: 119.
46. Barton RPE. Ann Otol Rhinol Laryngol 1976; 85: 74.
47. Davey TF. Lepr Rev 1974; 45: 97.
48. Rees RJW, McDougall AC, Weddell AGM. Lepr Rev 1974; 45: 112.
49. Davey TF, Rees RJW. Lepr Rev 1974; 45: 121.
50. Br Med J Annotation 1975; 2: 460.
51. Gil Tutor E. Acta Otorinolaryngol Iberoam 1971; 22: 366.
52. Hunter D. The diseases of occupations. 6th ed. London: Hodder & Stoughton, 1978; 350: 436.
53. Nicolas F. J Philippine Islands Med Ass 1924; 4: 140.
54. Fischman A, Mundt H. Br J Vener Dis 1971; 47: 91.
55. Cited by Friedmann I, Osborn DA. In: Symmers W St C, Systemic Pathology. 2nd ed. vol 1. Edinburgh: Churchill Livingstone, 1976; 205.
56. Toppozada H, Mazloum H, El-Sawy M, Malaty R, Yakout Y. J Laryngol Otol 1983; 97: 55.
57. Hoffmann EO. Int Pathol 1967; 8: 74.
58. Hoffmann EO, Duque E. Rev Latinoam Pathol 1971; 10: 57.
59. Rees TA, Gregory MM. Lancet 1977; i: 650.
60. Gumprecht TF, Nichols PW, Meyer PR. Laryngoscope 1983; 93: 627.
61. Mott FW. Proc Roy Soc B 1905; 76: 235.
62. Friedmann T. Trans Am Acad Opthalmol Otolaryngol 1963; 67: 261.
63. Thiery JP. In: Wolstenholme GEW, O'Connor M, eds. Cellular aspects of immunity. London: J & A Churchill, 1960; 59.
64. Friedmann I. Sci Basis Med 1963; 302.
65. Welsh RA, Correa P, Herran R. Exp Molec Pathol 1963; 2: 93.
66. Hoffmann EQ, Loose LD, Harkin JL. Am J Pathol 1973; 73: 47.
67. North ME, Newton CA, Wright DJM, Webster ADB. J Med Microbiol 1982; 15: 267.
68. Schwartz J. Hum Pathol 1982; 13: 519.
69. Smith H. Hosp Update 1976; 2: 573.
70. Osborn DA. J Laryngol 1963; 77: 39.
71. Martinson FD. Am J Trop Med Hyg 1971; 201: 449.
72. Joe LK, Eng NIT, Pohan A, van der Meulen H, Emmons CW. Arch Dermatol 1956; 74: 378.
73. Martinson FD, Clark BM. Am J Trop Med 1967; 16:
74. Emmons CW, Bridges CH. Mycolgia 1961; 53: 307.
75. Bras G, Gordon CC, Emmons CW, Prendegast KM, Sugar M. Am J Trop Med 1965; 14: 141.
76. Andrade ZA, Araujo PL, Sherlock IA, Cheever AW. Am J Trop Med 1967; 16: 31.
77. Grueber LE. J Christ Med Assoc India 1969; 44: 20.
78. Symmers W St C. Ann de la Soc Belg de Med Trop 1972; 52: 365.
79. Williams AO, Lichtenberg F, Smith JH, Martinson FD. Arch Pathol 1969; 87: 459.
80. Gregory GE, Golden A, Haymaker W. Bull Johns Hopkins Hosp 1943; 73: 405.
81. Stratemeier WP. Arch Neurol 1950; 63: 179.
82. Bauer H, Ajello L, Adams E, Hernandez DU. Am J Med 1955; 138: 822.
83. Baker RD. JAMA 1957; 163: 805.
84. Yanagisawa E, Friedmann S, Kundargi RS, Smith HW. Laryngoscope 1977; 87: 1319.
85. Kurrein F. J Clin Pathol 1954; 7: 141.
86. La Touche CJ, Sutherland CW, Telling M. Lancet 1963; ii: 811.
87. Bauer H, Flanagan JF, Sheldon WH. Am J Path 1955; 31: 600.
88. Pillsbury HC, Fischer MD. Arch Otolaryngol 1977; 103: 600.
89a. Case 38-1982. N Engl J Med 1982; 307: 806.
89b. Brennan RO, Crain BJ, Proctor AM et al. Am J Clin Pathol 1983; 80: 98.
90. Symmers W St C. In: Wolstenholme GEW, Porter R, eds. Ciba Foundation Symposium on Systemic Mycoses. London: J & A Churchill, 1968: 26.
91. Spens N, Tattersall WH. Br Med J 1965; 2: 862.
92. Turner KJ, Papadimitrious J, Hackshaw R, Wetherall JD. J Reticuloendothel Soc 1975; 17: 300.
93. Epstein SM, Miale TD, Moossy J, Verney E, Sidransky H. J Neuropathol Exp Neurol 1968; 27: 473.
94. Levine PA. Arch Otolaryngol 1977; 103: 560.
95. Br Med J 1977; i: 1291.
96. Stammberger H, Jakse R. HNO 1982; 30: 81.
97. Veress B, Malika OA, El Tayer AE. Am J Trop Med 1973; 22: 765.
98. Rudwan MA, Sheikh HA. Clin Radiol 1976; 27: 497.
99. Miglets AW, Saunders WH, Ayers L. Arch Otolaryngol 1978; 104: 47.
100. Blackmon JA. Am J Clin Pathol 1981; 75: 506.
101. Symmers W St C. J Clin Pathol 1960; 13: 287.
102. Nakamura T, Grant JA, Thrlkeld R, Wible L. Am J Clin Pathol 1972; 58: 365.
103. Kannan-Kutty M, Teh EC. Pathology 1974; 6: 63.
104. Kannan-Kutty M, Teh EC. Pathology 1974; 6: 183.
105. Kannan-Kutty M, Teh EC. Arch Pathol 1975; 99: 51.
106. Vanbreuseghem R. Dermatol Monatsschrift 1976; 162: 512.
107. Seeber GR. Thesis. Buenos Aires: Universidad Nacionale, 1900.
108. Ramachandra PV, Jain SN, Hanumantha RTV. Ann Soc Belge Med Trop 1975; 50: 119.
109. Lasser A, Smith HW. Arch Otolaryngol 1976; 102: 308.
110. Desmond AF. J Laryngol Otol 1953; 67: 51.
111. Kameswaran S, Jaiswal SL, Mahure MN. J Laryngol Otol 1970; 84: 1083.
112. Chatterjee PK, Khatua CR, Chatterjee SN, Dastidar N. J Laryngol Otol 1977; 91: 729.
113. Rajam RV, Viswanathan GS, Rao AR, Rangiah PN, Anguli VC. Indian J Surg 1955; 17: 269.
114. Subramanyam CSV, Ramano RAV. Br J Surg 1960; 47: 411.
115. Montgomery JZ, Becroft DMO, Croxson MC, Doak PB, North JDK. Lancet 1969; ii: 867.
116. Kernan JD. Laryngoscope 1936; 46: 483.
117. Voss HGW. J Am Dent Assoc 1939; 26: 260.
118. Hersch JH. Arch Otolaryngol 1945; 41: 204.
119. Stanton MB. J Laryngol Otol 1966; 80: 168.
120. Lewy RB, Manning EL. Arch Otolaryngol 1949; 49: 423.
121. Nocard E. Ann Institut Pasteur 1888; 2: 293.
122. Eppinger F. Beitr Pathol Anat Allg Pathol 1890; 9: 287.
123. Spencer H. Pathology of the lung. 3rd ed. Oxford: Pergamon Press, 1977: 255.
124. Friedmann I, Osborn DA. Pathology of granulomas and neoplasms of the nose and paranasal sinuses. Edinburgh: Churchill Livingstone, 1982: 79.
125. Katz P, Fauci AS. JAMA 1977; 238: 2397.
126. Manson-Bahr PEC, Winslow DJ. In: Marcial-Rojas

RA, Moreno E, eds. Pathology of protozoal and helminthic diseases with clinical correlation. Baltimore: Williams & Wilkins, 1971; 97.

127. Jaffe L. Arch Otolaryngol 1954; 60: 601.
128. Chance ML. Br Med J 1981; 283: 1245.
129. Emslie ES. Br Med J 1962; i: 299.
130. Woo Z-P, Reimann HA. J Am Med Ass 1957; 164: 1092.
131. Loveless MO, Winn RE, Campbell M, Jones SR. Am J Clin Pathol 1981; 76: 491.
132. Assal AM, Arafa MS. J Egypt Soc Parasitol 1983; 13: 509.

3

Non-healing nasal granulomas of unknown cause

THE MIDFACIAL GRANULOMA SYNDROME

The wide variety of granulomatous diseases of the nasal region includes a very important group of progressive necrotizing granulomas of unknown causation that have little or no tendency to heal spontaneously. The multiplicity of names that have been given to these conditions indicates the unresolved nature of the aetiological problem. Whilst two main and distinct forms of these non-healing granulomas are now widely recognized, Wegener's disease and the so-called Stewart type of necrotizing granuloma, these represent the ends of a spectrum of related conditions.

Stewart[1] gave a detailed account of destructive granulomas in the nose whilst another form of nasal granuloma was defined by Wegener[2, 3] who described it as a rhinogenic form of polyarteritis. Wegener's granulomatosis, in contrast to the 'Stewart type' of granuloma, was frequently found to exhibit widespread involvement, particularly of the lungs and kidneys, but, subsequently, a localized or limited form was reported.[4, 5]

These two conditions are histologically of quite different pattern, and typical cases of each are readily recognized and cannot be confused with one another: in the intermediate series of cases that do not fall clearly into one category or the other there is represented every shade of histological pattern, linking the two extremes.

Wegener's disease is a giant celled tuberculoid necrotizing granuloma that arises in the upper air passages and eventually involves the lungs, kidneys and small arteries throughout the body. The Stewart type of necrotizing granuloma, in contrast, is a non-tuberculoid histiocytic and lymphocytic granuloma, frequently confined to the nasal region and without accompanying visceral and vascular changes. Its granulomatous nature is less apparent than that of Wegener's disease and it has been much more often taken for a malignant tumour than the latter. Many attempts have been made to clarify the conflicting biological concepts and histological interpretations of these two forms of necrotizing granuloma of the nose. Their study has been hampered by unresolved aetiological problems and confusion has been added to by the introduction of a multiplicity of descriptive names.

Neither of these diseases is as rare as the comparatively small number of published cases might seem to indicate. Both have been recognized as entities only comparatively recently: yet they are already familiar to most pathologists and ear, nose and throat specialists from personal experience. In the past the Stewart type of necrotizing granuloma was generally mistaken for carcinoma, and most clinicians and pathologists of today can look back on cases of supposed cancers of the face or nose that, in the light of present knowledge, would probably be regarded as examples of this disease. It must be pointed out, however, that some cancers arising in the nose—particularly malignant lymphomas—may exactly reproduce the clinical features of the Stewart granuloma. This may cause serious practical difficulties, especially because it is often hard to distinguish confidently between the latter and these types of sarcoma on histological grounds, particularly in biopsy specimens from early lesions.

WEGENER'S GRANULOMATOSIS [2–6]

The disease takes the form of a necrotizing giant-celled granuloma that usually presents first in some part of the upper respiratory tract, with the subsequent development of confluent, necrotic lesions in the lungs. An arteritis of polyarteritic type affects the pulmonary and systemic vasculature.

The preventing symptoms may relate to the nose, or nasal manifestations may be trivial and overshadowed by purpura, haematuria, abdominal pain and renal failure. Malaise, fever and loss of weight may be out of proportion to other clinical findings, the significance of such local symptoms as 'catarrh' and 'sinusitis' being then readily overlooked. Sooner or later, signs that point to the respiratory system, and particularly to the upper respiratory tract, usually develop. Rarely, however, evidence of nasal or pulmonary involvement is not evident until necropsy. The more obtrusive symptoms of upper respiratory tract disease, such as bloodstained nasal discharge or frank epistaxis, hoarseness and deafness or earache are less likely to be neglected in diagnosis.

The earlier intranasal changes take the form of crusted, bleeding granulations on the septum and conchae, with thickening of the mucosa. Later protuberant granulomas form, especially on the septum, and become ulcerated with conspicuous destruction of the tissues. In our series of 25 cases the presenting lesion was in the nose in 11 cases, in a maxillary sinus in 6, in the hard palate in 2, in an ear in 3 and in an orbit in 3. As the disease advances external signs often appear; oedema of the orbits and face, proptosis, antroalveolar fistula and even collapse of the nasal bridge are among these. Spreading ulcers may develop in the mouth, pharynx and larynx. Prior to modern treatment death occurred within 6 months to 1 year of the onset of symptoms. It is generally the result of renal failure caused by the vascular changes in the kidneys: characteristically, there is a necrotizing glomerulitis as well as renal arteritis (Figs 3.1, 3.2). Necrotizing granulomas similar to those in the respiratory tract, but small and discrete, and sometimes mistaken for miliary tubercles, are found in the spleen (the 'speckled spleen' or *Fleckmilz* of the literature in German) and other viscera in some cases.

Histopathology

The presence of multinucleate giant cells, although not pathognomonic, is helpful in the correct interpretation of the significance of the presenting lesion in cases of Wegener's granulomatosis (Figs 3.3, 3.4, 3.5). In some cases giant

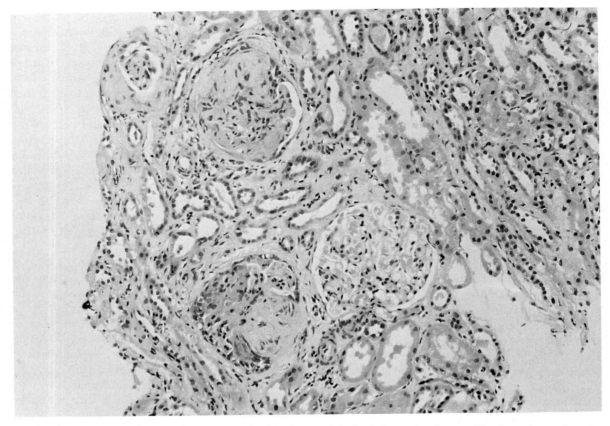

Fig. 3.1 Wegener's granulomatosis. Renal biopsy showing characteristic focal glomerular changes. The three glomeruli are in different stages of necrosis and hyalinization.

Haematoxylin–eosin   × 180

cells are found readily: in others, they are scanty, and tend to be grouped near to blood vessels. Sometimes they lie so close to the artery that the picture is very similar to that of giant cell arteritis, but the two conditions can be distinguished by the fact that in Wegener's granulomatosis the giant cell reaction is not related to the breakdown of the elastica in the vessel wall as it is in true giant cell arteritis (Figs 3.6, 3.7).

The giant cells may resemble those of tuberculosis, but their nuclei are often peculiarly compact, appearing dense, ovoid, and so intensely haematoxyphilic that they frequently look black (Fig. 3.5). The nuclei are often clustered in two sickle-shaped groups at opposite poles of the cell. The cytoplasm is generally more compact, more homogeneous and more eosinophilic than in the giant cells of other tuberculoid granulomas.

Attention to these cytological details can be helpful in diagnosis.

The differential diagnosis includes the specific infective granulomas and non-specific granulomas.

The destruction of tissue is not as extensive in Wegener's granulomatosis as in the Stewart type of necrotizing granuloma: in particular, there is less tendency for cartilage and bone to become involved.

The disease usually occurs in adults. There is no significant difference in the sex incidence. Little is known of its causation. Allergy to the bacteria that are associated with chronic infections of the nose, sinuses, throat and ears has been suggested and sensitization to drugs—particularly sulphonamides and antibiotics—has also been named as a possible factor, as in polyarter-

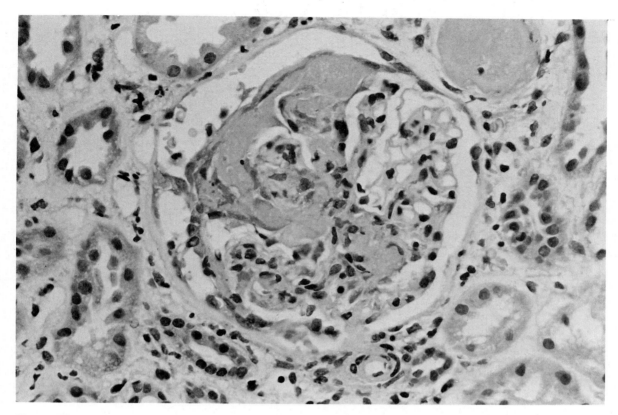

Fig. 3.2 Wegener's granulomatosis. Renal biopsy showing segmental hyalinization of a glomerulus. Haematoxylin–eosin   × 480

itis.[7] It is relevant that patients who develop the disease seem to be unusually liable to sensitivity reactions of one sort or another: this is indicated by the high incidence of urticarial drug reactions and of blood transfusion reactions of the 'serum sickness' type. However, the causal significance of an allergic factor has not been proved in any case. It is of interest that prednisolone acetate injected into the nasal mucosa for the treatment of allergic rhinitis may cause a destructive granuloma. It may be solitary or confluent, containing a central area of amorphous and/or birefringent crystalline material which leads to the formation of a foreign body granuloma.[8]

Others have regarded the disease as being due to an autoimmune reaction[9] or possibly to a deficiency of cell-mediated immunity.[10] Circulating immune complexes have been reported in Wegener's granulomatosis with varying frequency;[11] and it has been said that they can be found in about two-thirds of cases.[12] The immune complexes may be present during the active phase of Wegener's disease but tend to disappear during remission brought about by immunosuppressive therapy.[13] It has been observed that relapses that have occurred in patients with Wegener's granulomatosis have been provoked by bacterial or viral infection.[14] A possible explanation of this occurrence of relapse following infection is that immune complexes formed during infection reactivate the disease.

Limited Wegener's granulomatosis
The concept of limited Wegener's granulomatosis, in which the kidneys appear to be unaffected, is well recognized.[4, 5, 15] The most frequent site of the lesion is in the lungs, but the nose and/or larynx may be the only site affected. Early diagnosis of the disease has gained importance in

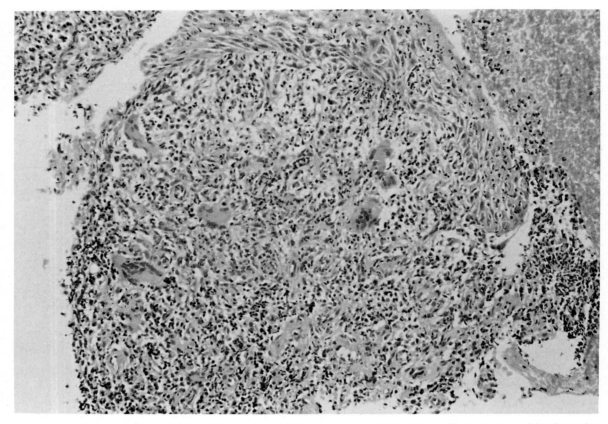

Fig. 3.3 Wegener's granulomatosis. Nasal biopsy showing inflammatory granulation tissue with numerous multinucleate giant cells and an area of necrosis (taken after renal biopsy: see Figs 3.1 and 3.2).   Haematoxylin–eosin   × 180

view of the success of treatment with cyclophosphamide and prednisolone.[16–20] It is therefore important to recognize the disease in its earlier limited form in the upper respiratory tract.[21]

Atypical Wegener's granulomatosis

Atypical cases of Wegener's granulomatosis have been described, presenting as rheumatoid arthritis, the nasal lesions developing subsequently.[22] The nervous system may be involved.[23] The genital organs may also be affected in both sexes.[17, 24]

THE STEWART TYPE OF NON-HEALING NECROTIZING GRANULOMA ('MALIGNANT GRANULOMA')

A plethora of terms has been introduced including 'malignant granuloma',[25] 'granuloma gangraenescens',[26] 'progressive lethal granulomatous ulceration',[1] 'lethal midline granuloma',[27] 'non-healing midline granuloma',[28] 'polymorphic reticulosis',[29] 'midline malignant reticulosis',[30] and 'idiopathic midline granuloma'.[31] Furthermore, the expression 'midfacial' is considered more acceptable than 'midline'. The substitution of 'reticulosis' for 'granuloma' has received support from other authors.[32, 33] The descriptive title '*rhino-sinusites nécrosantes léthales plurilésionelles*'[34] is the most comprehensive. Batsakis[35] uses the term 'idiopathic midline (non-healing) granuloma'. In the course of studying a number of patients presenting with destructive lesions of the upper respiratory tract, Tsokos et al[36] found 11 cases with the unique clinicopathological features, resembling the classical Stewart type of midfacial granuloma, calling it 'idiopathic midline destructive disease'.

The Stewart type of midline granuloma is al-

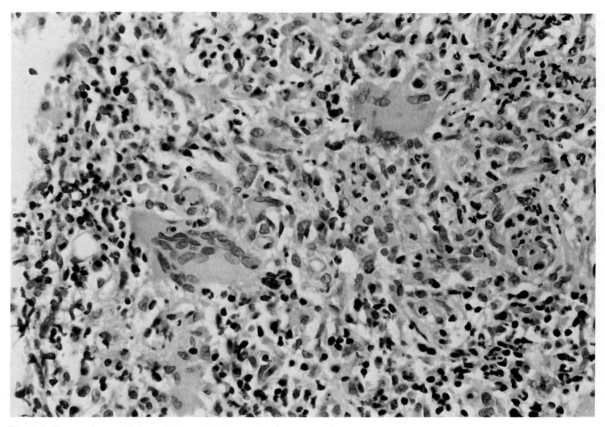

Fig. 3.4 Wegener's granulomatosis. Detail of Figure 3.3 showing giant cell granulation tissue in nasal biopsy. Haematoxylin–eosin × 480

most always preceded by a longstanding, non-specific infection of the nose or nasal sinuses. The initial manifestation of the developing granuloma is an indurated swelling of the tissues of some part of the nose: this may be the vestibule, the septum, or more rarely one of the conchae. Ulceration of the affected part follows and epistaxis may be the presenting symptom, often with some obstruction of the airway. In some cases the initial changes are in one of the maxillary sinuses. The ulcerated mucosa is covered by sticky, black or brownish-yellow crusts. Removal of the crusts reveals what looks clinically like simple granulation tissue. Cartilage and bone are eroded and as the condition progresses sequestra may form. Ulceration develops on the conchae and septum, spreading rapidly throughout the nose,[37] (Fig. 3.8) often involving the hard palate,

which may become perforated. Bacterial infection of the ulcerated tissues leads to inflammatory oedema of the lips, cheeks and eyelids and subcutaneous abscesses may follow. Extensive erosion and destruction of the nose, cheeks, lips and hard palate soon result and in some cases the entire roof of the nose and nasopharynx may be visible through the mouth, with exposure of the roof of the maxillary sinus after destruction of the lateral wall of the nose. Ulceration may occur at any stage in the maxillary or other sinuses, or in the oropharynx spreading to the nasopharynx and hypopharynx. Sometimes there is deep ulceration of the alveolar processes, with loss of teeth. Occasionally the larynx is involved.

Death may result from septic pneumonia following aspiration of infected material, from haemorrhage from erosion of a large vessel, from

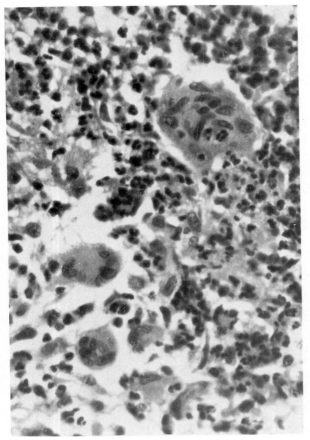

Fig. 3.5 Wegener's granuloma presenting as a nasal 'polyp' causing nasal obstruction and epistaxis. Histology of the excised polyp shows granulation tissue with characteristic giant cells.

Haematoxylin-eosin   × 225

meningitis following invasion of the cranial cavity, or from cachexia, due to the difficulty of getting adequate nutrition.

Histopathology
The essential picture is a dense accumulation of pleomorphic cells in the affected tissues (Fig. 3.9). The cells are predominantly lymphocytes; there is an admixture—often considerable—of plasma cells and there are also many peculiar elongated or spindle-shaped histiocytes with round or indented nuclei. Stimulated lymphocytes and immunoblasts may also be present.[38] Necrosis is not limited to the ulcerated surface, but characteristically affects a very considerable

part of the cellular tissue both superficially and in depth.

Various histological patterns can be recognized: a) non-specific pleomorphocellular granulation tissue with 'waves' of fibrous tissue alternating with cellular layers or seams (Fig. 3.10); b) non-specific granulation tissue with plasma cells and histiocytes predominating (Fig. 3.11); c) non-specific granulation tissue with necrotic changes predominating (Fig. 3.12).

These variants may represent stages of the same underlying process as implied in the term 'polymorphic'.[39]   Small   haemorrhages   are numerous. Dense fibrous granulation tissue is laid down in the deeper layers, alternating with cell infiltrates during periods of organization or

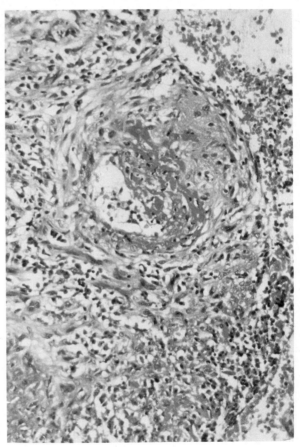

Fig. 3.6 Wegener's granulomatosis. Nasal biopsy showing necrotizing vasculitis. There is fibrinoid necrosis of the wall of a small vessel with inflammatory cell infiltration.

Haematoxylin-eosin   × 195

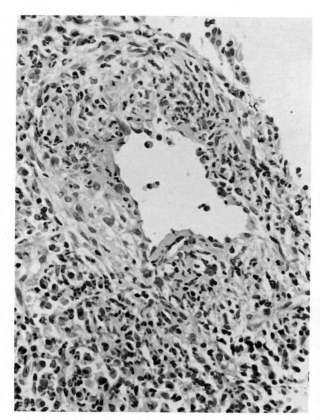

Fig. 3.7 Wegener's granulomatosis in a 41-year-old male. Nasal biopsy showing vasculitis. There is acute inflammatory cell infiltration of the vessel wall.

Haematoxylin–eosin   × 340

following treatment (Fig. 3.10). Vascular thrombosis and infarction of soft tissue and bones may occur.[40] The infiltrate has a pronounced tendency towards vascular orientation and to undergo necrosis (Figs 3.13, 3.14)[41] and may be indistinguishable from lymphomatoid granulomatosis.

Possible relationships to other diseases

Lymphomatoid granulomatosis

Lymphomatoid granulomatosis is an angiocentric and angiodestructive polymorphic lymphoreticular infiltration first described by Liebow, Carrington and Friedman involving the lungs.[38] A similar pattern of infiltrate has been noted by various authors in the Stewart type midfacial granuloma.[39, 42, 43] Although the original descrip-

tion of lymphomatoid granulomatosis did not include midfacial involvement, the association of lesions in the midfacial region with those in the lungs has since been reported.[42, 43] This microscopical resemblance has led some authors to the conclusion that the two diseases are identical.

Lymphomas

Interpretation of the nature of the disease is complicated by the fact that typical non-Hodgkin's malignant lymphomas may arise in the nose or sinuses, and behave in a manner clinically indistinguishable from the Stewart type of granuloma except that sooner or later foci of the tumour develop elsewhere—for example in the cervical lymph nodes, mediastinum or skeleton (particularly the cranial bones).

The distinction between tumour-like prolifera-

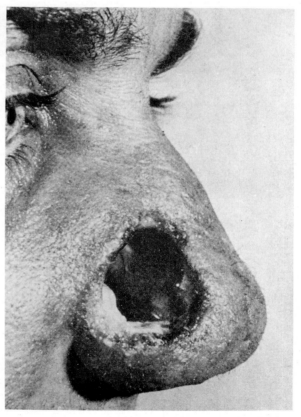

Fig. 3.8 Stewart type midfacial granuloma presenting as a large ulcerative lesion destroying the lateral wall of the nose.

Provided by Professor P. G. Gerlings, University of Utrecht, Netherlands.

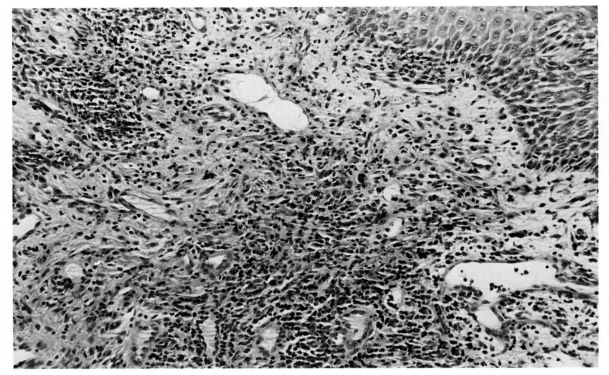

Fig. 3.9 Stewart type midfacial granuloma in a woman of 63 showing vascular stroma infiltrated by pleomorphic inflammatory cells.   Haematoxylin–eosin   × 160

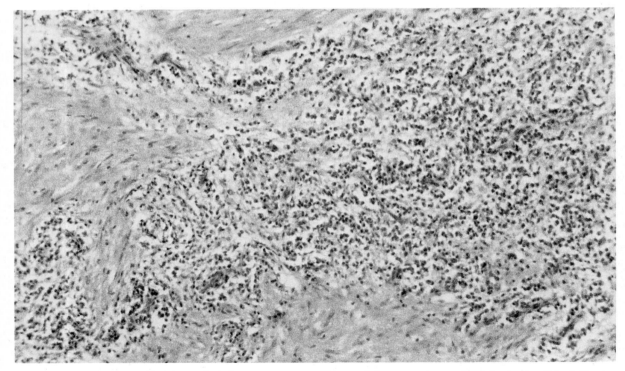

Fig. 3.10 Stewart type midfacial granuloma in a young woman. Characteristic pattern: layers of mainly plasmacellular infiltrate alternate with layers of fibrous granulation tissue. Original biopsy in case illustrated in Figure 3.15. Haematoxylin–eosin   × 100

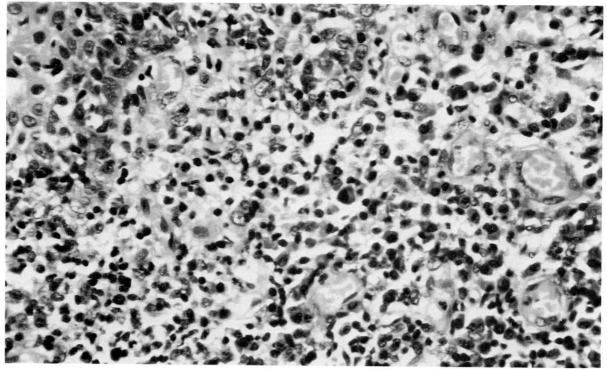

Fig. 3.11 Stewart type midfacial granuloma. There is a pleomorphic cellular infiltrate with plasma cells and scattered histiocytes in the subepithelial vascular granulation tissue.   Haematoxylin-eosin   × 500

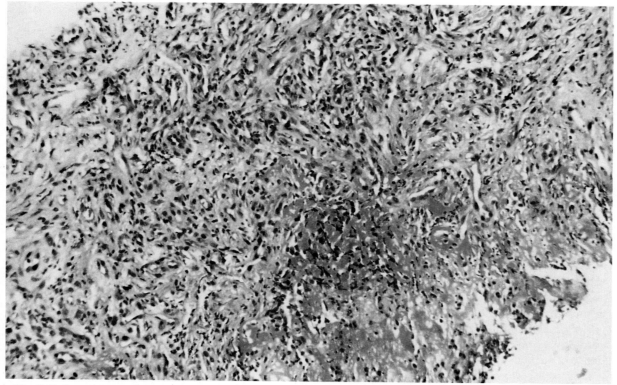

Fig. 3.12 Stewart type midfacial granuloma. Ulcerated nasal mucosa replaced by necrotizing granulation tissue. Haematoxylin-eosin   × 120

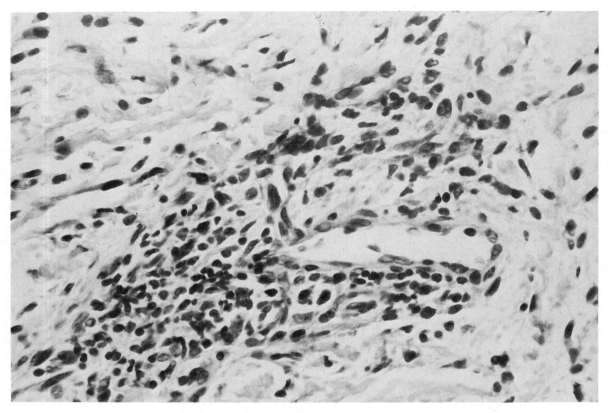

Fig. 3.13 Stewart type midfacial granuloma. Same case as illustrated in Figure 3.9 showing an area with a predominantly perivascular distribution of the infiltrate.   Haematoxylin-eosin   × 360

tive diseases and true neoplasms is nowhere less clear than in the lymphoreticular system. This is not to say that the Stewart type of granuloma is itself a neoplastic disease of the lymphoreticular system. It does mean, however, that the greatest care has to be taken to try to distinguish between non-Hodgkin's lymphomas of the nose and the Stewart type of granuloma.[44] The heterogeneity of the proliferating cells accompanying the histiocytic elements and the lack of well-defined neoplastic characteristics make it unlikely that the disease represents a true tumour. The presence of atypical cells in this lesion is not necessarily an indication of its neoplastic nature.[45] It has been suggested that some of the pleomorphic midfacial granulomas may ultimately become malignant lymphomas but follow up of cases that we have studied has not, so far, revealed convincing evidence of such an event.

It is well recognized that various drugs, viral infections and autoimmune diseases can cause lymphadenopathy which clinically resembles malignant lymphoma.[46] Two patients have been described with cryoglobulinaemia and necrotizing arteritis who developed severe lymphadenopathy.[47] Clinically, the diagnosis was thought to be malignant lymphoma but histological studies demonstrated a pseudolymphomatous reaction with vascular damage. The lesson of these two cases can be applied equally to any other lesion mimicking a lymphoma.

Non-Hodgkin's lymphoma referred to above and malignant histiocytosis affecting the nose and midfacial tissues should, therefore, be included in the differential diagnosis of midfacial granuloma, in common with specific lesions and other neoplasms.[48] Modern cytochemical methods can assist in distinguishing the different types of lymphoma, although the presence of scattered alpha-naphthyl-acetate-esterase-positive,

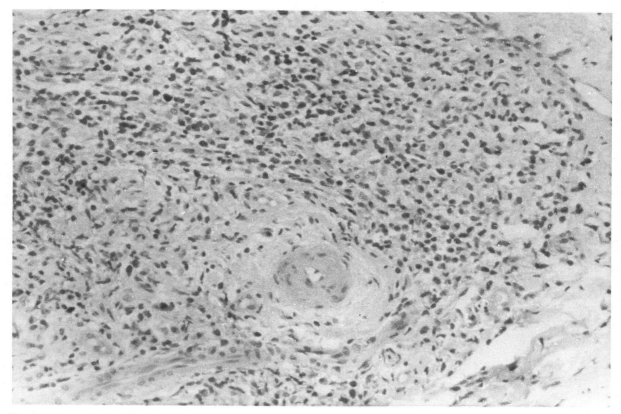

Fig. 3.14 Lymphomatoid granulomatosis. Illustrating the vasocentric pleomorphic cellular infiltrate similar to that seen in the Stewart type midfacial granuloma. Haematoxylin–eosin ×320

muramidase-positive histiocytes does not determine the diagnosis of malignant histiocytosis in the absence of the systemic features of the disease (contrasting with the localized character of Stewart type idiopathic midfacial granuloma). Moreover, the atypical cells, multinucleated cells and erythrophagocytosis described as characteristic of malignant histiocytosis[49] do not occur in the classic 'idiopathic midline destructive disease' as defined by Tsokos et al.[36] It has been suggested that the Stewart type of idiopathic midfacial granuloma is an early phase of T-cell lymphoma;[50] however the morphology of the nasal lesions described and the clinical symptoms and signs are not compatible with the Stewart type granuloma.

There is growing recognition of the fact that all the classic features of the Stewart type granuloma are not always present. The earlier concept was that of a strictly localized lesion but it has

become clear that remote involvement can occur.[51] A patient may present with the clinical and microscopical features of the Stewart type of lesion and develop, after a long intervening period, a giant cell lesion of the nose[16, 52–54] (Fig. 3.15).

Course

Without treatment the Stewart type granuloma leads to massive destruction of the nose and face and ultimately to the death of the patient, frequently as a result of intercurrent infection. The introduction of low-dosage irradiation[51, 55–58] transformed the survival pattern. Irradiation can produce rapid resolution, especially in the earlier stages of the disease. A disadvantage of low-dose radiotherapy is that in the event of a misinterpretation of the histological picture of a lymphoma as the Stewart type granuloma the former would be inadequately treated:[45] for this reason high-

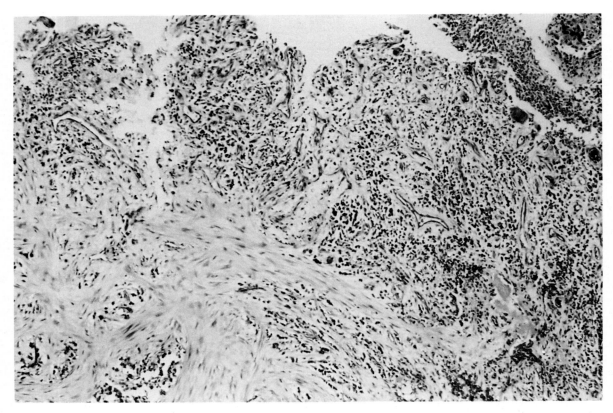

Fig. 3.15 Stewart type midfacial granuloma of 10 years' duration in a 28-year-old woman. The histology of the presenting lesion is illustrated in Figure 3.10. The disease progressed with gradual destruction of the nasal septum producing a 'saddle nose' deformity. Biopsy at this stage showed alternating fibrous and cellular layers in the deeper tissues, similar to the original biopsy, blending with vascular granulation tissue in which there were many giant cells, replacing the ulcerated mucosa.

Haematoxylin–eosin   × 140

dosage radiotherapy has become the treatment of choice.[45]

THE NATURE OF NON-HEALING NASAL GRANULOMAS OF UNKNOWN CAUSE[59]

At present, the cause and the nature of these conditions is obscure. The three supposed entities—the systemic and limited forms of Wegener's granulomatosis and the Stewart type granuloma—could conceivably be variants of a single disorder, probably vascular in its basis and possibly due to a disturbance that is immunologically-determined. It has been suggested that there are compelling considerations in favour of a unification incorporating all three conditions into a continuum.[60, 61]

A generic term 'respiratory vasculitis' has been

proposed to encompass the three conditions.[62] In this context it is interesting to note that rectal biopsies may provide evidence of vasculitis in systemic vasculitis and in the difficult area of overlap between the polyarteritis group and the systemic necrotizing vasculitis.[63] In certain disorders vasculitis is the predominant and most obvious manifestation, whereas other primary disorders may be associated with varying degrees of vasculitis. Within the entire spectrum of vasculitis any size or type of blood vessel in any organ system can be involved. There is now substantial evidence that most of the vasculitic syndromes are caused by, or are closely associated with, the deposition of immune complexes in blood vessel walls.[64]

There is often blurring of the distinction between the two main types of midfacial granuloma. Their correct histological identification in biopsy specimens of the presenting lesion may be difficult. Confusion may also arise in the interpretation of malignant lymphomas and malignant histiocytosis presenting in the nose with apparently similar histological features.[45, 65]

According to Spector[66, 67] the dynamic behaviour of granulomatous lesions cannot be interpreted through the histological pattern and varies greatly according to the nature of the causal agent. The cellular turnover in a granuloma—that is, the rate of replacement of cells either by emigration from the circulation or by mitosis in situ ranges from a high to a low order. High-turnover granulomas are dependent particularly on emigration from the circulation, whereas low- turnover granulomas are more self-sufficient and presumably depend for their continued existence on multiplication of macrophages within the lesion. This would seem to correlate well with the natural history of midfacial granulomas which are probably largely of low-turnover type. In so far as macrophages have the ability to transform into epithelioid and giant cells, it is possible that the Stewart type granuloma could evolve, enhanced by delayed hypersensitivity, into an epithelioid or giant-cell granuloma. Consideration of these basic principles may assist in a better understanding of the enigma of the midfacial granuloma syndrome.

REFERENCES

1. Stewart JP. J Laryngol Otol 1933; 48: 657.
2. Wegener F. Verh Dtsch Ges Pathol 1936; 29: 202.
3. Wegener F. Beitr Pathol Anat Allg Pathol 1939; 102: 36.
4. Fienberg R. Am J Clin Pathol 1953; 23: 413.
5. Carrington CB, Liebow AA. Am J Med 1966; 41: 497.
6. McDonald TJ, DeRemee RA, Kern EB et al. Laryngoscope 1974; 84: 2101.
7. Walton EW. Br Med J 1958; ii: 265.
8. Wolff M. Am J Clin Pathol 1974; 62: 775.
9. Blatt IM, Seltzer HS, Rubin P, Furstenberg AC, Maxwell JH, Schull WJ. Arch Otolaryngol 1959; 70: 707.
10. Shillitoe EJ, Lehner T, Lessof MH, Harrison DFN. Lancet 1974; i: 281.
11. Wolff SM, Fauci AS, Horn RG, Dale DC. Ann Int Med 1974; 81: 513.
12. Travers RL. Br J Hosp Med 1979; 22: 38.
13. Howell SB, Epstein WV. Maer J Med 1976; 60: 259.
14. Pinching AJ, Rees AJ, Pussell BA, Lockwood CM, Mitchison RS, Peters DK. Br Med J 1980; 281: 836.
15. Cassan SM, Coles DT, Harrison EG. Am J Med 1970; 49: 366.
16. Friedmann I. J Laryngol 1982; 96: 1.
17. Friedmann I. J Laryngol Otol 1971; 85: 631.
18. Fauci AS, Wolff SM. Medicine 1973; 52: 535.
19. Fienberg R. Hum Pathol 1981; 12: 458.
20. Fauci et al. Ann Int Med 1983; 98: 76.
21. Friedmann I. Proc R Soc Med 1976; 69: 785.
22. Pritchard MH, Crow PJ. Proc R Soc Med 1976; 69: 501.
23. Anderson JM, Jamieson DG, Jefferson JM. Q J Med 1975; 44: 309.
24. Matsudo S, Mitsukawa S, Ishii N, Shirai M. Tohoku J Exp Med 1976; 118: 145.
25. Woods R. Br Med J 1921; ii: 65.
26. Kraus EJ. Klin Wochenschr 1929; 8: 932.
27. Williams HL. Ann Otol Rhinol Laryngol 1949; 58: 1013.
28. Walton EW. J Laryngol Otol 1959; 73: 242.
29. Eichel BS, Harrison EG, Devine KD, Scanlon PM, Brown HA. Am J Surg 1966; 112: 597.
30. Kassel SH, Echevarria RA, Guzzo FP. Cancer 1969; 23: 920.
31. Fauci AS, Johnson RE, Wolff SM. Ann Int Med 1976; 84: 140.
32. Fechner RE, Lamppin DM. Arch Otolaryngol 1972; 95: 467.
33. Schafer RJ, Schuster HH. Zentralbl Allg Pathol 1975; 119: 111.
34. Moncades J, Hagege CE, Marchand J. J Otolaryngol Chirurg Faciale 1977; 94: 339.
35. Batsakis JC. Head Neck Surg 1979; 1: 213.
36. Tsokos M, Fauci A, Costa J. Am J Clin Pathol 1982; 77: 162.
37. Gurlings PG. HNO 1965; 13: 337.
38. Liebow AA, Carrington CRB, Friedman PJ, Hum Pathol 1972; 3: 457.
39. DeRemee RA, Weiland LH, McDonald TJ. Mayo Clin Proc 1978; 53: 634.
40. Moschella SL. Cutis 1973; 11: 650.
41. Friedmann I, Balkany T, Sando I. J Laryngol Otol 1978; 92: 601.
42. Stamenkovic I, Toccanier Marie-F, Kapanci Y. Virchows Arch (Pathol Anat) 1981; 390: 81.
43. Crissman JD, Weiss MA, Gluckman J. Am J Surg Pathol 1982; 6: 335.
44. Aozasa K, Ikeda H, Watanabe Y. Path Res Pract 1981; 172: 161.
45. Michaels L, Gregory MM. J Clin Path 1977; 30: 317.
46. Symmers W St C. In: Systemic Pathology. 2nd ed. Vol. 2 Edinburgh: Churchill Livingstone, 1978; 696.
47. Slater DN, Bleehan SS, Hancock BW, Messenger AG, Harvey L. J R Soc Med 1982; 75: 346.
48. Batsakis JG. Ann Otol Rhinol 1982; 91: 541.
49. Aozasa K. J Clin Pathol 1982; 35: 599.
50. Ishii Y, Yamanaka N, Ogawa K, Yoshida Y, Takami et al. Cancer 1982; 50: 2336.
51. Dickson RJ. J Chronic Dis 1960; 12: 417.
52. Byrd LJ, Shearn MA. Arthritis Rheum 1969; 12: 247.
53. Spear GS, Walker WG. Bull Johns Hopkins Hosp 1956; 99: 313.

54. Wetmore SJ, Platz CE. Ann Otol Rhinol Laryngol 1978; 87: 60.
55. Glass EJG. J Laryngol Otol 1955; 69: 315.
56. Howells GH. J Laryngol Otol 1955; 69: 309.
57. Ellis MP. Br Med J 1955; i: 1251.
58. Ardouin AP. Proc R Soc Med 1964; 57: 299.
59. Friedmann I, Osborn DA. Pathology of granulomas and neoplasms of the nose and paranasal sinuses. Edinburgh: Churchill Livingstone, 1982: 95.
60. DeRemee RA, McDonald TJ, Harrison EG, Coles DT. Mayo Clin Proc 1976; 51: 777.
61. Nieberding PH, Schiff M, Harmeling JG. Arch Otolaryngol 1963; 77: 512.
62. DeRemee RA, Weiland LH, McDonald TJ. Mayo Clin Proc 1980; 55: 492.
63. Tribe CR, Scott DGL, Bucon PA. J Clin Pathol 1981; 34: 843.
64. Fauci AS, Haynes BF, Katz P. Ann Intern Med 1978; 89: 660.
65. Aozasa K, Nara H, Kotoh K et al. Path Res Pract 1982; 174: 147.
66. Spector WG. In: Richter GW, Epstein MA, eds. Granulomatous inflammatory exudate. New York: Academic Press, 1969: 1.
67. Spector WG. Proc R Soc Med 1971; 64: 941.

4

Neoplasms of the nose and nasal sinuses

It cannot be urged too strongly that all tissues removed from the nose and nasal sinuses should be examined microscopically. Many nasal neoplasms present as polyps, and on clinical examination may exactly simulate simple polyps. Furthermore, tumours arising in the nasal sinuses and in the nasopharynx also frequently present as polyps. Unless all polyps are sectioned, the diagnosis of some cases of nasal cancer will inevitably be unnecessarily delayed. It is important to note, too, that for the histological examination to be adequate, all the pieces excised must be sectioned and not merely one or two supposedly representative samples of the tissue. Exfoliative cytology occasionally has a part in the recognition of the presence of cancer in the nasal region. Its potential is limited by the frequency of infection, which results in an inflammatory cellular exudate that confuses or totally obscures the cytological evidence of malignant disease.

Although there is no sharp anatomical division between the nasal cavities and the nasal sinuses, and in spite of a considerable similarity in the types of tumours that arise in the two situations, there are good reasons for paying attention to the distinction between the tumours of the nasal cavities and those of the nasal sinuses. First, among the great variety of tumours that occur in the upper respiratory tract there are some that tend to arise most frequently or even exclusively in one or the other of these regions. Second, the relative proportions of benign and malignant tumours differ markedly in the two regions. In our experience the ratio of benign to malignant tumours in the nasal cavities is about 6 : 1; in the nasal sinuses the ratio has been almost exactly the reverse of these figures. Third, tumours of similar histological type may differ in their behaviour in the two regions: for example, the survival rate in cases of squamous carcinoma of a nasal cavity is almost three times that of squamous carcinoma of equivalent differentiation arising in the sinuses.

However, it must be appreciated that the precise site of origin of a carcinoma in a sinus can seldom be determined, for by the time of diagnosis a large part of the sinus may be involved and the tumour may have extended into adjoining parts. It may, therefore, be impossible to tell whether a carcinoma within the nose has arisen in the nasal cavities or in the sinuses.

Classification

Classification of the tumours of the nasal region is often based on their behaviour. We believe that the close relationship between certain benign and malignant tumours makes it more convenient and more appropriate to adopt a classification based on tissue of origin.

EPITHELIAL TUMOURS

BENIGN

Squamous papilloma

The commonest benign tumour of the region is the squamous papilloma. It arises almost exclusively in the vestibule. Usually hyperkeratotic, it is often indistinguishable from the common skin wart.

Although there is a clearly defined peak age distribution of warts of the hands in the second decade of life, the age distribution of the vestibular wart shows a maximum occurrence in middle age.

The cauliflower-like growth may obstruct or project from the nostril and is usually solitary; multiple, bilateral tumours are occasionally encountered. The microscopical picture is that of an exophytic squamous proliferation in which all the normal layers of the epidermis are represented, usually with hyperkeratosis. The basal layer may exhibit some degree of epithelial dysplasia.

The electron microscope reveals typical squamous cells with their multiple desmosomes and tonofibrils. The presence of virus-like particles has been noted within the nuclei (Fig. 4.1): the significance of this observation remains questionable not only on morphological grounds but also because of the absence, to date, of any experimental technique for reproducing the human wart. It is clear, therefore, that although the viral aetiology of vestibular papillomas is strongly suspected, it remains for the present unproven.

Keratoacanthoma

This essentially cutaneous lesion which arises

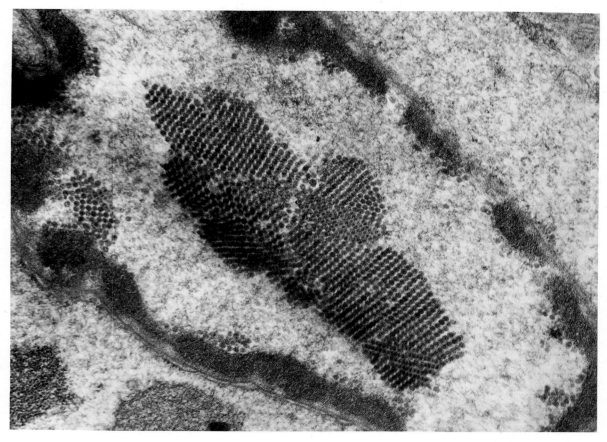

Fig. 4.1 Electron micrograph of a nasal wart showing 'crystalline' arrangement of viral bodies in the nucleus of a keratinized squamous cell.

× 52 500

from the wall of the upper portion of the hair follicle may occur in the region of the junction between the nasal vestibule and the skin of the nose. It is a rapidly growing dome-shaped lesion with a central crater filled by a plug of keratin. The keratin plug is surrounded by proliferating squamous epithelium which, in a biopsy, may be indistinguishable from well-differentiated squamous carcinoma. Knowledge of the short clinical history and gross appearance of the lesion are essential for correct diagnosis. Spontaneous regression occurs over a period of a few months.

The skin of the nose is one of the commonest sites of origin of the rare 'giant keratoacanthoma'.[1]

Transitional papilloma

The transitional papilloma is both the most important and the most interesting of the essentially benign tumours of the nasal region. It arises from epithelium of respiratory type but is characterized by squamous differentiation, its structure including a transition of epithelial types from columnar to fully-keratinized squamous. It was because those tumours that represent intermediate stages of squamous differentiation may mimic papillomas of the urinary tract in their appearances that this group as a whole came to be described as the transitional papillomas (transitional cell papillomas) of the nose.

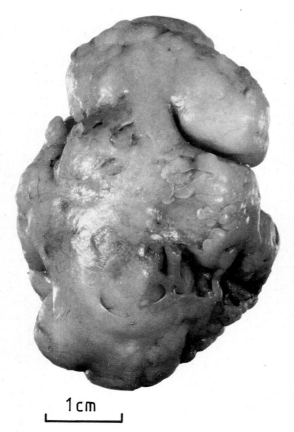

1 cm

Fig. 4.2 Transitional papilloma of the nose in a 54-year-old male showing a somewhat lobulated mass of solid consistency.

Terminology

A considerable variety of names have been applied to this lesion since Kramer & Som[2] introduced the term 'true papilloma of the nasal cavity'. These include 'cylindrical or transitional cell papilloma',[3] 'transitional cell papilloma',[4] 'inverting papilloma',[5, 6] and 'inverted papilloma'.[7–9] The term 'inverted papilloma' may be regarded as an attempt to emphasize the infolded character of the epithelial proliferation, which can be misinterpreted as downgrowths. In naming this lesion one may refer either to its character and pattern or to the behaviour of the epithelium.[10] We prefer the term 'transitional papilloma', which relates to the microscopical pattern of the tumour.

It is interesting that cells transitional from glandular to squamous were observed in the early stages of squamous metaplasia in the nasal res-

piratory epithelium of rats exposed to hexamethylphosphoramide by inhalation.[11] Similarly, in an interesting study of the pathogenesis of experimental lung tumours in the rat, 'transitional cells' formed the surface layer of the hyperplastic bronchial mucosa.[12] Papillary endobronchial tumours with a 'transitional cell pattern' also occur[13–15] and are classified as 'transitional' papilloma by the World Health Organization.[16]

Transitional papillomas account for about 25% of tumours of the nasal cavities. They occur over a wide age range with the peak in the fifth and sixth decades. Men are affected five times more often than women. The tumours are usually unilateral but affect the mucosa over a considerable area. Maxillary and ethmoidal sinuses are commonly involved and the frontal and sphenoidal sinuses much less frequently. The reported incidence of septal involvement varies greatly.[9]

Bilateral involvement is uncommon (4%). Bilateral tumours in one case presented first in one nasal cavity and about 6 months later in the other: when the second tumour appeared there was no evidence of recurrence of the tumour that had already been treated on the other side.[17]

Macroscopically, the transitional papilloma is polypoid (Fig. 4.2). It is usually firmer to the touch than a simple polyp, and liable to bleed

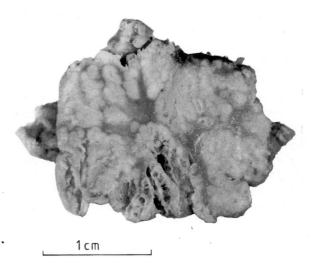

1 cm

Fig. 4.3 Transitional papilloma of the nose in a 65-year-old male. The cut surface presents a naked eye impression of infolding of the surface epithelium.

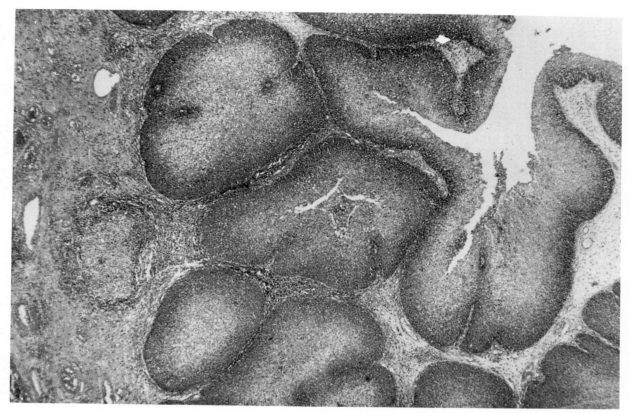

Fig. 4.4 Transitional papilloma of the nose. Characteristic pattern of complexly infolded hyperplastic epithelium. The tumour formed first in one nasal cavity followed 6 months later by a similar tumour in the opposite side.

Haematoxylin–eosin   × 40

during removal. Occasionally, a cut surface may reveal alternating solid and relatively translucent areas, corresponding to the epithelial and stromal components (Fig. 4.3).

Histopathology
Epithelial proliferation leads inevitably to an increase in surface area which is accommodated most readily by infolding into the soft oedematous stroma. Continuing epithelial proliferation may reduce the connective tissue element to narrow strips between the epithelial masses. The deep infolding may often give a false impression of down-growth. The original surface cells may degenerate and come to lie at the centres of apparently isolated masses, thereby producing a picture simulating central necrosis and invasion. The epithelial pattern is essentially that of pro-

liferation and metaplasia, producing a characteristic spectrum that ranges from pseudostratified columnar through true stratified columnar and transitional type to completely metaplastic squamous epithelium (Figs 4.4, 4.5, 4.6, 4.7).

The proliferated epithelium, more particularly in the absence of complete squamous metaplasia, often contains numerous spaces presenting a 'moth-eaten' appearance. Some of these spaces are due to incarceration of goblet cells but many are intercellular and these often contain polymorphonuclear leucocytes which commonly infiltrate the epithelium (Fig. 4.8).

In spite of the variation from columnar to squamous-cell type, the arrangement of the cells is generally regular. The nuclei in the basal layer may be hyperchromatic and somewhat variable in appearance, and mitotic figures are not infre-

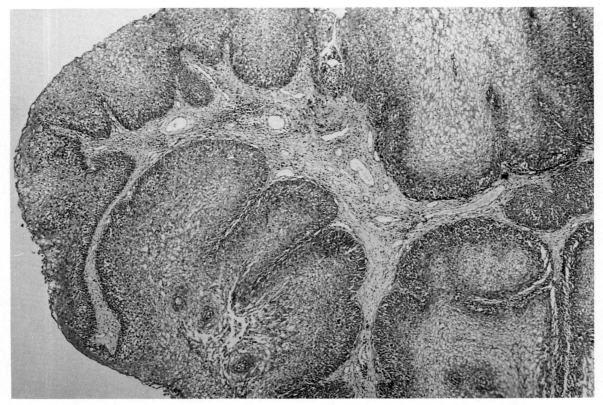

Fig. 4.5 Bilateral transitional nasal papilloma. Same patient as Figure 4.4. Similar pattern of papilloma on other side. Haematoxylin–eosin × 50

quent. Cholesterol granulomas may form in the stroma, particularly when infection has led to breaking down of some of the epithelial masses.

Nature and course

The nature of these tumours is controversial. A broad histological spectrum can be drawn, ranging from what appears to be strictly local epithelial hyperplasia in an otherwise typical simple nasal polyp to solid growths of unquestionably neoplastic epithelium. The fact that there is a notable tendency for the lesions to recur over a long period of time has led many to regard the transitional type papilloma as at least premalignant.

There is recurrence in about one-third of cases.[18] Multiple recurrences are not infrequent and their incidence is probably underestimated. The greater number of such cases have one or two recurrences only, but in a few the event is repeated annually over a period of many years.

Except in the event of malignant change, the histological picture shows no significant alteration. An increase in infolding with consequent reduction of the stroma is not uncommon in recurrent tumours but in itself does not have any sinister implication. Papillomas undergoing malignant change show increased nuclear irregularity and disorientation of cells; invasive squamous carcinoma may ensue. It is essential that all material from this type of papilloma should be examined histologically (Figs 4.9, 4.10).

Malignant change

On the subject of malignant change, the issue has been confused by the application of different criteria. The simultaneous finding of a papilloma and a carcinoma at the first histological examination is a not uncommon experience.[3, 5, 9, 19–22] Whilst such an observation constitutes strong circumstantial evidence it is not proof.

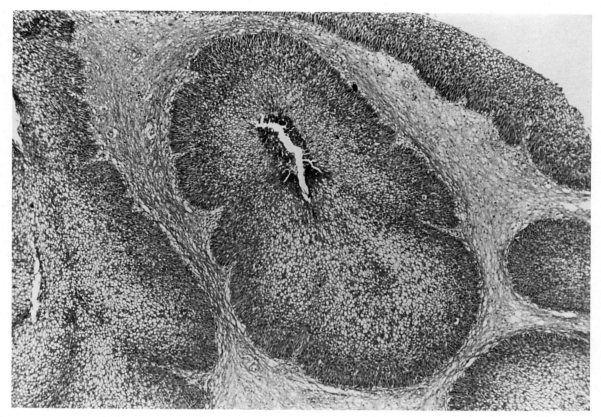

Fig. 4.6 Transitional papilloma of the nose showing infolded epithelium which gives the impression of an isolated cell mass with pseudocentral necrosis.

Haematoxylin–eosin   × 90

Malignant change developed in four out of 200 cases (2%) under controlled observation, the interval ranging from 5–25 years.[18] This corresponds quite closely to the total of 12 cases among between 700 and 800 cases of papilloma published in the literature. It is justifiable to state here that the great majority of transitional papillomas of the nasal passages show no evidence of malignant change, even after there have been multiple recurrences over a period of many years. However, the difficulty of prognostication in individual cases is real.

CARCINOMA

Squamous carcinomas, transitional carcinomas, anaplastic carcinomas and adenocarcinomas account, perhaps surprisingly, for only about 50% of malignant tumours of the nasal cavities.

The many classifications which have appeared in the literature were based on histological subdivision.[23–27] The expression 'Schneiderian carcinoma'[28] has no specific meaning beyond indicating the origin of a carcinoma from the lining mucosa of the region (the Schneiderian membrane—see p. 4): the term is now obsolete.

Carcinoma of the nose and sinuses is relatively rare and in most geographical regions it is generally accepted as accounting for substantially less than 1% of all malignant tumours in all sites. According to the Registrar General's statistics for 1980, in the United Kingdom, deaths from cancer of the nose and sinuses were found to be 0.15% of all malignancies.[29] In the material collected at the Institute of Laryngology and Otology, London, between 1948 and 1974, all types of carcinoma accounted for 24% of all tumours in the nose and sinuses and 72% of all malignant

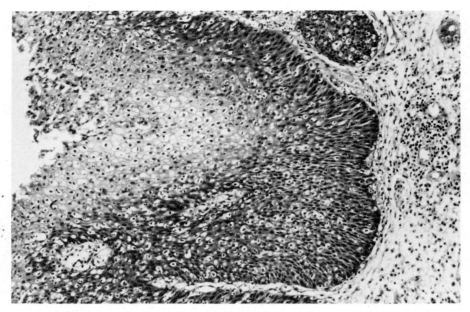

Fig. 4.7 Transitional nasal papilloma. Detail showing transitional epithelium composed of three layers of cells of different appearance—basal, transitional and squamous.
Haematoxylin–eosin   × 180

neoplasms in the region.[30] In the nasal sinuses carcinomas account for about 80% of malignant tumours. A higher incidence of paranasal carcinoma has been observed amongst Africans[31] and in Mexico.[32] The age distribution in both nasal and paranasal carcinoma shows a peak in the sixth decade and there is no significant difference between the various histological types. The sex ratio shows a predominance of males ranging from 1.5:1 in paranasal to 2:1 in nasal carcinomas.

Aetiology
Contrary to what is sometimes said, no correlation has been established between carcinoma and chronic sinusitis. The former high incidence of nasal and paranasal carcinoma amongst nickel workers appears to have been related to exposure to flue dust produced by the extraction process. This hazard seems to have been eliminated in Wales but not satisfactorily in Norway.[30, 33] Woodworker's adenocarcinoma is discussed below (p. 74).

Site of origin
In the nasal cavity about 75% of carcinomas are squamous and arise anteriorly. Because of their situation these tumours are diagnosed earlier and have a better prognosis than those arising in the nasal sinuses. The carcinomas that arise farther back in the nasal cavities are about equally divided between transitional and anaplastic growths, with only an occasional adenocarcinoma. In contrast, in the sinuses squamous tumours account for about 45% of the carcinomas, transitional for about 20%, anaplastic for about 20% and adenocarcinomas arising from seromucinous glands for the rest. The site of origin of the tumours of the sinuses may be difficult to determine: two-thirds or so appear to arise in the maxillary sinus, especially its antroethmoidal angle, and most of the others are ethmoidal. Carcinoma of the frontal sinus is rare and carcinoma of a sphenoidal sinus even rarer.[30]

Spread
The spread of a carcinoma of the nasal region depends to some extent on its site of origin. Most nasal carcinomas tend to remain localized for a considerable time. In contrast, antral and ethmoidal tumours frequently involve the lateral nasal wall and the nasal cavity at a comparatively

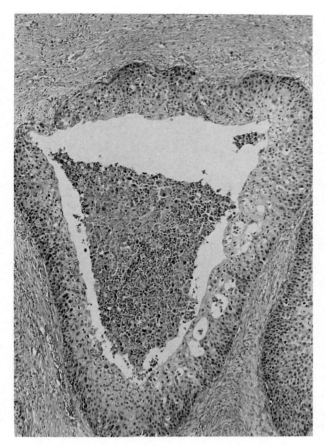

Fig. 4.8 Transitional nasal papilloma. Purulent focus in the stroma surrounded by vacuolated transitional epithelium.
Haematoxylin–eosin   × 70

early stage. The orbital cavity is much more frequently invaded by carcinomas arising in the antro-ethmoidal angle than by those strictly of ethmoidal origin. Invasion of the anterior and lateral walls of the maxillary sinus by carcinoma arising there often leads ultimately to involvement of the soft tissues of the cheek, sometimes with ulceration of the skin; the palate may also be invaded. Less frequently, there is extension from the antrum to the sphenoidal or frontal sinuses and the anterior cranial fossa. This may also occur, less rarely, in cases of ethmoidal carcinoma.

In the cases studied at the Institute of Laryngology and Otology, London, haematogenous spread occurred in 14% of cases, principally to the lung. Histologically confirmed lymph node involvement was much less frequent.

Recurrence

The recurrence rate of paranasal carcinoma is of the order of 40% whereas that of primary nasal carcinoma in less than 20%. In spite of its less aggressive behaviour in other ways, transitional carcinoma exhibits a greater tendency to local recurrence as compared with the squamous and anaplastic types.

Squamous carcinoma

Squamous carcinoma of the nasal cavities and sinuses is usually moderately well differentiated (Fig. 4.11). There is often great variation within a single tumour and it is important to note that the malignancy of a given tumour is usually determined by its least differentiated part.

Anaplastic carcinomas

These account for approximately 20% of paranasal carcinomas but less than 10% of those arising in the nasal cavity. Ethmoidal carcinomas are more likely to be of this type. Microscopically they may be pleomorphic or of spindle-cell or spheroidal-cell types and are liable to be confused with amelanotic malignant melanoma, plasmacytoma or lymphoma. An admixture of lymphocytes sometimes presents the picture of the so-called lympho-epithelioma (see p. 147 — nasopharyngeal carcinoma). The 'oat cell' type of anaplastic small-cell carcinoma is rarely seen in the nasal region.

Transitional carcinoma

The transitional carcinoma is of particular interest because it resembles and may be related to the transitional type papilloma and also because of its distinctive behaviour. The histological resemblance to the papilloma is readily apparent in the better differentiated tumours and the two have all too often been confused. The pattern of surface proliferation is the same, leading to infolding of the neoplastic epithelium: this is delineated by long stretches of basal lamina which appears to be intact even when the polarity of the cells is disturbed and dedifferentiation marked. The persistence of the basal lamina results in the 'ribbon' or 'garland' appearance that has been considered characteristic (Figs 4.12, 4.13). In many areas the appearance is essentially that of

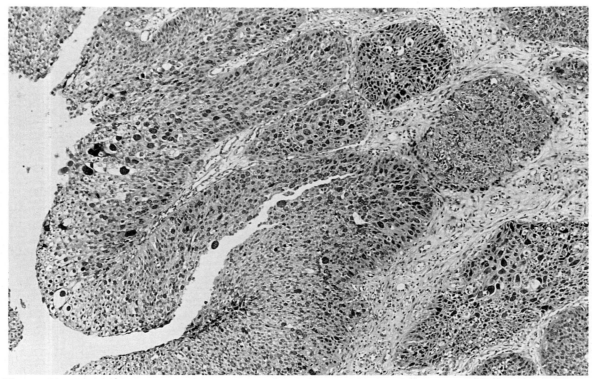

Fig. 4.9 Transitional nasal papilloma showing intra-epithelial malignant change. There is loss of polarity of the cells and marked nuclear pleomorphism. Haematoxylin–eosin × 90

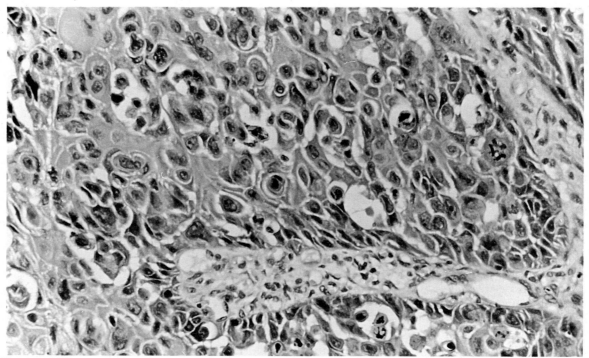

Fig. 4.10 Malignant change in a transitional type papilloma of the nose in a 66-year-old male. Higher magnification showing disturbed polarity and atypical mitoses. Haematoxylin–eosin × 225

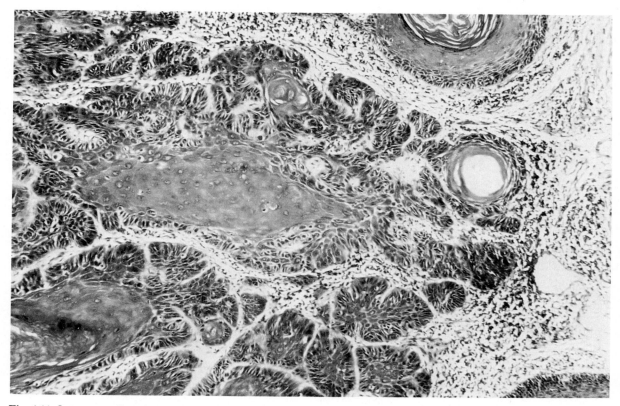

Fig. 4.11 Squamous cell carcinoma of the nose invading the underlying tissue.   Haematoxylin–eosin   × 100

an intra-epithelial carcinoma: careful search may be necessary to establish the presence of areas of invasion, which are always present.

It is noteworthy that the tendency for the basal lamina to persist in cases of transitional carcinoma indicates a relative inability of the tumour to grow invasively and so implies a better outlook. The 5-year survival rate in cases of transitional carcinoma of the nasal cavities (36%) is about twice that of squamous carcinoma and anaplastic carcinoma arising in these situations.

Adenocarcinoma

This rare tumour, which takes its origin from the columnar epithelium, occurs in the sixth to seventh decade with a marked predominance of males.[34, 35] Patients may present with nasal obstruction, epistaxis, pain or local swelling; extension of the growth may lead to epiphora, proptosis and disturbance of vision.

Histopathology

The tumour presents as a polypoid mucosal mass. Microscopy shows tubulocystic structures lined by usually well differentiated cubical or columnar epithelium with varying numbers of interspersed mucus-secreting cells (Fig. 4.14). Papillary processes may be present, sometimes projecting into cyst-like spaces (Fig. 4.15); a high degree of differentiation may suggest an initial diagnosis of 'papillary cystadenoma'. Evidence of invasion may be found in the presence of irregular clumps of tumour cells in the stroma, though in many areas the basal lamina appears to be intact.

Under the electron microscope mucous secretory granules can be identified as either discrete or semiconfluent structures as in the cells of normal mucous glands. Less specific features include accumulations of glycogen, swollen mitochondria and lipochondria which should not be confused with secretory granules such as may be found in

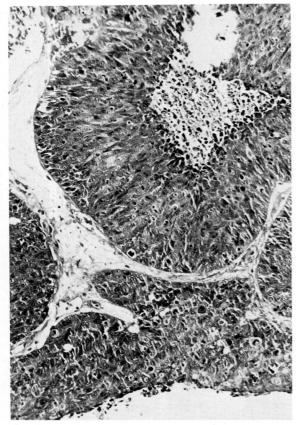

Fig. 4.12 Detail of transitional carcinoma of maxillary antrum showing the characteristic ribbon-like arrangement of neoplastic cells with intact basal lamina.

Haematoxylin–eosin   × 120

an acinic cell tumour. Occasionally, basally located cells may be found showing myoepithelial differentiation.

Aetiology and pathogenesis
The relationship between nasal adenocarcinoma and the furniture industry was established, in 1967, by Hadfield and her colleagues.[36–40] Their observations were based on a geographical area in Southern England, covering the adjacent parts of the counties of Buckinghamshire and Oxfordshire. Subsequently, confirmation of this hazard appeared in reports from France,[41] Belgium,[42] Denmark,[43] Australia[35] and the United States[44] and Sweden.[44a] In the United Kingdom, nasal adenocarcinoma has now been officially recognised as an industrial disease. In woodworkers

who have been employed for 10 years or more, an impairment of mucociliary clearance was found, probably related to the development of squamous metaplasia at the site of deposition of wood dust.[45] It is suspected that the influence might be chemical rather than mechanical, though the effect of simple drying of respiratory type epithelium cannot be entirely excluded.

Woodworker's adenocarcinoma probably arises primarily in the middle concha on the anterior end of which the wood dust is most abundantly deposited.[40] Spread to the paranasal region occurs subsequently. Local spread between the nasal and paranasal cavities is common but dissemination by the lymphatics or blood stream is less frequent, occurring in under a quarter of cases. Local recurrence is encountered in about half the cases.

MUCOSAL GLAND TUMOURS

The various types of mucosal gland tumour of the nose and paranasal sinuses differ greatly in incidence and importance.[46]

Tubulocystic adenoma
This tumour is less common in the nasal region than in the larynx. It consists of simple tubules and cysts lined by cubical or columnar epithelium which may sometimes be mucus-secreting. Frequently, the cells have the intense eosinophilic granularity seen in 'oncocytes'[47] the result of packing of the cytoplasm with enlarged mitochondria. Difficulty may sometimes be encountered in distinguishing between adenoma, well-differentiated adenocarcinoma and, occasionally, metastatic renal carcinoma.

Microcystic papillary adenoma
The bizarre microcystic pattern of the epithelial component of this tumour has been erroneously interpreted as protozoa. The columnar papillary structure has prompted an equally incorrect suggestion that it is variant of the transitional papilloma.

The microcystic papillary adenoma is a relatively rare tumour. Its peak age incidence is in the seventh decade; there is no significant sex

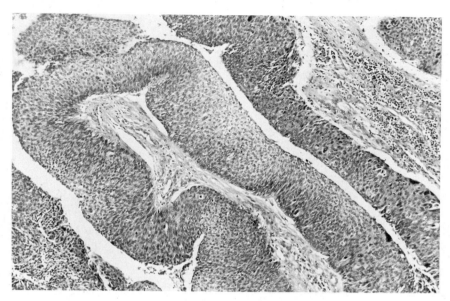

Fig. 4.13 Cervical lymph node metastasis from transitional carcinoma reproducing the characteristic ribbon-like pattern and intact basal lamina. Haematoxylin–eosin ×75

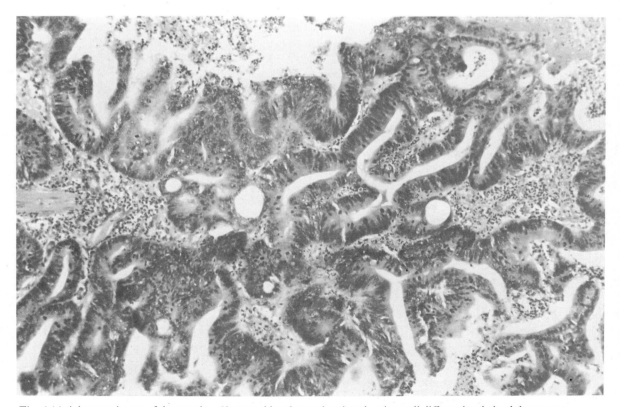

Fig. 4.14 Adenocarcinoma of the nose in a 69-year-old male woodworker showing well differentiated glandular pattern. Haematoxylin–eosin ×135

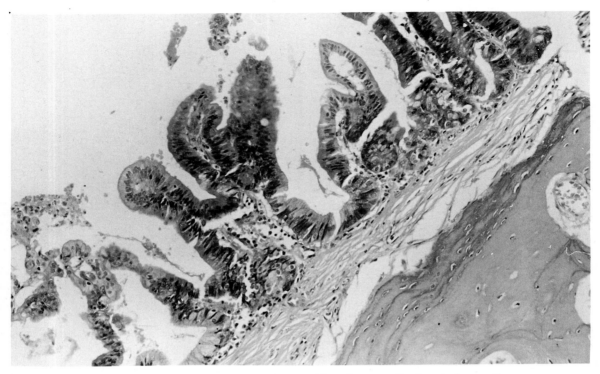

Fig. 4.15 Well differentiated papillary adenocarcinoma of the maxillary sinus spreading into the bony wall.
Haematoxylin–eosin   × 100

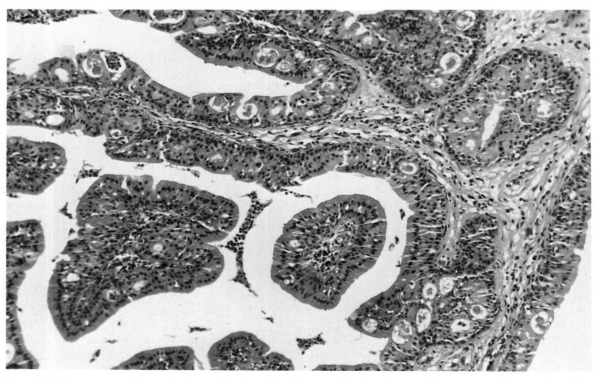

Fig. 4.16 Microcystic papillary adenoma of the nose in a 47-year-old male. Note papillary pattern with pseudostratified columnar epithelium containing microcysts filled with mucous secretion or pus cells.
Haematoxylin–eosin   × 135

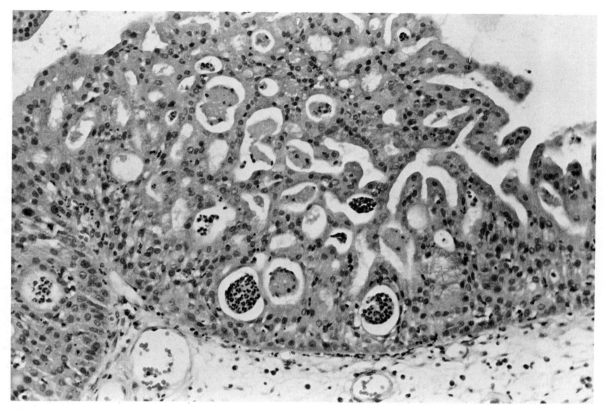

Fig. 4.17 Microcystic papillary adenoma of the nose. Higher magnification showing numerous microcysts, many containing polymorphonuclear leucocytes.
Haematoxylin–eosin   × 225

difference. It usually presents as a polypoid lesion causing nasal obstruction. About three-quarters of the tumours occur in the nasal cavity; the remainder involve the maxillary and ethmoid sinuses. Following removal local recurrence is not uncommon. There may sometimes be repeated recurrences but malignant transformation has not been encountered.

Histopathology
Microscopy shows pseudostratified epithelium forming many papillary structures projecting into cystic spaces which often contain mucus. The constituent cells vary in size but are mainly tall and cylindrical with abundant eosinophilic granular cytoplasm resembling that of oncocytes. A prominent feature is the presence of numerous intra-epithelial microcysts which often contain epithelial type mucin (Figs. 4.16, 4.17). Under

the electron microscope, many of the cells are seen to contain greatly enlarged mitochondria, mucous secretory granules or a mixture of both.

Oncocytoma (eosinophilic granular cell tumour)
The oncocytoma is rare in any location; it is least rare in the major salivary glands.[48] Four nasal oncocytomas have been reported.[49–51] It occurs only in the older age groups; all the patients with nasal oncocytoma were over 60. There is no evidence of sex predilection. The tumour presents with nasal obstruction, epistaxis or discharge.

Histopathology
The characteristic microscopical feature is the presence of large, closely-packed cells possessing an abundant coarsely granular cytoplasm which is intensely eosinophilic. The rounded nuclei are

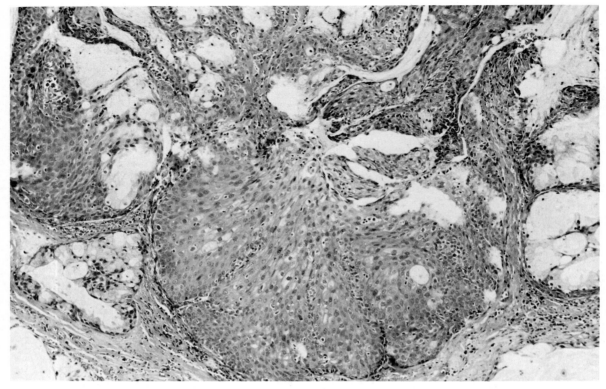

Fig. 4.18 Muco-epidermoid tumour showing solid areas of squamous cells and cysts lined by clear columnar cells containing mucous secretion.
Haematoxylin–eosin   × 125

well stained with fairly abundant heterochromatin but nuclear irregularity and hyperchromatism may occur. The occasional formation of tubular structures confirms its glandular origin.

Although originally regarded as a benign tumour, oncocytomas of the salivary gland have been known to metastasize.[52, 53] Three of the four published nasal tumours[49, 50] showed malignant features.

Acinic cell tumour

The acinic cell tumour is extremely rare in the nose and sinuses.[54] It is composed of round to polygonal cells with a granular basophilic cytoplasm, resembling the serous cells of salivary glands. The small hyperchromatic nuclei are frequently peripherally located. There is some scanty, occasionally more abundant, vascular stroma which may be hyalinized. Scattered lymph follicles may be present and patchy calcification may be seen. Acinic cell tumours may

originate from the serous cells of seromucinous glands or from the cells of intercalated ducts.

Despite the slow rate of growth this tumour may recur and metastasize to regional lymphnodes and distant sites.[54b] There is no sharp distinction between its benign and malignant varieties.

Muco-epidermoid tumour

This is one of the rarer glandular neoplasms in the nose.[51, 55] Its age distribution is broadly based and there is no significant sex difference in its incidence. It is found more frequently in the maxillary region than in the nasal cavity.[51, 56]

Histopathology (Figs 4.18, 4.19)
Microscopy shows greatly varying combinations of solid cellular masses of epidermoid cells and tubulocystic structures of varying size, lined by cuboidal columnar mucus-secreting cells or even by squamous cells. The lumina usually contain

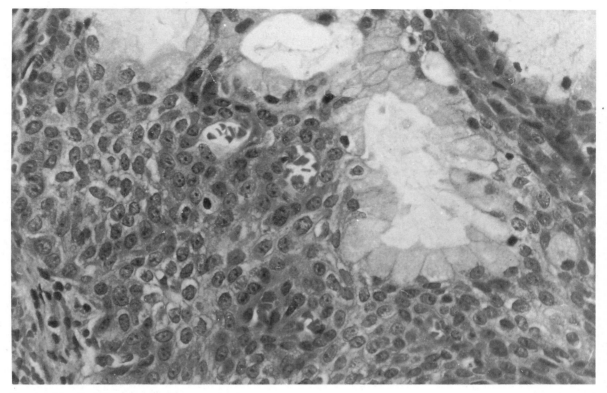

Fig. 4.19 Detail of Figure 4.18.　Haematoxylin–eosin　×450

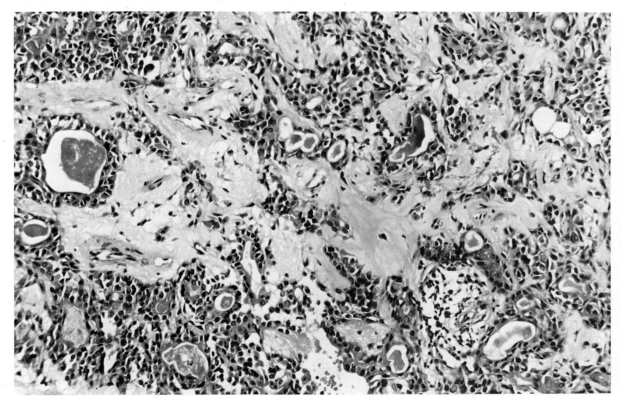

Fig. 4.20 Pleomorphic adenoma of the nasal cavity showing tubular structures with an outer layer of myoepithelial cells tending to become detached and lying free in the myxoid stroma.　Haematoxylin–eosin　×180

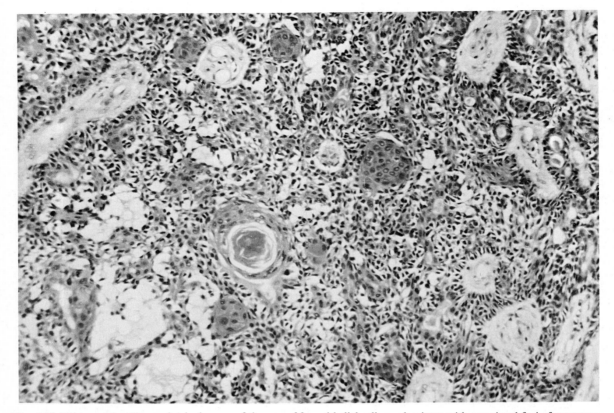

Fig. 4.21 Pleomorphic salivary gland adenoma of the nose. Myoepithelial cells predominate with occasional foci of squamous metaplasia in this example.   Haematoxylin–eosin   × 180

mucous secretion of epithelial type. Occasionally the squamous cells may produce keratin.

Muco-epidermoid tumours may be subdivided into low-grade, intermediate and high-grade malignancy, based on the relative proportions of cystic structures and solid cellular areas and on the degree of anaplasia.[56]

Pleomorphic adenoma ('mixed tumour')

Pleomorphic adenomas comprise less than 10% of all glandular tumours in the region.[51, 57] The age distribution is broadly based and in the published cases has ranged from the second to the eighth decade without any significant sex difference. Local swelling leads to nasal obstruction which may be present for many years before the patient seeks advice. The commonest location is in the nasal cavity; rarely the tumour arises on the nasal septum or in a maxillary sinus.[51, 57–62]

Histopathology (Figs 4.20, 4.21)

The tumours form firm sessile slightly lobulated masses that appear sharply circumscribed and the microscopical picture is no different from that of the major salivary gland tumours of this type.

Adenoid cystic carcinoma (cribriform adenocarcinoma)

In 1952, Reid[62] proposed the term 'adenoid cystic carcinoma' and the WHO Sub-Committee on the classification of salivary gland tumours has recommended its adoption.[63]

In the ear, nose and throat region it occurs at least as frequently as the pleomorphic adenoma. It occurs more frequently in mucosal than in major salivary glands, the ratio probably being of the order of 4:1.[58] The commonest sites are the maxillary sinus and the nasal cavity.

There is a wide age distribution with a peak in

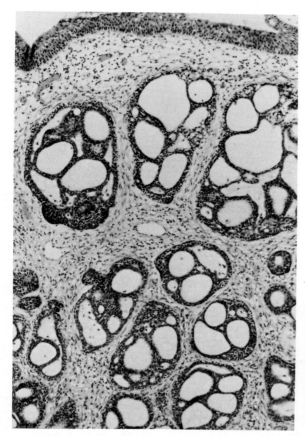

Fig. 4.22 Adenoid cystic carcinoma of the lateral wall of the nose showing the characteristic cribriform pattern.

Haematoxylin–eosin   × 75

the fourth decade.[64] There is no significant sex difference. The common forms of presentation are local swelling and pain whilst epistaxis is not uncommon. Orbital involvement results in proptosis and disturbance of vision.

Histopathology

The tumour forms a firm, opaque whitish mass of tissue indistinguishable from other forms of carcinoma. The microscopical appearances are well known.[65, 66] The classic cribriform pattern is pathognomonic of this neoplasm (Figs 4.22, 4.23). Sometimes a tubuloglandular appearance predominates (Fig. 4.23) and this can cause confusion with the pleomorphic adenomas which may occasionally contain pseudocribriform areas.

The stroma, which may be hyaline, is characteristically sharply delineated from the epithelial component, in contrast to the pleomorphic adenoma.

Local invasion is invariable and 60% of the paranasal tumours invade the orbit.[62] Systemic spread occurs in nearly 40% of cases and is much more common than lymph node metastasis.[51] Recurrence is common.[64, 67] A sinister feature of this tumour is its propensity to infiltrate perineural spaces (Fig. 4.24).

Basal cell tumour

Basal cell adenoma[68, 69] and other monomorphic salivary gland adenomas are extremely rare in the nose and sinuses.[70] The tumour is so called because of its resemblance to cutaneous basal cell carcinomas.

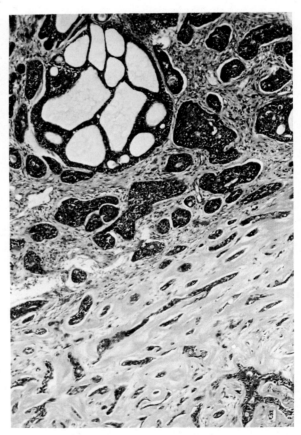

Fig. 4.23 Adenoid cystic carcinoma. Same case as Figure 4.22 showing mixed cribriform basiloid and tubular patterns with hyaline stroma.

Haematoxylin–eosin   × 75

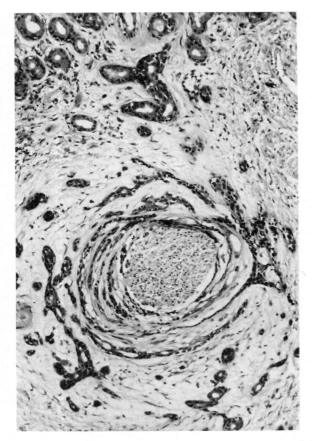

Fig. 4.24 Characteristic perineural spread in an adenoid cystic carcinoma Haematoxylin–eosin   × 120

Histopathology

The tumour has a lobulated pattern composed of sharply demarcated compact masses of spindle-shaped or ovoid cells which have indistinct cytoplasm. A palisaded border to the cell masses is not uncommon and small tubular structures may be present. Occasional foci of calcification and necrosis have been noted.

Necrotizing sialometaplasia

This condition, first reported in the palate,[71] is a benign inflammatory condition affecting the mucosal glands which can be confused with the mucoepidermoid tumour. Three cases of necrotizing sialometaplasia occurring in the nasal region have been reported.[72, 73] The lesion is characterized by infarction or necrosis of gland lobules, maintenance of the general lobular pattern, squamous metaplasia of mucous acini and ducts, and considerable acute and chronic inflammatory infiltration around the affected glands (Fig. 4.25).

MALIGNANT MELANOMA

Malignant melanoma is second only to squamous carcinoma among the cancers that arise in the nasal region.[74] Its incidence is highest in the sixth decade. There is no significant sex difference. Most of the tumours arise in the nasal cavities, few in the sinuses.

The pathogenesis—particularly the cytogenesis—of these tumours has recently been clarified by the recognition, with the aid of silver staining methods, that melanin-containing dendritic cells are normally present in the nasal mucosa. For long it has been generally believed that melanin is not found in the normal nasal mucosa except in the olfactory area, the natural brownish colour of which is due to the presence of this pigment in the supporting cells; in contrast it was recognized that melanocytes are a regular constituent of the squamous epithelium of the nasal vestibule. It seemed a paradox that melanomas should be exceptionally rare in the vestibule, where melanocytes occur, and arise in the great majority of cases in a part of the mucous membrane where melanocytes were thought to be absent under normal circumstances. The demonstration of melanocytes in the respiratory epithelium of Blacks and Asians, and in nasal glands and the stroma of the septum and conchae in Blacks, Asians and Whites, has indicated that the seeming paradox was based on inaccurate observation of the normal condition: it may be concluded that the melanocytes of the mucosa are the source of the malignant melanomas that arise in these parts. In our experience, melanocytes are relatively seldom seen in the general run of biopsy specimens of the nasal respiratory mucosa: in contrast, they are conspicuously numerous in the respiratory mucosa adjacent to a primary melanoma. The explanation of this observation is obscure. It has been shown that melanogenesis in the oropharyngeal and nasal mucosa may be activated in the presence of a malignant melanoma of the oral cavity. The relation that exists in the skin be-

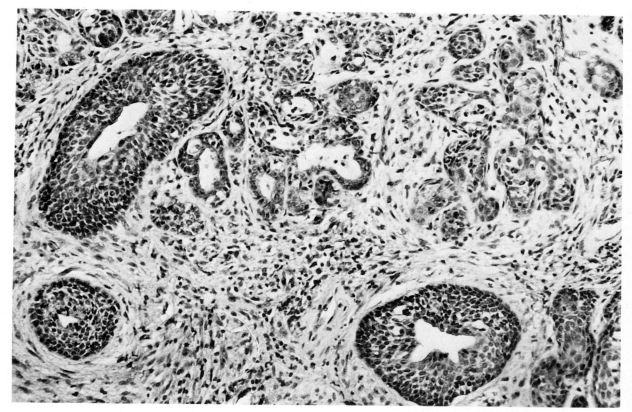

Fig. 4.25 Necrotizing sialometaplasia. Excision biopsy of palatal ulcer showing squamous metaplasia of mucous acini and ducts surrounded by inflammatory granulation tissue.

Haematoxylin–eosin   × 160

tween malignant melanoma and junctional naevus has no counterpart in the nose, where the occurrence of junctional naevi has not been demonstrated nor is there any clinical or histological evidence for the occurrence of any benign pigmented lesion in the nasal cavity.[75, 76] However, examination of malignant melanomas of the nose often reveals conspicuous changes in the immediately adjoining surface epithelium that may be compared with junctional activity in skin.[76, 77]

Histopathology
Macroscopically, malignant melanomas of the nose are usually polypoid and may be ulcerated (Fig. 4.26). They may be pigmented or unpigmented. Microscopically, they show the pleomorphism characteristic of these tumours wherever they arise. The sarcoma-like spindle-celled form is the most frequent (Fig. 4.27). Me-

lanin is usually abundant (Fig. 4.28) but when it is scanty or absent the tumour is liable to be mistaken for an anaplastic carcinoma or sarcoma.

Electron microscopy has shown that the ultrastructure of malignant melanomas of the nose is essentially the same as that of malignant melanomas arising in the skin.[78-80] Neoplastic melanocytes are characterized by the presence of varying numbers of pigmentary organelles (melanosomes) which tend to be scattered diffusely throughout the cytoplasm. The melanosomes present a pleomorphic pattern, ranging from elongated or cigar-shaped to short oval or rounded bodies, whilst ring forms or irregular masses are not uncommon. When melanization is incomplete, the internal structure of the premelanosomes is visible in varying degree, in the form of crystalloid cross-banding (Fig. 4.29). The prognosis is bad.

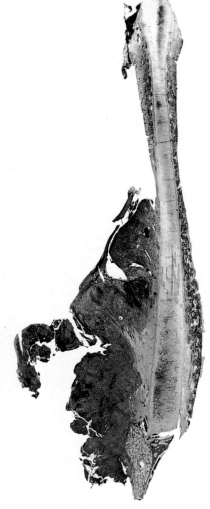

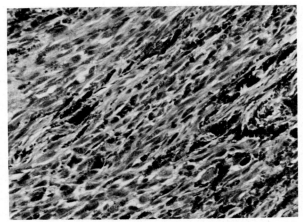

Fig. 4.27 Malignant melanoma of the nose in a 43-year-old male showing spindle cell structure.

Haematoxylin–eosin   × 140

Fig. 4.26 Malignant melanoma of the nasal septum in a 55-year-old male.

Haematoxylin–eosin   × 3.5

Involvement of regional lymph nodes occurs at an early stage and there is often early and widespread dissemination through the blood stream.

NEUROGENIC TUMOURS

Peripheral nerve tumours

Peripheral nerve tumours are not very common in the nose and sinuses. One of the earliest refer-ences to neurogenic tumours in this location was by Weinhold[81] who, in 1810, briefly mentioned a nerve swelling which involved the maxillary sinus. When they occur in this situation they are usually of the Schwannoma type. In one series of 50 cases there was only one,[82] and there was only one in a series of 152 cases of neurilemmoma arising in the head and neck.[83] In a review[84] 15 examples of peripheral nerve tumours in the paranasal sinuses were found: most were Schwannomas, but two were neurofibromas and two showed a mixed pattern. There were only seven neurogenic tumours among 646 tumours of the nasal cavities collected at the Institute of Laryngology and Otology, London.[85]

In the nose and paranasal sinuses the age distribution of neurogenic tumours tends to be concentrated in early middle life, being maximal in the third and fourth decades. There is a slight predominance of males but the sex difference is not significant. The symptoms include pain, nasal obstruction, epistaxis and unilateral exophthalmos. Pain is common in tumours of the maxillary antrum and epistaxis occurs when the tumour is located in the nasal fossa or ethmoid air cells. Surgical removal may be accompanied by severe bleeding because of the rich vascularity of Schwannomas. Recurrence has been observed, even after many years, but frankly malignant behaviour is very rare.

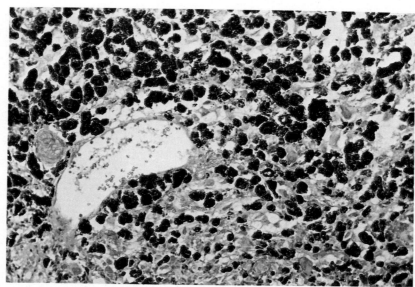

Fig. 4.28 Malignant melanoma of the nose in a 47-year-old male showing heavily pigmented polygonal cells.
Haematoxylin–eosin   × 160

Histopathology

The light microscopic features of peripheral nerve tumours are somewhat variable. There is a tendency to consider them as belonging to a single group, Schwannoma or neurilemmoma. Benign Schwannomas are generally defined as encapsulated neoplasms of Schwann cell origin composed of two readily distinguishable types of tissue (Fig. 4.30), a compact spindle cell pattern with nuclear palisading—the Verocay bodies (Antoni-A) (Fig. 4.31)—admixed in variable proportions with a looser and often more pleomorphic spindle cell tissue with foam cells (Antoni-B).[86, 87]

Neurofibromas, diffuse or plexiform, are tumours derived from the fibroblasts of the perineural tissue; they are unencapsulated and do not contain Verocay bodies. They may be solitary or form part of von Recklinghausen's neurofibromatosis in which Schwannomas may also occur.

Electron microscopy[88–91] has confirmed that the neurilemmomas are composed almost entirely of Schwann cells whilst neurofibromas contain, in addition, variable numbers of fibroblasts. The Schwann cells possess elongated cytoplasmic processes surrounded by a basal lamina, in con-

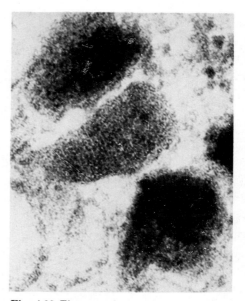

Fig. 4.29 Electron micrograph of a malignant melanoma of the nose in a 50-year-old male showing melanosomes and paler laminated premelanosomes.

× 168 000

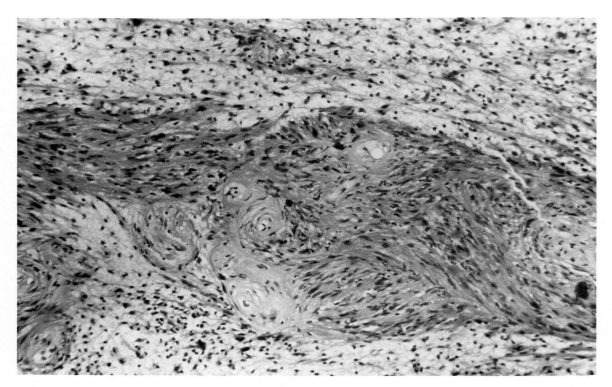

Fig. 4.30 Schwannoma of the nose showing Antoni A type tissue composed of compact bundles of spindle shaped cells surrounded by oedematous Antoni B type tissue.   Haematoxylin–eosin   × 200

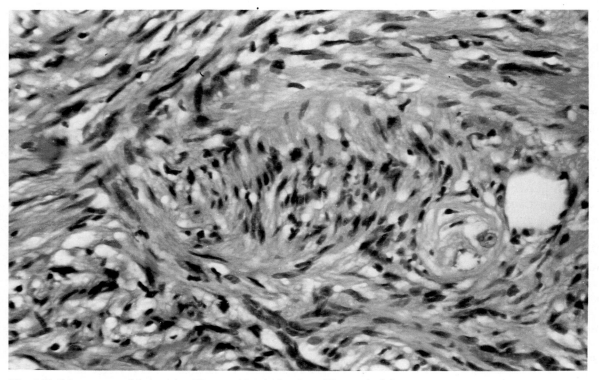

Fig. 4.31 Schwannoma of the nose in a 59-year-old male showing a 'Verocay body'.
Haematoxylin–eosin   × 500

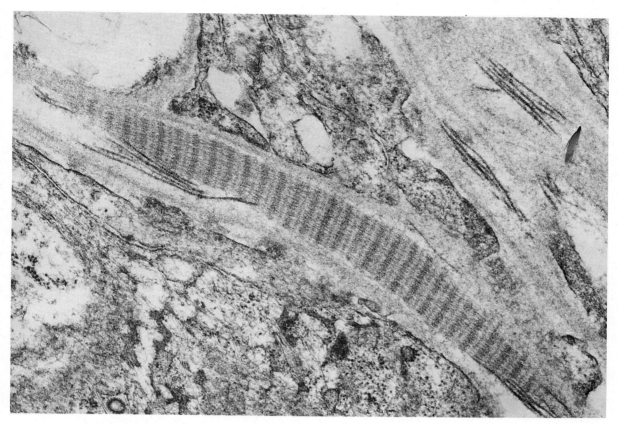

Fig. 4.32 Schwannoma of the nose. Electron microscopy of the tumour in Figures 4.30 and 4.31. Note characteristic structure of long spacing collagen (Luse body).

× 38 000

trast to the fibroblasts which present no such structure. The collagen fibrils of neurofibromas have the normal periodicity of about 64 nm; in contrast, as was first described by Luse,[88] Schwannomas frequently contain banded fibrils with the periodicity of 100 nm or more (Fig. 4.32)—these 'Luse bodies' are almost certainly procollagen and have been described as a type of long-spaced collagen.[92]

Melanin may be present in peripheral nerve tumours[90, 93] and has also been observed in tissue culture of these tumours.[94] Electron microscopy[93] has shown the presence of melanosomes and pre-melanosomes confirming that there is intracellular pigment production.

Schwannomas often show marked nuclear irregularity but this does not necessarily imply malignant change. Malignant change may occur in von Recklinghausen's disease and is then usually confined to a single tumour. In a review of 115 cases of malignant peripheral nerve tumours[95] 30% were associated with von Recklinghausen's disease.

Peripheral nerve tumours occasionally display foci of glandular differentiation and it has been suggested that such tumours have a better prognosis.[96] This feature has not been observed in tumours of the nasal region.

Nasal glioma

The so-called 'glioma' of the nose, a tumour-like lesion seen almost exclusively in young children, is not a true tumour but a congenital lesion arising during early embryonic development in the area of juxtaposition of the upper respiratory tract and the prosencephalon.[97] The WHO

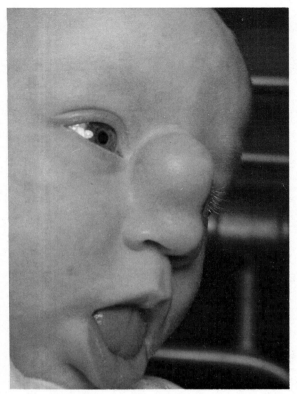

Fig. 4.33 Nasal glioma ('nasal glial heterotopia') in an infant, showing the characteristic location beneath the skin at the root of the bridge of the nose.

classification refers to the lesion as 'nasal glial heterotopia'.[98] However, in deference to clinical usage it is probably justified to retain the diagnostic term 'glioma'. The condition is rare: reports are either of single cases or of small series of six cases or less.[99–102]

About 60% present as external swellings beneath the skin on one side or other of the bridge of the nose (Fig. 4.33). About 30% are intranasal, beneath the mucosa of the upper part of the nasal cavity, and cause obstruction. The lesion, which is readily mistaken for a simple nasal polyp, may present at the anterior nares[103] and simple excision may have fatal consequences.[104] The remaining 10% exhibit a combination of the two presentations. Sometimes a stalk is found passing through a defect in the nasal wall or, rarely, into the cranium. Intranasal lesions may have a pedicle extending through a bony defect in the roof of the nose, often involving the cribriform plate. Macroscopically they are formed of firm greyish tissue. Intranasal lesions are less translucent and firmer than simple nasal polyps.

Histopathology
The nasal glioma consists of mature glial tissue composed of astrocytes and a profusion of glial fibres interspersed with collagenous fibrous tissue (Fig. 4.34). The astrocytes may show the normal characteristic disposition around blood vessels; sometimes they have a vesicular appearance and contain multiple nuclei, and occasionally they may be swollen and of gemistocytic appearance. Very occasionally a few nerve cells and their axons may be found;[105] spaces lined by ependymal cells have also been reported.[99, 102, 106]

The fact that many of these lesions appear isolated led to the view that they were heterotopic brain tissue. It is now generally accepted that they are all initially encephaloceles. The external 'glioma' results from protrusion of brain through the fonticulus frontonasalis, the membrane-filled gap (fontanelle) between the frontal and nasal bones in early embryonic life. Subsequent bony closure of this fontanelle obliterates the connection with the brain, leaving an isolated mass of nervous tissue beneath the skin. Protrusion of brain substance through the fronto-ethmoidal suture at the position of the foramen caecum gives rise to the intranasal 'glioma': communication with the intracranial contents is then less likely to be obliterated.

The majority of cases present during the first year of life. A few are encountered up to the age of 10 years and very occasionally even as late as middle life.[100, 107] Sex incidence is equal. Growth of the lesion is usually slow and generally commensurate with the growth of the patient. Excision can be expected to effect a complete cure. When an intracranial connection persists, simple intranasal removal may be followed by leakage of cerebrospinal fluid and the risk of meningitis. Frontal craniotomy may therefore be necessary to deal with the dural and cerebral connection and to repair the bony defect. Recurrence due to incomplete removal is not unknown but a second excision usually results in cure.

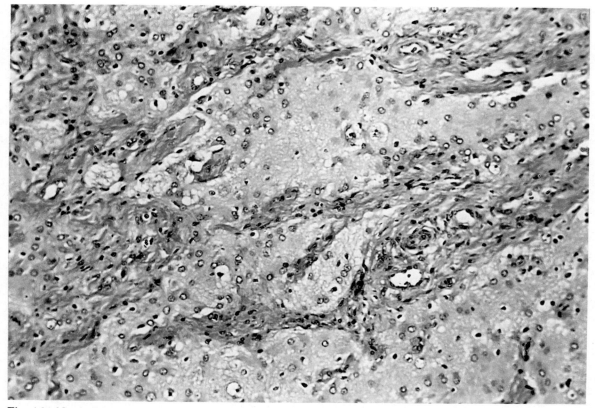

Fig. 4.34 Nasal glioma ('nasal glial heterotopia') composed of fibrillary neuroglial tissue intersected with bands of vascular connective tissue.
Haematoxylin–eosin   × 200

Olfactory neuroblastoma (olfactory neuro-epithelial tumour)

This relatively uncommon nasal tumour was first recognized and reported by Berger et al in 1924.[108] Although its identity has now been established for 60 years, it is still noteworthy for errors in diagnosis owing to the unfamiliarity of the general pathologist with this type of neoplasm. In the 42 years following the first report over 100 cases were published.[109]

A variety of terms for the designation and sub-classification of this tumour have been introduced, but unfortunately their usage has been far from consistent. Berger and his colleagues[108] described the first case under the title of *esthésioneuroépithéliome olfactif*, indicating the presence of an epithelial component. Subsequently, Berger & Coutard[110] reported another case in which there did not appear to be any

epithelial derivative and they labelled it *esthésioneurocytome*. Lindstrom & Lindstrom[111] while recognizing the Berger subtypes of neuro-epithelioma and neurocytoma, recommended 'olfactory neuroblastoma' as a generic term.

The age distribution is broadly based; the greatest frequency is in the second decade. The youngest patient on record was a 3-year-old boy; the oldest was 70 years old.[112] The tumour presents in the upper part of a nasal cavity, often as a haemorrhagic mass with evidence of bone destruction.

Histopathology

Microscopically, the tumour is characterized by rounded, compact, cellular foci: these are often discrete, and separated by very vascular stroma. The nucleus of the tumour cell is oval or round and stains deeply (Figs 4.35, 4.36). The growth

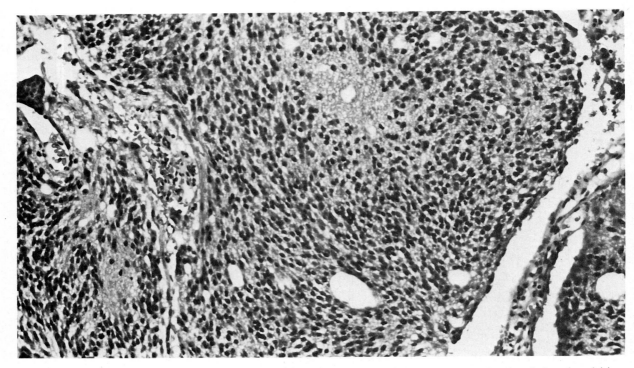

Fig. 4.35 Olfactory neuroblastoma composed of well defined compact cellular masses with round and oval shaped nuclei in a fibrillary matrix.   Haematoxylin–eosin   × 200

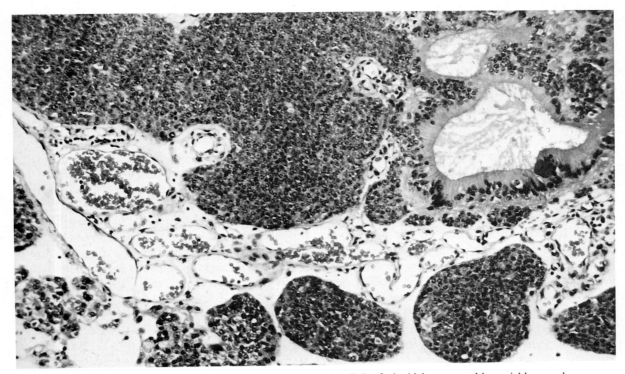

Fig. 4.36 Olfactory neuroblastoma composed of rounded compact cellular foci widely separated by a richly vascular stroma. A very rarely observed feature of olfactory epithelial differentiation is shown in the upper right corner (see Fig. 4.37).

Haematoxylin–eosin   × 180

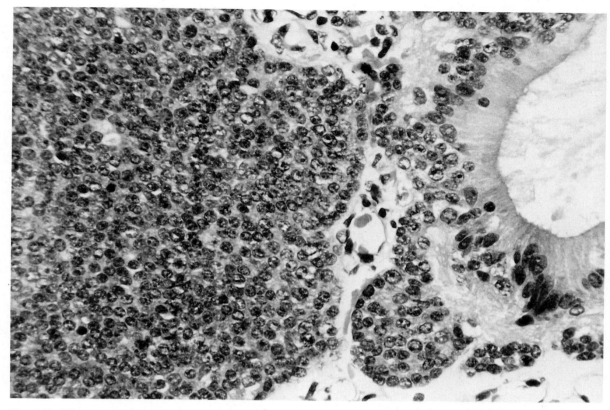

Fig. 4.37 Olfactory neuroblastoma. Higher power of Figure 4.36 showing the neoplastic tissue composed of predominantly spheroidal cells, many with apparently 'naked' nuclei. There are several small poorly formed rosettes present. Well formed olfactory-type epithelium blends with the tumour. Haematoxylin–eosin   × 450

can be confused with other types of small-cell tumour. In general, the cells have more cytoplasm than lymphocytes, though it may be so poorly defined that the appearances are those of 'naked' nuclei (Figs 4.35, 4.37). The presence of rosettes is diagnostically helpful but is far from a constant feature. The rosettes may be of the type conventionally referred to as 'true rosettes', consisting of cuboidal or columnar cells about a central space, thus resembling a glandular structure (Flexner rosette) (Fig. 4.38); alternatively the cells enclose fibrillary or granular material (Homer Wright rosette) (Fig. 4.39). These are not to be confused with non-diagnostic pseudo-rosettes where the cells are arranged around vessels. Flexner rosettes are uncommon in olfactory tumours but when present the lesion is often referred to as an olfactory neuro-epihelioma. Very occasionally both types of true rosette may be

present.[109, 113] True olfactory epithelial differentiation has been observed[114] (Figs 4.36, 4.37). Calcification may occur (Fig. 4.40) and the presence of melanin has been reported.[115]

Electron microscopy. The principal cells are polygonal or spherical and contain a large rounded nucleus which often has finely distributed chromatin. Nucleoli may be present but are often inconspicuous. There is a profuse network of neurites attached to the cells and forming synaptic connections. Many of the cells contain neurosecretory granules characterized by dense centres separated from the limiting membrane by a narrow clear zone. The granules range in size from about 100–200 nm in diameter. They may also be found in the neurites (Fig. 4.41).

Catecholamines and other biological amines

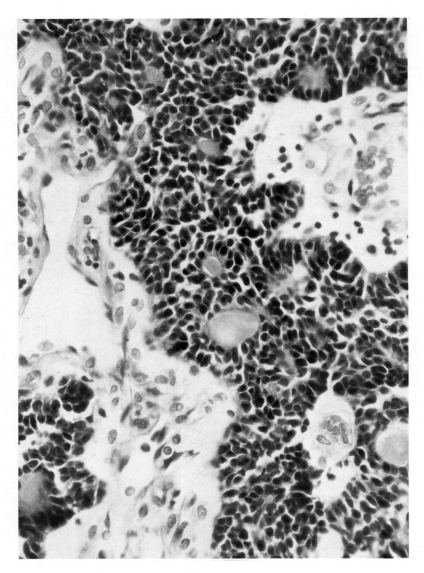

Fig. 4.38 Olfactory neuroblastoma to show Flexner type rosettes formed by cuboidal cells around a central space containing some secretion.   Haematoxylin–eosin   × 450

produced by the cells form highly fluorescent condensation products with formaldehyde:[117] the technique of formaldehyde-induced fluorescence has been applied to the histological diagnosis of olfactory tumours.[118]

Diagnosis

The histological diagnosis of these tumours is not always easy. Neither true rosettes nor pseudo-rosettes are commonly present and care has to be

taken not to confuse the former with true glandular structures which may have become infiltrated by tumour tissue. In some cases the neurofibrils are not very obvious and the diagnostic difficulties are then greatly increased. Confusion with transitional or anaplastic carcinoma, malignant lymphoma or even plasmacytoma may arise and the application of immunohistological techniques may prove helpful in the differential diagnosis.[119] Small-cell carcinomas with neurosecre-

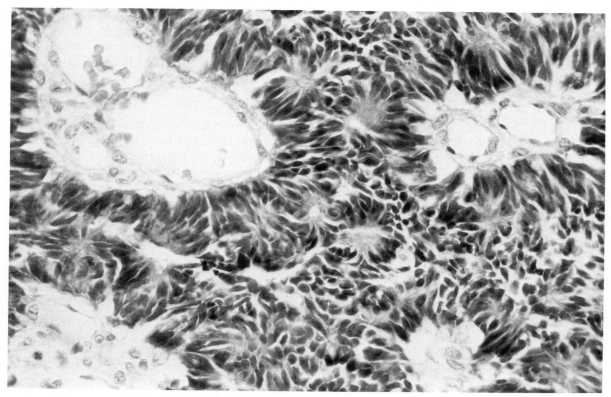

Fig. 4.39 Olfactory neuroblastoma composed of cells with round and elongated nuclei surrounding vascular spaces (pseudo-rosettes) and forming Homer–Wright rosettes with a central core of fibrillary material.
Haematoxylin–eosin   × 450

tory granules but lacking rosette or pseudorosette formation have recently been described in the paranasal sinuses under the term neuroendocrine carcinoma.[114, 120]

Causation
No clue to the causation of these tumours in man has so far emerged. Olfactory tumours have been produced in Syrian hamsters by the injection of diethyl nitrosamine.[121] The origin of the olfactory neuroblastoma has been variously ascribed to the olfactory placode, the organ of Jacobson, the sphenopalatine ganglion, the olfactory bulb and the olfactory mucosa.

Course
In many cases the olfactory neuroblastoma is slowly growing. It may recur after surgical removal or radiotherapy. Local spread to the paranasal sinuses, the palate and the orbit is com-

mon.[111, 122–125] Intracranial involvement has been reported.[126–128] Metastasis occurs in over 20% of cases,[129] the usual sites being lymph nodes (especially cervical), lungs and bones, in that order of frequency. Other sites, such as skin, liver and spleen may occasionally be involved. Increased urinary excretion of catecholamines has been observed in some cases of olfactory neuroblastoma. A patient with a nasal neuroblastoma was found to have hypertension and severe hyponatraemia:[130] the assay of tumour tissue post mortem revealed high levels of arginine vasopressin.

In contrast with adrenal neuroblastomas or retinoblastomas, survival rates are much better in the case of the olfactory tumour: they correspond more closely to other extra-adrenal tumours of this type. 5-year survival rates of over 50% have been reported.[129, 131] The most effective form of treatment for nasal neuroblastoma appears to be a combination of surgery and radiotherapy; the

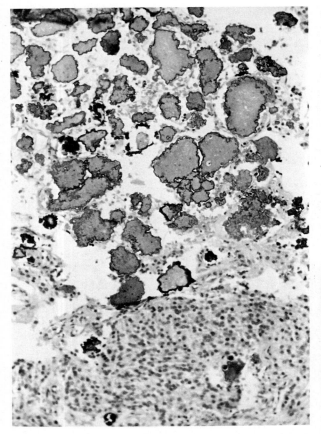

Fig. 4.40 Olfactory neuroblastoma from an elderly woman who survived about 25 years after the diagnosis. Note extensive calcification of the tumour.

Haematoxylin–eosin   × 170

contribution that chemotherapy may offer must still be assessed.

Meningioma

Meningioma occurs very rarely in the nose and sinuses. The patient may present with nasal obstruction, proptosis, epiphora, pain or epistaxis. The nasal cavity and the maxillary, ethmoidal and frontal sinuses are more likely to be involved than the sphenoidal sinus. The tumours take origin in the orbit or intracranial cavity and extend into the nasal cavity or sinuses.[132, 133] Tumours originating in the nose, maxillary and frontal sinuses have also been reported.[134, 135]

The tumours are of rubbery consistency and in the nasal cavity may give the impression of simple polyps.[134] The microscopical picture is variable and may be subdivided into syncytial, transitional, fibroblastic and angioblastic subtypes,[136] but essentially it is made up of two types of cell, polyhedral and spindle, the latter often arranged in whorls which may contain some calcified matter.[137]

Most meningiomas are benign in that they do not metastasize, but local permeation of crevices and foramina and pressure erosion may result in spread from one cavity to another. Recurrence is not uncommon, even after apparently complete removal,[133] but long survival is usual. It is clearly important to watch for evidence of intracranial involvement which may cause epilepsy.

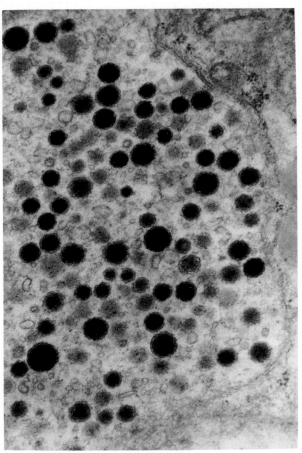

Fig. 4.41 Electron micrograph of an olfactory neuroblastoma in a 40-year-old female showing dense-cored neurosecretory granules.

× 36 750

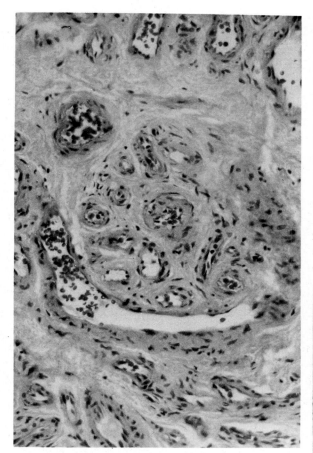

Fig. 4.42 Capillary haemangioma of the nose showing the lobular structure of the tumour.

Haematoxylin–eosin ×225

VASCULAR TUMOURS

The vascular tumours comprise both true tumours and malformations.

Haemangiomas

Tumours or tumour-like proliferations of blood vessels are important in ear, nose and throat practice since they are a source of bleeding. Many of these lesions occur on the nasal septum and have long been recognized clinically under the title 'bleeding polyp of the septum'. They are common, and constitute about 20% of all benign neoplasms of the nasal cavity.[138]

Many tumour pathologists regard all benign vascular growths as hamartomatous malforma-tions, a view presupposing their presence in some form at the time of birth. As so many of these lesions in most parts of the body occur in young patients this view would seem in general to be acceptable. In the nasal region, however, the angioma has its peak incidence in the fifth and sixth decades, and its history is usually short—less than 6 months in most of our cases: such a lesion is more easily explained as of recent origin than as a result of activation in middle life of a congenital condition. Confusingly, these nasal angiomas are often referred to as angio-fibromas, although in structure they resemble haemangiomas of other parts of the body. They must not be confused with juvenile angiofibroma, another benign condition, but of totally different origin and presentation (see p. 96).

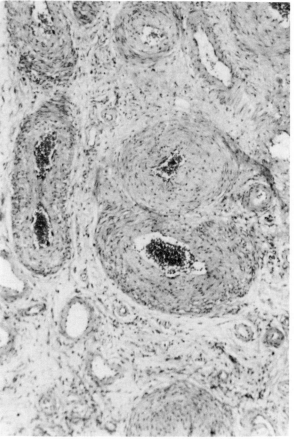

Fig. 4.43 Capillary haemangioma of the nose showing greatly thickened vessels.

Haematoxylin–eosin ×85

There is no sex difference in the occurrence of nasal haemangiomas. In most cases the complaint is epistaxis, with or without attendant nasal obstruction. The patient commonly presents with a reddish-blue polypoid swelling with a smooth surface which may sometimes be ulcerated. The tumours are almost invariably confined to the nasal cavity and the septum is the most frequent site.[139] The usual site of the septal angioma is Little's 'bleeding area'—the antero-inferior part of the septum where the main septal branch of the sphenopalatine artery anastomoses with the septal branch of the superior labial artery. In exceptional instances the angioma becomes a large, tense and very hyperaemic mass that protrudes from the nostril.

Histopathology
Most of these tumours have the classic structure of capillary haemangioma, consisting of closely-set collections of well formed capillaries separated by loose connective tissue giving an impression of lobularity (Fig. 4.42). In some instances irregular thick-walled vessels are also present (Fig. 4.43). The intervening connective tissue is of varying density and is often rather oedematous. Some of the vessels may be obliterated by thrombosis: different stages in organization and scarring will then be seen. Iron pigment may be scattered in the tissue, usually sparsely. Inflammatory cells are scanty or absent unless ulceration has occurred. It is those lesions in which there is a heavy inflammatory infiltrate that acquired the name 'pyogenic granuloma', 'telangiectatic granuloma' or 'haemangiomatous granulation tissue', all misleading terms. Recently the designation 'lobular capillary haemangioma' has been introduced.[140]

Juvenile angiofibroma
The condition known as juvenile angiofibroma is less common and more serious than the capillary haemangioma. The two conditions are unrelated and confusion has been caused by the occasional designation of the latter as angiofibroma (see above). While the juvenile angiofibroma is often said to be a nasopharyngeal growth, it is more appropriately discussed here. The first recorded description of this fibrovascular tumour-like

lesion, involving predominantly the postnasal region, was by Chelius in 1847[141] but it seems that surgeons had endeavoured to deal with growths of this nature even before the nineteenth century[142] and it has been asserted that their removal was practised by Hippocrates.[143]

The condition is relatively rare in the western world but impressions of a higher incidence in the Middle East and Far East have not always been borne out by the published facts.[138, 143–146] This growth may be found in patients in any part of the world and of any race. It is a disease pre-eminently of boys. It is rare before the age of 10 years; most cases present at about the time of puberty. Sometimes the disease is familial. Contrary to a frequently expressed view, there is no doubt that the disease may occur in girls, although this is exceptionally rare.

The first symptoms are nasal obstruction and, less constantly, bleeding. Severe epistaxis is unusual, except as a complication of surgery: bleeding following a biopsy operation has occasionally been uncontrollable and followed by death. As the tumour grows it tends to fill the nasal and postnasal cavities. Its bulk may cause those bones of the base of the skull that have not yet completed osseous union to be forced apart. Although the tumour does not invade the bones its mass may lead to extensive local destruction of the cranium through pressure atrophy, and in rare cases this has been complicated by suppurative meningitis. As the space between the orbits gradually widens to accommodate the growing tumour, the characteristic 'frog-face' deformity results: this has been described particularly among Chinese patients and occurs only rarely among patients of other races.

Anatomical site of origin
The location of the attachment or origin of this lesion is important both to the surgeon and to the pathologist. It has already been noted that the lesion tends to fill the nasopharynx, and, in so far as a proportion of cases exhibit unequivocal adherence to the roof of that cavity, it is understandable that the condition came to be regarded as a nasopharyngeal tumour. Careful assessment, however, reveals that in many cases the principal attachment is around the margins of the

Histopathology

Microscopically, the angiofibroma consists of numerous vascular channels embedded in fibrous tissue (Fig. 4.45). The latter varies in texture from a compact, hyaline mass to an oedematous granulation tissue: in general it has a laminar pattern, reminiscent of scar tissue, rather than the whorled and fascicular arrangement more characteristic of fibromas. The wall of many of the vessels is no more than a layer of endothelium, thus the liability to bleeding is readily understood. Some vessels, however, have a muscular wall, which may vary remarkably in the degree of its development, with abrupt transitions between stretches where there is a thick well-defined muscle coat and those with no more than the simple endothelial layer between lumen and fibrous tissue (Fig. 4.46). These vessels probably

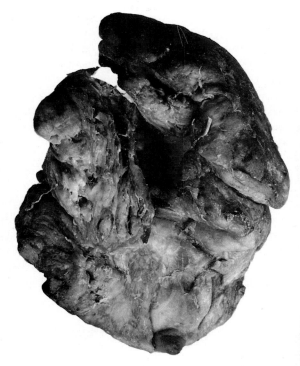

Fig. 4.44 Juvenile angiofibroma of the nasopharynx. Gross appearance showing solid lobulated polypoid mass with areas of haemorrhage on the surface.

choanae.[147] Less commonly a paranasal origin of the tumour has been described.[148–151]

Macroscopically, the lesion appears fibro-vascular, oedematous and often haemorrhagic (Fig. 4.44). It is usually symmetrically disposed but rarely the condition is confined, or largely so, to one side and the resultant disfiguration is correspondingly unilateral. Occasionally it arises in a maxillary sinus.[148, 152] Although the growth may have some attachment to the postnasal region, this is generally trivial in comparison with the involvement of the structures of the nasal wall and it is for this reason that the disease is better considered in the context of the nose than among diseases affecting the nasopharynx primarily. In exceptional cases the growth spreads so far forward within the nasal cavity that it presents at the nostril on one or both sides.

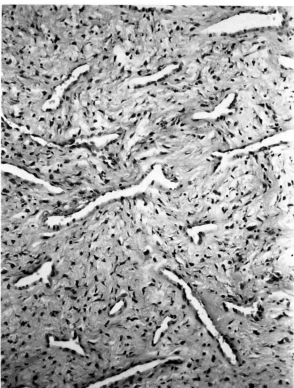

Fig. 4.45 Juvenile angiofibroma in a 15-year-old boy showing numerous thin-walled vessels embedded in dense fibrous tissue.

Haematoxylin–eosin   × 200

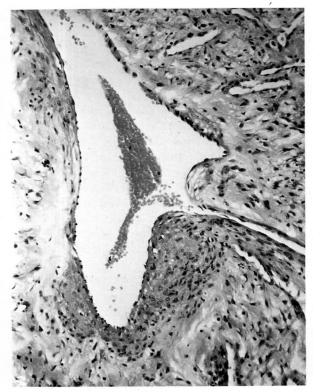

Fig. 4.46 Juvenile angiofibroma. Same case as Figure 4.45 showing anomalous vessel with abrupt change in the wall from muscular to mere endothelial thickness.

Haematoxylin–eosin   × 200

represent a malformation of the structures concerned in the formation of the nasal erectile tissue.[147] Other microscopical features of the lesions are more or less extensive foci of reparative granulation tissue, haemorrhages and scattered clusters of mast cells. Atypical stromal cells (Fig. 4.47) may occur as in some nasal polyps (see p. 23).

Nature
Earlier views of the nature of juvenile angiofibroma of the nose were coloured by preoccupation with the fibrous component and the possibility that the condition might be related to the various forms of fascial and aponeurotic 'fibromatosis'. Osborn[147] drew attention to the similarity between the anomalous vessels in the nasal angiofibroma and the vascular elements of

nasal erectile tissue, suggesting that the condition is a vascular hamartoma. Coincidentally, Schiff[152] studied the stromal component and came to the conclusion that the lesion was a desmoplastic response to malformed erectile tissue, probably mediated by hormonal activity. The nasal erectile tissue, because of its complex development and its concentration toward the back of the nasal cavities, is the likeliest source.

The sex incidence of juvenile angiofibroma could be thought an impediment to accepting the malformation theory. The explanation of the remarkable preponderance of boys among patients with the disease remains obscure. The possible relation between the nasal erectile tissue and the erectile tissue of the genital organs may have some potential aetiological significance, perhaps in terms of an anomalous hypertrophic response

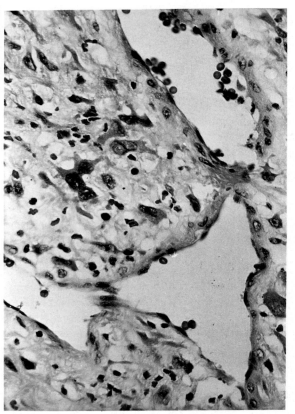

Fig. 4.47 Juvenile angiofibroma in a boy of 16. There are atypical pleomorphic stromal cells present.

Haematoxylin–eosin   × 210

to the physiological hormonal changes associated with puberty.[153]

Sarcomatous change
A case of fibrosarcoma arising from a recurrent juvenile angiofibroma 18 years after radiation therapy has been described. This was the third documented case of sarcomatous transformation of juvenile angiofibroma.[154] Sarcomatous transformation occurred after local radiation therapy in all three cases, suggesting a cause and effect relationship.

MALIGNANT VASCULAR TUMOURS

Angiosarcomas are rare in the nose. They include the haemangiopericytoma and, even rarer, the angiosarcoma (malignant haemangioendothelioma).

Haemangiopericytoma

Although the incidence of the haemangiopericy-toma in the head and neck region is high it is rare in the nose and nasal sinuses.[155, 156] It can occur at any age but usually in older adults. Its malignant potential is often low.

Histopathology
The tumour is composed of spindle-shaped and polyhedral cells arranged around narrow slit-like or dilated vascular spaces lined by normal endothelial cells (Fig. 4.48). The nuclei of the tumour cells vary in shape and size. Occasional mitotic figures may be seen. Reticulin impregnation (Fig. 4.49) outlines the basal lamina, demarcating the comparatively normal endothelial lining of the vascular channels from the neoplastic cells; the latter form processes bulging into the vascular lumen. The extravascular location of the tumour cells assists in distinguishing between haemangiopericytoma and angiosarcoma (see below).

Stout[157] has emphasized the variable histological picture. The degree of pleomorphism and variable ultrastructural features of the tumour

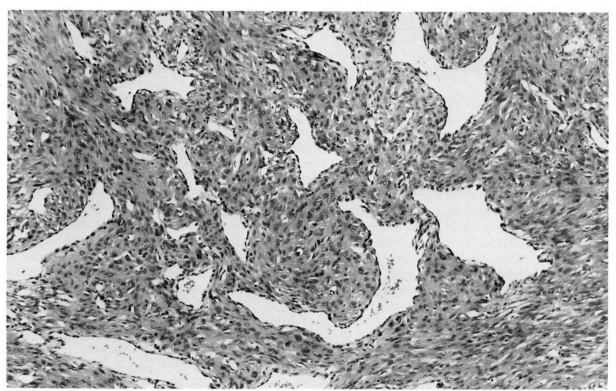

Fig. 4.48 Haemangiopericytoma of the nose in a 35-year-old man showing numerous dilated vascular spaces separated by masses of spindle and polyhedral shaped tumour cells. Haematoxylin–eosin × 120

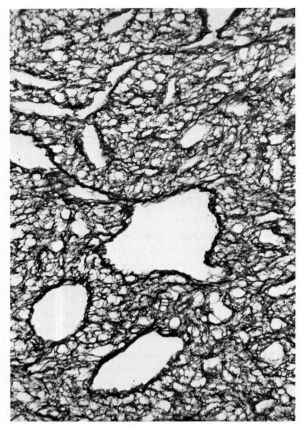

Fig. 4.49 Haemangiopericytoma. Reticulin impregnation reveals dense reticulin meshwork surrounding the tumour cells and outlining the basal lamina separating the vascular channels from the neoplastic cells.

Haematoxylin–eosin   × 325

make the histological distinction between benign and malignant varieties often difficult. Differential diagnosis from glomus tumour (see below) is based on the concentric organoid perivascular arrangement of the cells in the latter, which are usually spheroidal, contrasting with the elongated or stellate cells of the haemangiopericytoma.

The behaviour of haemangiopericytoma is variable though more favourable than that of angiosarcoma. Recurrence has been reported in about a quarter of the published cases of nasal or paranasal tumours. However in contrast to haemangiopericytoma in other sites, metastasis of a nasal or paranasal primary is exceptional.[158, 159]

Angiosarcoma (malignant haemangioendothelioma)

This tumour is very rare in the nasal region.[155, 160] Its occurrence is evenly spread between the second and eighth decades. There is no sex difference in its incidence.

Histopathology

The neoplasm is composed of weakly cohesive cells forming vascular channels. The latter are lined by large pleomorphic, often multinucleated endothelial cells (Fig. 4.50). Numerous mitotic figures are seen and necrosis may be present. Reticulin impregnation shows well defined sheaths containing atypical neoplastic cells. The differential diagnosis from haemangiopericytoma and Kaposi's sarcoma is important because of the poorer prognosis of the angiosarcoma, which tends to metastasize to distant organs. Electron microscopy may assist in the differential diagnosis.[159]

In the breast three types of angiosarcoma have been distinguished according to their degree of differentiation.[161] The vascular nature of the neoplasms was demonstrated by utilizing immunoperoxidase stains with factor VIII-related antigen. Factor VIII-related antigen has been shown to be synthesized by endothelial cells, and recently this antigen has been used to help in the identification of tumours of vascular origin. Those cases classified as well-differentiated angiosarcomas showed marked reaction in the endothelial cells lining the well-formed vascular channels. Moderately- and poorly-differentiated angiosarcomas stained less intensely. The histological pattern correlated closely with the prognosis, four of the five patients with well-differentiated tumours remaining free of disease. Therefore angiosarcomas should not all be considered highly aggressive neoplasms associated with a dismal prognosis.

Glomus tumour of the nose and sinuses

This tumour is extremely rare in the nasal region, only two cases having been reported.[155, 162] The general microscopical structure is not unlike that of the haemangiopericytoma, normal endothelium-lined vascular channels being surrounded by tumour cells. However, the tumour

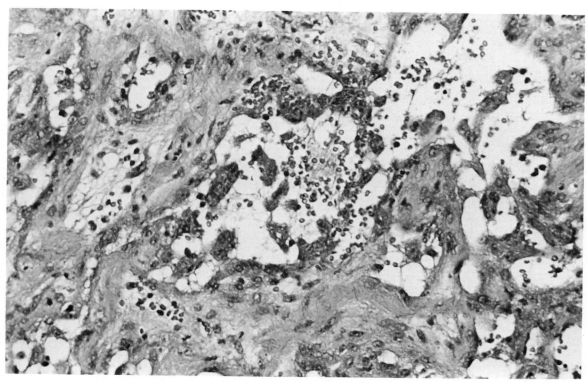

Fig. 4.50 Angiosarcoma of the nose in a 91-year-old man showing multinucleated neoplastic endothelial cells lining irregular anastomosing vascular channels.

Haematoxylin–eosin   × 575

cells are of a regular polyhedral shape, imparting an epithelioid appearance. The more organoid appearance together with the presence of numerous neurofibrils serve to distinguish this neoplasm from the haemangiopericytoma. Most glomus tumours are benign in their behaviour.

Paraganglioma (chemodectoma) of the nose and sinuses

Although comparatively rare, the chemodectoma or non-chromaffin paraganglioma is well recognized, particularly in the head and neck region. The more common sites of such tumours are the carotid body, the vagal body and the jugulotympanic bodies (glomus jugulare and glomus tympanicum). Other locations include the larynx and the orbit. The first report of a genuine paraganglioma of the nasal cavity was by Moran.[163] Since then a small number of cases have been recorded.[164]

TUMOUR-LIKE LESIONS AND TUMOURS OF SKELETAL TISSUES

The maxillary sinuses, and less often the nasal cavities, may be involved by generalized disorders of the bone that affect the maxilla and may grossly resemble neoplasms. These include Paget's disease, osteogenesis imperfecta, fibrous dysplasia, ossifying fibroma, aneurysmal bone cyst, reparative granuloma, eosinophilic granuloma and solitary bone cyst. The histological distinction between these conditions is not always straightforward, particularly when only small biopsy specimens are available, and particularly when inflammatory changes have been added in consequence of ulceration and infection. The disfiguring appearance that is sometimes described as *leontiasis ossea* may result from the presence of some of these disorders, including Paget's disease of bone and fibrous dysplasia.[165]

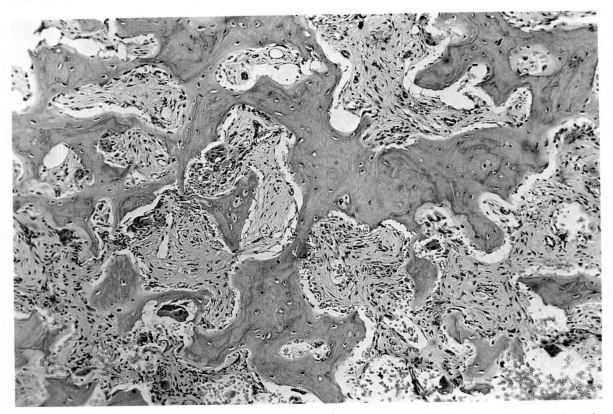

Fig. 4.51 Paget's disease involving the turbinate of a 64-year-old female showing osteoblastic and osteoclastic activity and a highly vascular stroma.

Haematoxylin–eosin   × 130

Paget's disease

Paget's disease[166] has attracted fresh interest in recent years, engendered by the biochemical changes that the overactive bone produces and their modification by treatment.[167]

Paget's disease of the bones of the nose is usually a manifestation of general skeletal involvement. The disease may be monostotic or generalized. The nasal conchae when involved may be mistaken for nasal polyps. The skull and face undergo gradual deformity accompanied by pain caused by nerve compression. The temporal bone may also be involved[168] and sarcoma may develop.

The incidence of paranasal involvement by Paget's disease is about 3%. Those affected are usually over 40 years old.[169] So-called juvenile Paget's disease is exceedingly rare.

Histopathology

There is in the early stage of the disease enhanced osteoclastic activity, causing extensive bone resorption and disorganization, followed by reorganization of the bone pattern by means of osteoblastic activity. A great amount of woven bone is laid down, with richly vascular bone marrow containing many multinucleated osteoclasts. The osteoblastic regeneration and successive waves of resorption lead to replacement of the normal structure by trabecular bone showing the characteristic mosaic-pattern of irregular cement lines (Fig. 4.51).

The cause of Paget's disease has remained obscure. Paracrystalline inclusions were noted in multinucleated osteoclasts from iliac crest biopsies studied under the electron microscope.[170] These inclusions have been interpreted as suggesting a virus infection.[171]

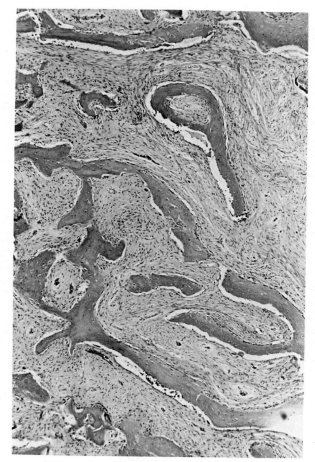

Fig. 4.52 Fibrous dysplasia of the maxilla showing irregular curved trabeculae of immature woven bone embedded in vascular fibrous tissue.

Haematoxylin–eosin   × 60

The alkaline phosphatase concentration in the plasma is greatly increased, consequent upon the intensive osteoblastic activity. The structure and metabolism of collagen have been extensively studied in Paget's disease.[167] The excretion of total hydroxyproline in the urine is increased due to enhanced osteoclastic activity and the breakdown of collagen.

Fibrous dysplasia

This non-neoplastic disease of unknown aetiology can affect the nasal structures. Fu & Perzin[155] noted 9 cases among 256 cases of benign non-epithelial tumours involving the nasal cavity.

There are monostotic[172] and polyostotic forms. They usually present in early adult life and the facial bones may be affected. The maxilla is more often affected than the mandible. The maxillary sinus, the orbital floor and the zygomatic arch may be affected. There is gradually increasing swelling of the jaw; in some patients the increase occurs more rapidly. Facial asymmetry may be striking and associated with unilateral exophthalmos.

Histopathology
Slender curved trabeculae of woven bone are surrounded by a stroma of delicate fibrous tissue (Fig. 4.52). There is some osteoclastic and osteoblastic activity. The microscopical features in the more active lesion merge with those of ossifying fibroma.

Ossifying fibroma

This lesion of the nose has been considered as a variant of fibrous dysplasia but is probably a neoplasm. It can present as a swelling of the maxilla or as a nasal 'polyp'. It occurs more commonly in females; the average age of the patients is about 15 years.[155]

Histopathology
The lesion consists of cellular fibrous tissue, with osteoblasts enveloping relatively uniform calcified bodies (calcospherules) showing varying degrees of ossification (Figs 4.53, 4.54). Lesions in which calcospherules predominate have been called 'ossifying cementomas' because of the resemblance to cementicles (Fig. 4.55). Whorl formation may be present and the lesion can then be mistaken for meningioma.

The histological distinction between ossifying fibroma and fibrous dysplasia affecting the bones of the head remains a source of considerable controversy.[155, 173]

Aneurysmal bone cyst

Aneurysmal bone cyst is rare in the jaw but in this site may involve the maxillary sinus. It has been reported in association with other giant cell lesions such as reparative granuloma, fibrous dysplasia and ossifying fibroma (Figs 4.55, 4.56).[174]

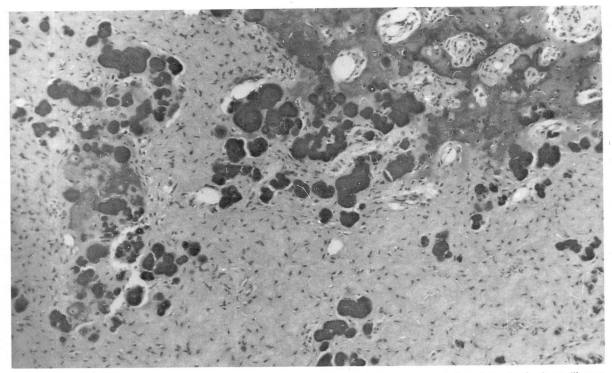

Fig. 4.53 Ossifying fibroma. There are scattered calcospherules and some immature cancellous bone in the loose fibrous stroma. Haematoxylin–eosin × 120

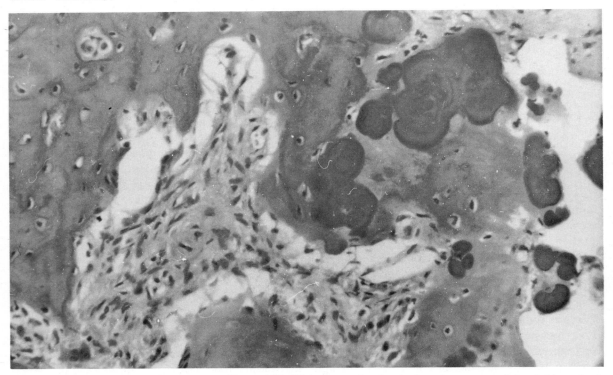

Fig. 4.54 Ossifying fibroma. Same case as Figure 4.53. High power showing laminated structure of the darkly stained calcospherules. Haematoxylin–eosin × 300

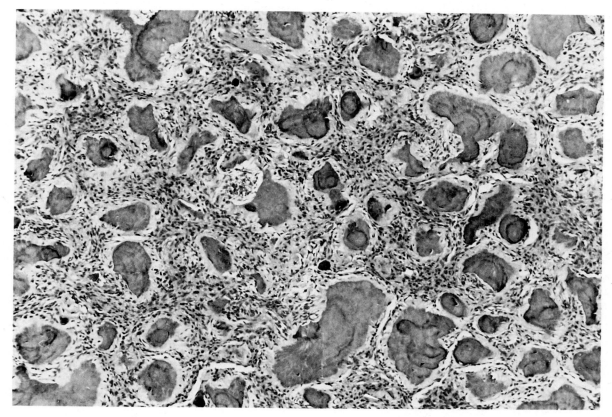

Fig. 4.55 Ossifying fibroma of maxilla in a man of 24 showing predominance of calcospherules resembling cementicles.
Haematoxylin–eosin   × 120

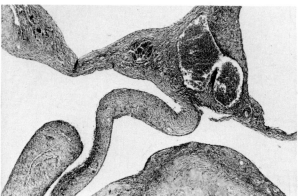

Fig. 4.56 Aneurysmal bone cyst. Same case as Figure 4.55. Recurrent tumour 2 years later bulging into maxillary antrum, now presenting the microscopical features of an aneurysmal bone cyst composed of irregular dilated vascular spaces.

Haematoxylin–eosin   × 23

Histopathology (Figs 4.56, 4.57, 4.58)

The aneurysmal bone cyst consists of anastomosing cavernous spaces usually filled with blood. The walls of these spaces lack the normal features of blood vessels and an endothelial lining is unusual. Between the cysts there is fibrous tissue which may contain osteoid trabeculae. Giant cells are often present, sometimes in large numbers. The histopathology of aneurysmal bone cyst therefore overlaps that of the other giant cell lesions and that of a simple bone cyst.

Reparative granuloma of the jaw

The so-called reparative giant cell granuloma of the jaw[175] is a rare disease, mainly affecting children and young people, particularly females, aged from 8 to 25 years. Some patients first present at a later age. The lesion affects the mandible more commonly than the maxilla. It may involve the

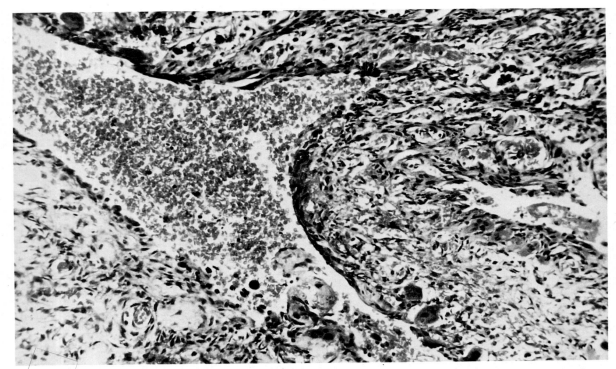

Fig. 4.57 Aneurysmal bone cyst. Detail of Figure 4.56 showing irregular vascular spaces separated by fibrovascular tissue with scanty giant cells. Haematoxylin–eosin ×200

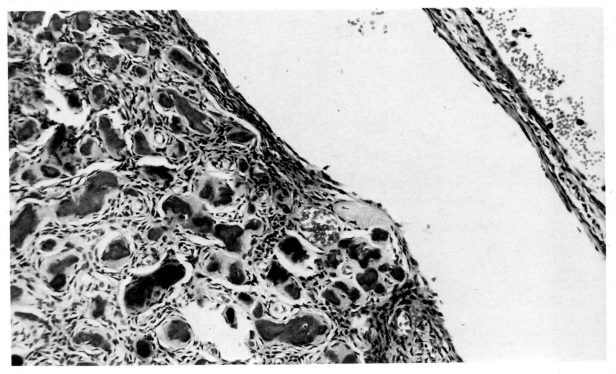

Fig. 4.58 Same specimen as Figures 4.56 and 4.57 showing an area of ossifying fibroma in the wall of one of the aneurysmal cysts. Haematoxylin–eosin ×200

maxillary sinus and can simulate a neoplasm both clinically and histologically.

Histopathology
Macroscopically the tissue of the reparative granuloma is friable and haemorrhagic. Microscopically it consists of a loose, vascular connective tissue stroma with haemorrhages or deposits of blood pigment surrounded by giant cells (Fig. 4.59). Giant cells are not a dominant feature and are usually small and widely scattered (Fig. 4.60). Here and there osteoid trabeculae of metaplastic origin are present. The differential diagnosis of giant cell reparative granuloma includes the 'brown tumour' of hyperparathyroidism, giant cell tumour, eosinophilic granuloma and fibrous dysplasia. There is less collagen, osteoid or bone present than in fibrous dysplasia. Giant cell reparative granuloma of the jaw is a benign lesion which seldom recurs after surgical removal.

Eosinophilic granuloma
Eosinophilic granuloma is generally regarded as the localized form of the clinical spectrum of histiocytosis X.[176] Although there is a particular tendency for the lesions to occur in the skull and facial bones, involvement of the nose and sinuses is extremely rare.

Most eosinophilic granulomas have their origin in bone though lesions also occur in soft tissue. About 40% of published cases have involved the head, particularly the bones of the jaw and the frontal, parietal and temporal bones.[177]

Histopathology
Eosinophils are always present, either as a diffuse infiltration or as more localized masses and are noteworthy for their relative maturity. Interspersed are larger characteristic histiocytic cells with large palely staining, ovoid and indented nuclei; the cytoplasmic boundaries of these cells show variable definition, some cells being sharply delineated whilst others present a syncytial appearance. These histiocytes are either diffusely scattered or concentrated in small groups. Some may show evidence of phagocytosis and multinucleate forms are not uncommon.

A large proportion of eosinophilic granulomas are, and remain, solitary. They may cause local bone destruction, giving rise to a clinical and radiological impression of a malignant tumour. Treatment by local surgery or irradiation usually results in cure without recurrence; some lesions undergo spontaneous resolution.

SARCOMAS

Sarcomas of the nose and sinuses are much less frequent than carcinomas. The surprisingly high incidence reported by earlier workers probably reflected misinterpretation of anaplastic carcinomas as sarcomatous. The least rare varieties, in descending order of frequency, are fibrosarcoma and malignant fibrous histiocytoma, chondrosarcoma, osteosarcoma and rhabdomyosarcoma. Overall, they account for about 15% of all malignant tumours of the nasal region. They arise in the sinuses more frequently than in the nasal cavities. They occur at any age and are about equally distributed between the sexes. The fibrosarcomas grow comparatively slowly. For this reason patients survive appreciably longer with a fibrosarcoma of the nasal region than with most forms of nasal carcinoma. Confusion with juvenile angiofibroma has to be avoided.

Fibrosarcoma
Fibrosarcoma affects mainly children and young adults and there is a moderate male preponderance.[155, 178] The most common presenting sign is a mass, either superficially palpable or deep and often associated with pain.

Histopathology
Microscopy shows spindle-celled tissue. This may be well-differentiated, with few mitotic figures and a dense collagenous matrix devoid of bone or cartilage formation. The poorly-differentiated fibrosarcomas show marked pleomorphism and irregularity of nuclear size and shape. Mitotic figures are frequent and only sparse reticulin and collagen fibres separate the tumour cells. The histological distinction from malignant fibrous histiocytoma may be difficult (see below).

Prognosis
Fibrosarcomas of the nose have a better prognosis than squamous cell carcinomas. However,

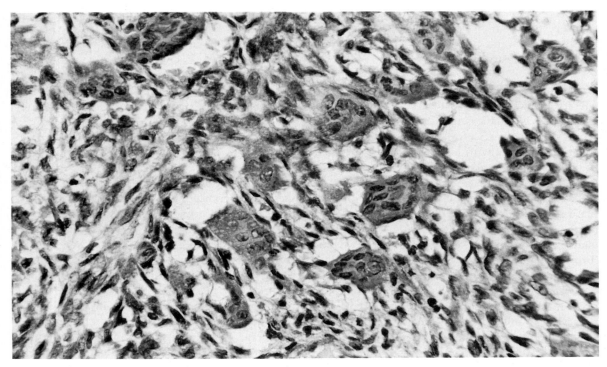

Fig. 4.59 Giant cell reparative granuloma of the maxilla showing loose vascular connective tissue stroma with haemorrhage and giant cells.   Haematoxylin–eosin   × 200

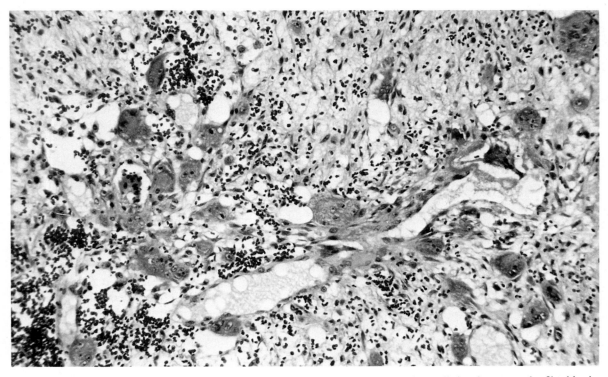

Fig. 4.60 Giant cell reparative granuloma showing the relatively small multinucleate giant cells in a loose vascular fibroblastic stroma.   Haematoxylin–eosin   × 500

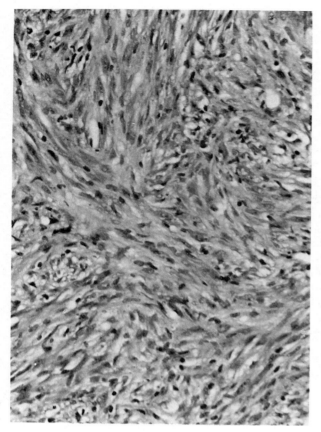

Fig. 4.61 Malignant fibrous histiocytoma showing spindle cells arranged in a storiform pattern.

Haematoxylin–eosin   × 300

local recurrence is the rule and metastasis is frequent.[179, 180]

Post-irradiation fibrosarcoma

Fibrosarcoma may arise in irradiated tissues,[181, 182] usually many years after treatment of other conditions, including retinoblastoma and—in the nasal region—angiofibroma[155] (p. 99).

Malignant fibrous histiocytoma

The term 'fibrous histiocytoma' proposed by Kauffman and Stout[183] replaces at least 21 synonymous terms. However, the unitarian hypothesis of Stout and his co-workers is not universally accepted.

Only 32 cases of malignant fibrous histiocytoma of the deep structures of the head and neck were reported up to 1977.[184] Malignant fibrous histiocytoma of the nose and paranasal sinuses, though rare, has been described more often.[185–187]

The tumour is usually of fibrous consistency. It may occur at any age and is more frequent in males.

A case of malignant fibrous histiocytoma of the maxillary sinus in a 65-year-old man, who died 6 months after the primary diagnosis with metastatic involvement of regional and other lymph nodes and of organs elsewhere, has been reported.[188] A case of malignant fibrous histiocytoma of the ethmoid sinus was recently described and the literature reviewed.[189] The histopathological diagnosis of these tumours may be difficult and both the natural history and response to various treatment modalities are unpredictable. It was noted that only five cases arising primarily from the ethmoid sinuses have previously been described[185, 186] whilst in another four cases secondary extension to this site from adjacent anatomical regions occurred.[186]

Histopathology

The microscopical picture is variegated. The tumour is composed characteristically of spindle cells in a storiform pattern (from the Latin *storea* = a rush mat) (Fig. 4.61).[190] Myxoid areas and pleomorphic giant cells may be present (Fig. 4.62), inflammatory cells and xanthoma cells are sometimes prominent and malignant fibrous histiocytoma has been subdivided into 'storiform-pleomorphic', 'myxoid', 'giant cell', 'inflammatory' and 'angiomatoid' variants.[191]

Surgical excision combined with chemotherapy is recommended.[192]

Giant cell tumour

Giant cell tumours of the nose and paranasal sinuses are rare.[193] The tumour consists of many large multinucleated giant cells surrounded by sheets of rather uniform small mononuclear cells. Differential diagnostic difficulties may be caused by the so-called 'brown tumour' of hyperparathyroidism and the giant cell reparative granuloma (p. 105). Giant cell tumours are locally aggressive and recur unless radically removed.

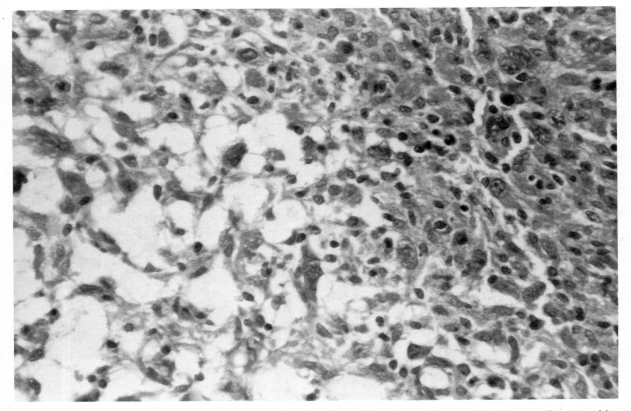

Fig. 4.62 Malignant fibrous histiocytoma of the nose showing pleomorphic and myxoid areas. Note bizarre cells scattered in both areas.
Haematoxylin–eosin   × 400

CARTILAGINOUS AND OSSEOUS NEOPLASMS

BENIGN

Chondroma

Although chondromas are relatively common in other locations, doubt has been cast on the existence of truly benign chondromas in the nasal region. They are usually located in the nasal cavity, mainly arising from the septum. Cartilaginous tumours of the paranasal sinuses are essentially sarcomatous even when slowly growing.

Chondromas in the nasal region tend to occur at a somewhat earlier age than their malignant counterparts and males tend to be affected more commonly than females. Seven chondromas were found amongst 256 non-epithelial tumours of the nose, nasal sinuses and nasopharynx;[193] three arose in the nasal septum, the other four being in the nasopharynx.

Histologically they resemble normal cartilage so closely that differentiation from the latter may be difficult.

Osteoma

Osteomas occur most frequently in the frontal sinuses and may reach a large size, filling the sinus and leading to its considerable distention. Pneumocephalus may develop as a complication.[194] They present as a sessile or pedunculated mass, often with a coarsely-lobulated surface; the overlying mucosa may be intact although atrophic, or ulcerated if infection has developed.

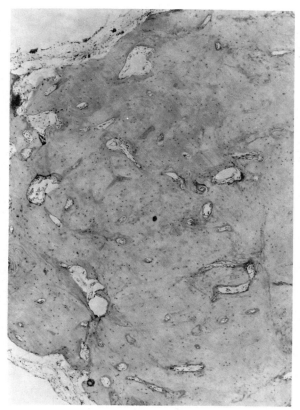

Fig. 4.63 Compact ('ivory') osteoma of the frontal sinus.
Haematoxylin–eosin   × 38

Microscopically, they range from the dense 'ivory' osteoma to the rarer cancellous osteoma, which may be finely or coarsely trabeculated. The structural differences may reflect the degree of osteoblastic activity. The *ivory osteoma* is composed of hard, dense, mature, lamellar bone, containing only a small amount of fibrous tissue (Fig. 4.63). The *cancellous osteoma* is composed of mature cancellous bone (Fig. 4.64) and may contain some active haemopoietic marrow.

Gardner's syndrome
Osteomas of the facial bones form part of Gardner's syndrome. This not uncommon inherited autosomal-dominant syndrome[195] comprises multiple osteomas of the jaws, epidermoid cysts of the skin and multiple polyps of the large intestine. The intestinal lesions have a marked tendency to malignant change.

MALIGNANT

Chondrosarcoma
Chondrosarcoma is a rare tumour in the nose and sinuses. The first paranasal chondrosarcoma to be reported as such was described by Mollison in 1916;[196] it was an antroethmoidal tumour that had invaded the orbit of a 19-year-old girl; the patient died shortly after operation. A review of

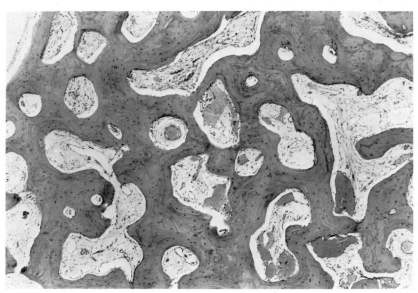

Fig. 4.64 Cancellous osteoma of maxillary sinus.
Haematoxylin–eosin   × 38

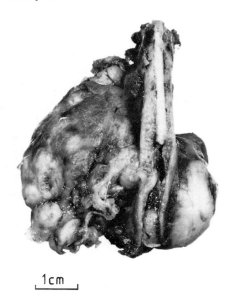

1cm

Fig. 4.65 Chondrosarcoma of the nasal septum showing the coarsely lobular tumour arising from the septal cartilage.

256 non-epithelial tumours of the nose, nasal sinuses and nasopharynx included 10 examples of chondrosarcoma of the nose and sinuses.[193] In a review of 82 patients presenting at the Mayo Clinic between 1950 and 1975 with sarcoma of the nasal cavity, nasal sinuses and nasopharynx, there were 13 with chondrosarcoma.[197]

Chondrosarcomas may arise in the nasal cavity (septum, floor, lateral wall or cribriform plate), the ethmoidal sinuses, maxilla and maxillary sinuses, and the sphenoid region. However at the time of presentation there is frequently extensive involvement of cavities of the nose and sinuses.

The gross appearance may show a resemblance to normal cartilage, though often composed of coarsely-lobulated, bluish-white masses (Fig. 4.65). The consistency may be hard with varying degrees of calcification and ossification, or it may be soft and gelatinous.

Histopathology
The appearance may resemble normal cartilage. When many cells with plump nuclei form clusters, or more than an occasional multinucleated cell is present, malignancy is to be suspected (Fig. 4.66). Nuclear irregularity and prominence of nucleoli are additional features that suggest

malignancy. Invasion of adjacent bone is of diagnostic significance (Fig. 4.67). Myxoid changes are less significant. Mitotic figures are usually scanty.

Behaviour
Chondrosarcomas vary greatly in behaviour, which in general reflects the apparent degree of malignancy indicated by the histological picture. Three grades of chondrosarcoma have been distinguished on the basis of mitotic rate, cellularity and nuclear size.[198]

Many of the more slowly-growing chondrosarcomas are distinguishable only with difficulty from benign cartilaginous tumours of the region.

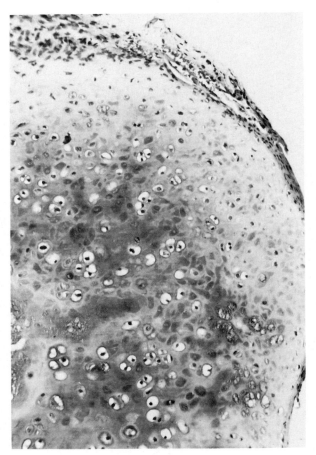

Fig. 4.66 Chondrosarcoma of the nose showing the lobular structure and greatly enhanced cellularity (in contrast to normal cartilage).

Haematoxylin–eosin   × 140

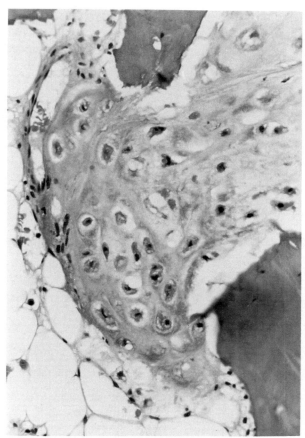

Fig. 4.67 Chondrosarcoma of the nose in a middle-aged man showing the cartilaginous tumour breaking through the bone.
Haematoxylin–eosin   × 270

Osteosarcoma

The term 'osteosarcoma' is preferred to 'osteogenic sarcoma' since the latter can be taken to imply a wider variety of sarcomas in bone.[199, 200] Osteosarcoma of the nose and sinuses (Fig. 4.68) is generally regarded as occurring much less frequently than fibrosarcoma and chondrosarcoma. The maxillary sinus is the most common site.[201, 202] Osteosarcomas of the bones of the jaw differ from those in other parts of the skeleton in that the average age of patients is higher and that approximately half of the tumours are predominantly chondroblastic.[199] A biopsy specimen may therefore show little or no osteoid formation: this explains why a small but significant proportion of tumours initially diagnosed as chondrosarcoma

turn out to be osteosarcomas (Figs 4.69, 4.70, 4.71, 4.72). In this site osteosarcomas tend to show much less anaplasia and on occasion may be difficult to differentiate from a benign lesion. Haematogenous spread occurs less frequently, wide resection offers a reasonable chance of cure, and the prognosis is better than for osteosarcoma elsewhere.

MUSCLE TISSUE TUMOURS

Leiomyoma and leiomyosarcoma

Smooth-muscle tumours of the nose and paranasal sinuses are extremely rare. There were only 8 cases in a series of 256 non-epithelial neoplasms of this region: 2 were benign leiomyomas and 6 were leiomyosarcomas.[203]

As with other neoplasms of the region these tumours usually present with nasal discharge and pain or as apparently simple 'nasal polyps'. Superficial biopsy specimens may contain only inflammatory granulation tissue, the underlying lesion escaping detection.

Histopathology

Microscopy shows interlacing bundles of spindle cells with blunt-ended vesicular nuclei (Fig. 4.73). Palisading of the nuclei is sometimes present and myofibrils may be demonstrable in the cytoplasm when stained with phosphotungstic acid haematoxylin. The number of cells containing fibrils varies and electron microscopy can be helpful in their demonstration. Reticulin fibres form parallel bundles and surround individual tumour cells. There are often vascular areas, and some of the irregular vascular channels may be enveloped by tumour cells.

It may be difficult to predict the behaviour of these tumours from their histological appearance, but in the presence of enhanced mitotic activity malignancy is to be suspected and metastasis is not uncommon.

Rhabdomyoma and rhabdomyosarcoma

Skeletal-muscle tumours of the nose and sinuses are extremely rare[204] and no example of rhabdomyoma has been reported as occurring in the nose and sinuses.

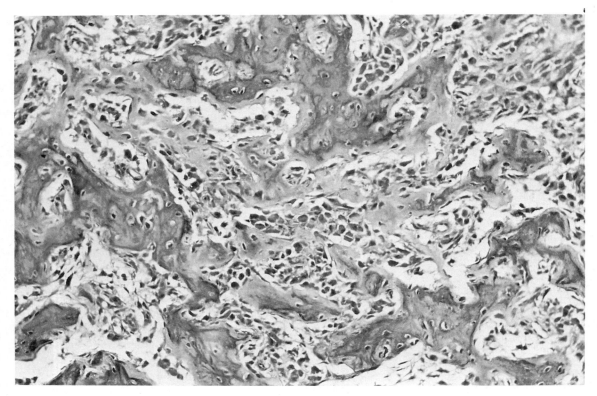

Fig. 4.68 Osteosarcoma of the maxillary sinus composed of pleomorphic osteoblastic cells associated with an irregular network of osteoid and immature woven neoplastic bony trabeculae.

Haematoxylin–eosin   × 180

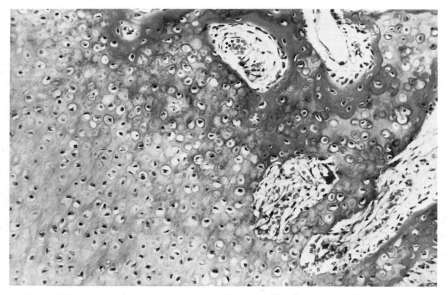

Fig. 4.69 Biopsy of well differentiated chondroblastic tumour from maxilla of a 20-year-old man.

Haematoxylin–eosin   × 120

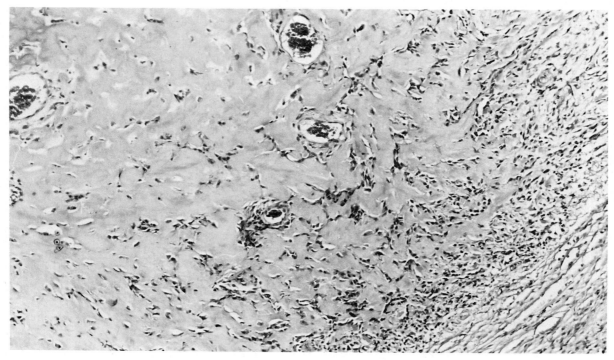

Fig. 4.70 Resection specimen of same tumour as Figure 4.69 most of which displayed the features of a moderately differentiated osteosarcoma. Haematoxylin–eosin   × 112

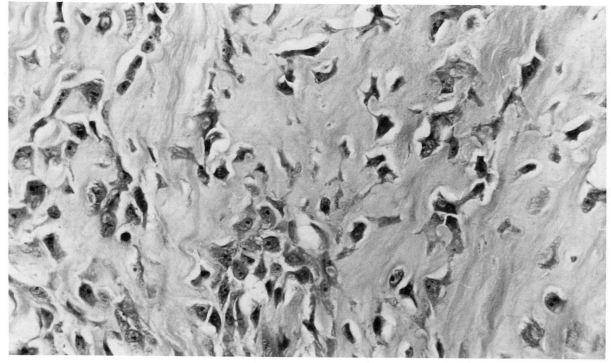

Fig. 4.71 Detail of Figure 4.70 showing an area of moderately differentiated osteosarcoma. Note irregular osteoblasts in a poorly formed osteoid matrix. Haematoxylin–eosin   × 450

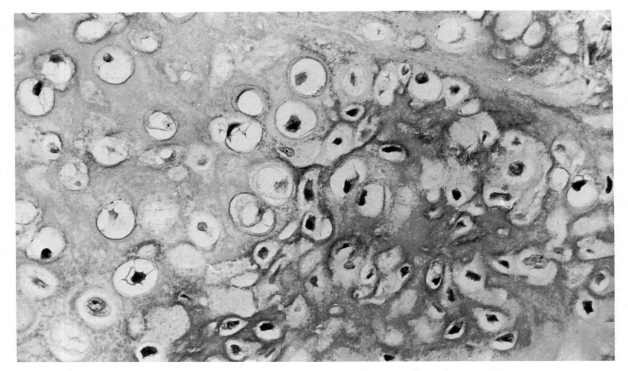

Fig. 4.72 Same specimen as Figure 4.70 showing a chondroblastic area.   Haematoxylin–eosin   × 450

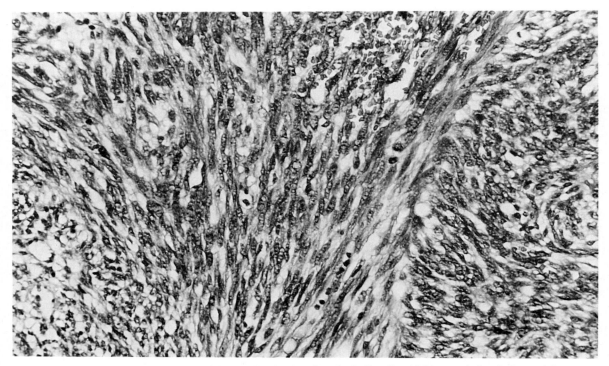

Fig. 4.73 Leiomyosarcoma of the nose and sinuses showing bundles of spindle cells with blunt ended vesicular nuclei.
Haematoxylin–eosin   × 275

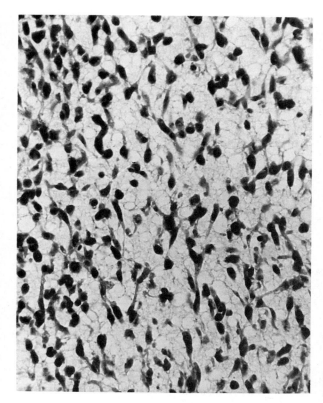

Fig. 4.74 Embryonal rhabdomyosarcoma in the upper nasal cavity from a boy aged four composed of small spindle-shaped cells, a few with straplike cytoplasm, in an unusually loose myxoid stroma.

Haematoxylin–eosin   × 450

Rhabdomyosarcomas arising in the head and neck are most frequent in children in the first decade and there is a slight male preponderance. In contrast, rhabdomyosarcomas of the peripheral musculature are seen mainly in the fifth and sixth decades.

Histopathology
Rhabdomyosarcomas recapitulate the embryonic development of muscle, but in a disorganized manner (Fig. 4.74). The malignant myoblast may assume various shapes in accordance with its resemblance to developing muscle cells (Fig. 4.75).[205, 206] Cross-striation is often difficult to demonstrate.

The diagnosis of rhabdomyosarcoma by conventional methods is sometimes very difficult, especially when large rhabdomyoblasts are not detected. For this reason pathologists often try to support a diagnosis of rhabdomyosarcoma by other methods, including electron microscopy, histochemistry and immunological techniques. By electron microscopy the diagnosis of rhabdomyosarcoma is only possible if thick (myosin), thin (actin) and Z-line material can be demonstrated (Fig. 4.76).[207, 208] Immunocytochemistry can be of diagnostic value: tumour cells of rhabdomyosarcomas stain clearly by antibodies to desmin, the intermediate filament type characteristic of muscle.[209] The presence of myoglobin may be demonstrated in a similar manner.[210]

Teratocarcinosarcoma (malignant teratoma?)
In a recent report 'a unique type of sinonasal tract neoplasm' was described by Heffner & Hyams.[211] This tumour displayed some histological features of a rhabdomyosarcoma and of both a carcinosarcoma and of a teratoma. The term *teratocarcinosarcoma* has been proposed for this highly malignant neoplasm.

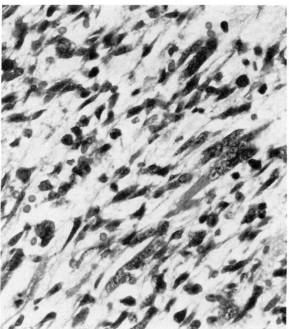

Fig. 4.75 Embryonal rhabdomyosarcoma in a girl of 10 presenting as a botryoid mass in the postnasal space. There are pleomorphic rhabdomyoblasts with eosinophilic strap-like cytoplasm among the primitive spindle cells.

Haematoxylin–eosin   × 340

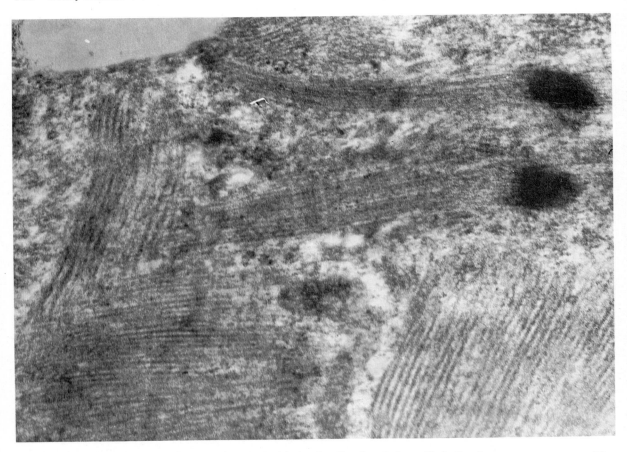

Fig. 4.76 Rhabdomyosarcoma. Electron micrograph showing bundle of typical myofibrils forming sarcomeres, some with dark condensations of Z band material. × 87 500

Prognosis

Treatment by surgery, irradiation and chemotherapy has considerably improved the prognosis:[212] previously most patients died within 2 years of diagnosis.

PLASMACYTOMA OF THE NOSE AND SINUSES

Although the term 'myeloma' has been used for both medullary and extramedullary plasma-cell tumours, it seems appropriate to reserve the term for plasma-cell tumours of the bone marrow.

Extramedullary plasmacytomas are uncommon. About 80% of them occur in the region of the head and neck, the most frequent sites being the nose and paranasal sinuses.[213-216] In the material studied at the Institute of Laryngology and Otology, London, there were seven cases, representing 2% of all malignant tumours in the nose and sinuses,[217] a similar incidence to that reported by Ringertz from the Karolinska Institute in Stockholm.[218]

The majority occur in the age range 40–70 years, with a peak incidence in the fifth and sixth decades. Men are affected twice as frequently as women. The tumour may present with nasal obstruction, discharge, epistaxis and facial swelling. Pain is less common. About 60% arise in the nasal cavity; most of the remainder arise in a maxillary sinus.

Usually solitary, the tumour may be polypoid, sessile or lobulated and is usually firm and deep red in colour. Ulceration is uncommon. Polypoid tumours usually remain confined to the soft

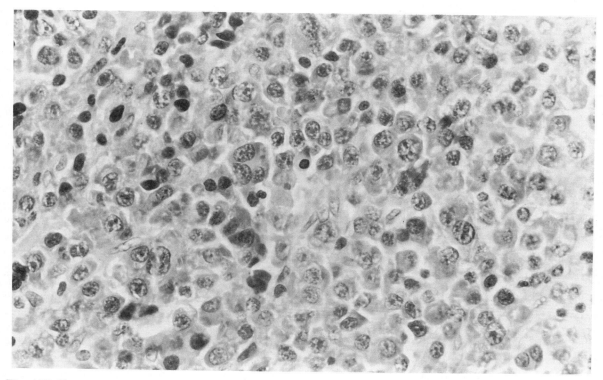

Fig. 4.77 Plasmacytoma of the nose composed of immature plasma cells with eccentric nuclei. There are also scattered multinucleate cells present. Haematoxylin–eosin × 500

tissues. Sessile tumours are generally more aggressive, are softer and more friable, and tend to invade the underlying bone.

Histopathology
Microscopically plasmacytomas are composed of closely packed cells with a fine vascular connective tissue stroma which may impart a packeted appearance to groups of cells, more easily seen with reticulin impregnation. The tumour cells may be so well differentiated that they closely resemble normal plasma cells or they may be so primitive that the growth may be confused with malignant lymphoma or anaplastic carcinoma. Characteristically the cells have an eccentric nucleus and their cytoplasm includes a pale paranuclear zone (the 'hof') (Fig. 4.77). There is often an element of pleomorphism and cells with two and three nuclei are common. Amyloid is present in the stroma in about 15% of cases.

Differential diagnosis
Distinction must be made between plasmacytoma and an intense plasmacytic inflammatory infiltrate (plasma-cell granuloma). The inflammatory lesions usually show an intermingling of other inflammatory cells, predominance of normal plasma cells and the presence of Russell bodies, which are very rarely seen in plasmacytomas. However, in difficult cases immunoperoxidase staining for immunoglobulins can be very helpful since inflammatory lesions will show polyclonal staining whereas plasmacytomas are monoclonal, staining for only one class of light chain immunoglobulin. Since the majority of cells in a plasmacytoma will show this monoclonal staining pattern the technique can also be of value in the differentiation from anaplastic carcinoma and malignant lymphoma. Electron microscopy may also be helpful in making this distinction.[219]

Prognosis

Extramedullary plasmacytoma must always be regarded as a malignant tumour. In a small proportion of cases it is a manifestation of myelomatosis, usually antedating the symptoms of the latter. It is essential therefore, to carry out biochemical, radiological and bone-marrow investigations in every case of extramedullary plasma cytoma. Only when the results of these examinations remain negative over several years can the prognosis be regarded as favourable. Myelomatosis has been known to appear as long as 15 years after the initial diagnosis of a nasal extramedullary plasmacytoma. The nasal lesion itself may give rise to widespread metastasis, usually to extraskeletal sites. Localization and the gross appearance of the tumours are more reliable prognostically than their histology.[220-222] Although the tumours are radiosensitive, recurrence and invasion of bone are bad prognostic signs.

LYMPHOMA

Lymphomas may arise in the nose or nasal sinuses but are rare.[223] They account for well under 10% of all malignant tumours in this region and in the material studied at the Institute of Laryngology and Otology, London,[224] they represented fewer than 3% of cases. This reflects the relative paucity of lymphoreticular tissue in the nose and sinuses in contrast to its abundance in the nasopharynx, where lymphomas are relatively much more frequent (see p. 152).

Lymphomas occur most commonly between 50 and 70 years of age and present with non-specific symptoms of nasal obstruction, swelling of the cheek, proptosis or pain; epistaxis is relatively uncommon. A paranasal origin seems to be more common,[225] but some tumours arise primarily in, and may remain confined to, the nasal cavity. Within the nasal cavity they may arise from the septum, floor or lateral wall; paranasal lymphomas are usually of antroethmoidal origin.

Histopathology

Although there have been several reports of Hodgkin's disease involving the nose and sin-

uses,[226-229] there is no convincing example of Hodgkin's disease arising primarily in the nasal region. Follicular lymphomas do not appear to arise in this site. Almost all the lymphomas of the nasal and paranasal region are diffuse non-Hodgkin's lymphomas, mostly of high-grade malignancy and mainly of large-cell type (British National Lymphoma Investigation Classification),[230] 'histiocytic' in the Rappaport classification[231] (Figs 4.78, 4.79).

Compared with nodal lymphomas a major difficulty in classification is a result of the nature of the tissue available for examination. This is often small and fragmented, with necrosis, secondary infection and inflammatory infiltration, and thus introducing the possibility of the mid-facial granuloma syndrome (p. 551) and malignant histiocytosis (p. 581) into the differential diagnosis. However, the polymorphic pattern characterizing the infiltrate in the Stewart type of granuloma is not usually seen in the malignant lymphomas, in which areas of more uniform cytology within the range of recognized types of lymphoma are discernible. This is also true of the nasal lymphomas of peripheral T-cell origin reported from Japan.[232]

Course and prognosis

Although initially localized, primary malignant lymphoma of the nasal region may spread to adjacent regions. Regional lymph node involvement occurs in approximately 20% of cases and distant nodal or systemic involvement is seen in about 50% of cases. However, although the majority of nasal lymphomas are of high-grade type, a considerable proportion of patients do not die directly of their lymphoma.[224, 227, 233a]

A review of 420 extra-nodal malignant lymphomas treated at Mount Vernon Hospital, Middlesex, England, between 1955 and 1979 showed that only 15 (3.5%) arose in the nose or sinuses.[233] Of these, 2 involved the nasal cavity, 12 involved the sinuses and one involved nasal cavity, sinus and tonsil. 14 were Stage I at the time of presentation (that is, limited to one site); only one had cervical node involvement (Stage II). Review of the histological material revealed 11 large-cell lymphomas, 2 lymphoblastic lymphomas and one each of small cleaved follicle-cell

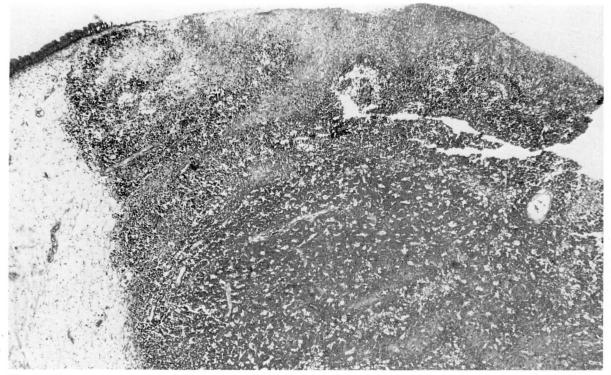

Fig. 4.78 Large cell lymphoma of maxillary antrum. Note ulceration and extensive necrosis in the more superficial part of the tumour. Biopsy from this part could be misleading or non-diagnostic.   Haematoxylin-eosin   × 50

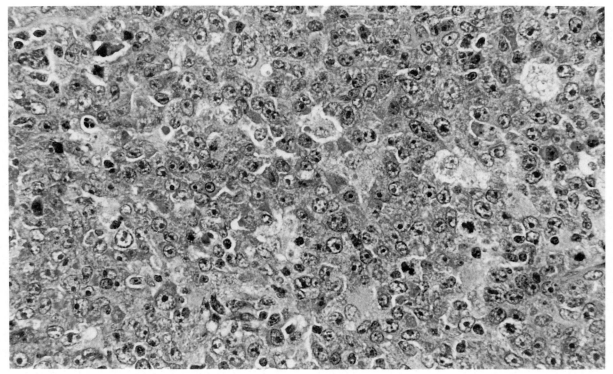

Fig. 4.79 Large cell lymphoma of maxillary antrum. Detail of deep part of Figure 4.78 showing the cells with large rounded nuclei and prominent nucleoli. There are scattered macrophages present.   Haematoxylin-eosin   × 500

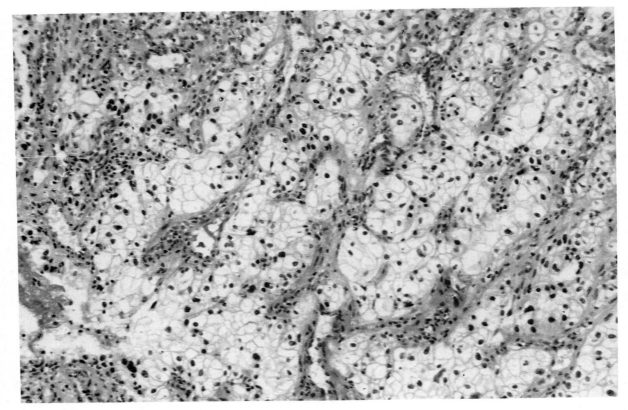

Fig. 4.80 Metastasis of renal carcinoma presenting as 'nasal polyp'. Note trabeculae composed of typical clear cells separated by vascular tissue. Haematoxylin–eosin × 160

and well-differentiated small lymphocytic types. All achieved complete remission with radiotherapy. 8 recurred within 2 years, 7 of these patients dying of generalized lymphoma. No patient remaining disease-free for 2 years has subsequently had a recurrence. Compared with other primary extra-nodal sites, the pattern of spread was unusual, being predominantly extra-nodal and with testicular involvement in 3 cases. This is of particular interest since spread to the nasal region from primary lymphomas of the testis has been reported.[234-236]

Malignant histiocytosis

Malignant histiocytosis (histiocytic medullary reticulosis) may affect the nose and mid-facial tissues[237, 238] and should be separated clinically and pathologically from malignant lymphoma and mid-facial granuloma of the Stewart type.[239] Malignant histiocytosis is a neoplastic systemic

proliferation of morphologically atypical histiocytes. In the nasal lesion the atypical histiocytes may be largely obscured by inflammatory cell infiltration, as in malignant histiocytosis of the intestine.[240] The demonstration of alpha-naphthyl acetate esterase or alpha-1-antitrypsin in the cytoplasm of morphologically malignant cells is confirmatory evidence of the diagnosis.[241, 242]

SECONDARY TUMOURS

A too-frequent cause of misdiagnosis is failure to consider the possibility that a tumour in the nasal region may be a secondary deposit from a cancer arising elsewhere in the body. Metastatic tumours in the nose may present as polyp-like lesions, a fact that justifies reiteration of our view that all polyps and polyp-like lesions removed from the nose must be examined histologically.

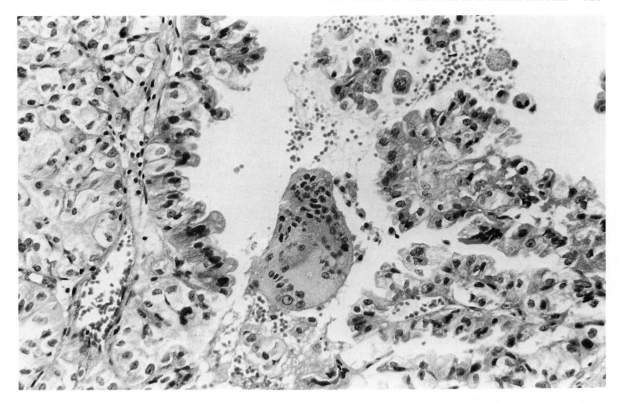

Fig. 4.81 Metastatic papillary carcinoma in the nasal cavity from a primary carcinoma of the thyroid gland. Haematoxylin–eosin   × 550

Secondary tumours in the nasal or paranasal region are uncommon.[243, 244] Although none were included in several reviews of metastatic tumours in the jaws,[245–248] there have been numerous single case reports of metastatic tumours in the region.

In the material studied at the Institute of Laryngology and Otology, London,[249] it. was noted that nearly 50% of secondary tumours in the ear, nose and throat region involved the nose and sinuses. Of these, nearly 80% were derived from primary renal carcinoma, though the nose and nasal sinuses are not a common site for metastatic deposits of renal carcinoma.[250, 251]

Secondary deposits of renal carcinomas present a variety of histological problems. The papillary adenomatoid structure has sometimes led to an erroneous diagnosis of 'papillary cystadenoma',[252] the clear-cell structure (Fig. 4.80) may be confused with a variant of acinic-cell tumour, and an occasional angiomatoid pattern may be mis-

taken for a haemangioma. The marked vascularity of the secondary tumours often results in presentation with profuse epistaxis.[253] It should be emphasized that primary renal carcinoma may remain occult until the patient presents with a metastatic deposit.[254, 255] Conversely a secondary tumour in the nasal region may not appear until after the primary neoplasm has been removed.[256, 257]

Secondary tumours from the alimentary tract are very uncommon in the nose and nasal sinuses.[246, 258] The possibility of confusion with primary adenocarcinoma has to be borne in mind. Similarly, tumours arising in breast or bronchus seldom metastasize to the nose and sinuses.[258–260]

Occasional cases of metastasis from the thyroid (Fig. 4.81)[261a, 261b] and from the genital tract,[252] including seminoma of the testicle[258] and choriocarcinoma,[262–264] have been reported.

REFERENCES

1. Rapaport J. Arch Dermatol 1975; 111: 73.
2. Kramer R, Som ML. Arch Otolaryngol 1935; 22: 22.
3. Ringertz N. Acta Otolaryngol (Stockh) 1938; Suppl 27, 4: 31.
4. Osborn DA. Cancer 1956; 25: 50.
5. Norris HJ. Laryngoscope 1963; 73: 1.
6. Trible WM, Lekagur S. Laryngoscope 1971; 81: 663.
7. Lampertico P, Russell WO, McComb WS. Arch Pathol 1963; 75: 293.
8. Fechner RE, Alford DO. Arch Otolaryngol 1968; 88: 507.
9. Hyams VS. Ann Otol Rhinol Laryngol 1971; 80: 192.
10. Perzin KH, Lefkowitch JH, Hui RM. Cancer 1981; 48: 2375.
11. Lee KP, Trochimowicz HJ. Am J Pathol 1982; 106: 8.
12. Reznik-Schuller HM, Gregg M. Virchows Arch 1981; 393: 333.
13. Assor D. Am J Clin Pathol 1971; 55: 761.
14. Spencer H. Pathology of the lung. 3rd ed. Oxford: Pergamon Press, 1977: 797.
15. Smith PS, McClure J. Arch Pathol Lab Med 1982; 106: 503.
16. Yesner R, Sobel J. Histologic typing of lung tumours. Geneva: World Health Organization, 1977.
17. Chatterji P, Friedmann I, Soni NK, Solanki RL, Ramdeo IN. J Laryngol Otol 1982; 96: 281.
18. Friedmann I, Osborn DA. Pathology of granulomas and neoplasms of the nose and paranasal sinuses. Edinburgh: Churchill Livingstone, 1982: 113.
19. Reuys H. Z Hals-Nasen-Ohrenheilk 1932; 30: 421.
20. Osborn DA. Cancer 1970; 25: 50.
21. Marcial-Rojas RA, DeLeon E. Arch Otolaryngol 1963; 77: 634.
22. Snyder RN, Perzin KH. Cancer 1972; 30: 668.
23. Kummel W. In: Heymann P, Holder A, eds. Handbuch der Laryngologie Rhinologie. Wien 1900.
24. Citelli S, Calamida U. Arch Laryngol 1903; 13: 273.
25. Harmer L, Glas E. Dtsch Z Chir 1907; 89: 433.
26. Hautant A, Monod O, Klotz A. Ann Otolaryngol 1933; 385.
27. Quick D, Cutler M. J Surg Gynec Obstet 1927; 45: 320.
28. Ewing J. Radiology 1927; 9: 359.
29. Registrar General's statistical review, England, Wales. London: HMSO, 1980.
30. Friedmann I, Osborn DA. Pathology of granulomas and neoplasms of the nose and paranasal sinuses. Edinburgh: Churchill Livingstone, 1982: 118.
31. Keen F, De Moor NG, Shapiro MP, Cohen L, Cooper RL, Campbell JM. Br J Cancer 1955; 9: 528.
32. Hendrick JW. Arch Otolaryngol 1958; 68: 604.
33. Magnus K, Andersen A, Hogetveit A Chr. Int J Cancer 1982; 30: 681.
34. Gamez-Araujo JJ, Ayala AG, Guillamon O. Cancer 1975; 36: 1100.
35. Ironside P, Matthews J. Cancer 1975; 36: 1115.
36. Macbeth RG. J Laryngol Otol 1965; 79: 592.
37. Acheson ED, Hadfield EH, Macbeth RG. Lancet 1967; i: 311.
38. Acheson ED, Cowdell RH, Hadfield E, Macbeth RG. Br Med J 1968; ii: 587.
39. Hadfield EH. Ann R Coll Sur Engl 1970; 46: 301.
40. Hadfield EH, Macbeth RG. Ann Otol Rhinol Laryngol 1971; 80: 699.
41. Gignoux M, Bernard P. J Med Lyons 1969; 50: 731.
42. Debois JM. Tijdschr Geneeskd 1969; 25: 92.
43. Mosbech J, Acheson ED. Dan Med Bull 1971; 18: 34.
44. Brinton LA, Blot WJ, Stone BJ, Fraumeni JF. Cancer Res 1977; 37: 3473.
44a. Klintenberg C, Olofsson J, Hellquist H, Sokjer H. Cancer 1984; 54: 482.
45. Black A, Evans JC, Hadfield EH, Macbeth RG. Br J Ind Med 1974; 31: 10.
46. Seifert G, Rieb H, Donath K. Zschr Laryngol Rhinol 1980; 59: 379.
47. Hamperl H. Z Mikrosk Anat Forsch 1931; 27: 1.
48. Blanck C, Eneroth CM, Jakobsen PA. Cancer 1970; 25: 919.
49. Hamperl H. Z Krebsforsch 1962; 64: 427.
50. Cohen M, Batsakia JG. Arch Otolaryngol 1968; 88: 71.
51. Spiro RH, Koss LG, Hajdu SI, Strong EW. Cancer; 1973: 31: 117.
52. Bauer WH, Bauer JD. Arch Pathol 1953; 55: 328.
53. Bazaz-Malik G, Gupta DN. Z Krebsforsch 1968; 70: 193.
54a. Abrams AM, Cornyn J, Scofield HH, Hanse LS. Br Med J 1965; ii: 587.
54b. Lucas RB. Pathology of tumours of the oral tissues. 3rd ed. Edinburgh: Churchill Livingstone, 1976: 327.
55. Bergman F. Cancer 1969; 23: 538.
56. Healey WV, Perzin KH, Smith L. Cancer 1970; 26: 368.
57. McDonald JR, Havens FZ. Surg Clin N Am 1948; 28: 1087.
58. Russell H. Br J Surg 1955; 43: 248.
59. Potdar GG, Paymaster JC. Oral Surg 1969; 28: 310.
60. Martis CS, Karakasis DT. Plas Reconstr Surg 1971; 47: 290.
61. Compagno J, Wong RT. Am J Clin Pathol 1977; 68: 213.
62. Reid JD. Cancer 1952; 5: 685.
63. Thackray AC, Sobin LH. Histological typing of salivary gland tumours. Geneva: World Health Organization, 1972.
64. Osborn DA. J Clin Pathol 1977; 30: 195.
65. Thackray AC, Lucas RB. Br J Cancer 1960; 14: 612.
66. Thackray AC, Lucas RB. Tumours of the major salivary glands. Atlas of Tumour Pathology, Second Series, Fascicle 10. Washington DC: Armed Forces Institute of Pathology, 1974.
67. Perzin KH, Gullane P, Clairmont AC. Cancer 1978; 42: 265.
68. Kleinsasser O, Klein HJ. Arch Klin Exp Ohren-Nasen- Kehlkopfheilk 1967; 189: 302.
69. Christ TF, Crocker D. Cancer 1972; 30: 214.
70. Alterman, Hutton, Isikio 1982.
71. Abrams AM, Melrose RJ, Howell FV. Cancer 1973; 32: 130.
72. Maisel RH, Johnston WH, Anderson HA, Cantrell AW. Laryngoscope 1977; 87: 429.
73. Johnston WH. Hum Pathol 1977; 8: 589.
74. Friedmann I, Osborn DA. Pathology of granulomas and neoplasms of the nose and paranasal sinuses. Edinburgh: Churchill Livingstone, 1982: 162.
75. Mayoux R, Perron R. Rev Laryngol Otol Rhinol 1939; 60: 245.

76. Freedman HM, Desanto LW, Levine KD, Weiland LH. Arch Otolaryngol 1973; 97: 322.
77. Holdcraft J, Gallagher JC. Ann Otolaryngol Rhinol Laryngol 1969; 78: 1.
78. Curran RC, McCann BG. J Pathol 1976; 119: 135.
79. Friedmann I. Proc R Soc Med 1961; 54: 1064.
80. Wright JWL, Heenan PJ. Otol Rhinol Laryngol 1975; 37: 233.
81. Weinhold CA. In: Ideen über die abnormen Metamorphosen der Hyghmorshöhle. Leipzig: Rein W, 1810; ch 3, 183.
82. Stout AP. Am J Cancer 1935; 24: 751.
83. Kraigh LV, Soule EH, Masson JK. Surg Gynecol Obstet 1960; 111: 211.
84. Robitaille Y, Seemayer TA, El Deiry A. Cancer 1975; 35: 1254.
85. Friedmann I, Osborn DA. Pathology of granulomas and neoplasms of the nose and paranasal sinuses. Edinburgh: Churchill Livingstone, 1982: 173.
86. Das Gupta TK, Brasfield RD, Strong EW et al. Cancer 1969; 24: 355.
87. Asbury AK, Johnson PC. Maj Prob Pathol 1978; 9: 1.
88. Luse SA. Neurol 1960; 10: 881.
89. Cravioto H, Lockwood R. Acta Neuropathol (Berl) 1969; 12: 141.
90. Mandybur TI. J Neurosurg 1974; 41: 187.
91. Lassmann H, Jurecka W, Lassmann G, Gebhart W, Matras H, Watsek G. Virchows Arch (Pathol Anat) 1977; 375: 197.
92. Friedmann I, Cawthorne T, Bird ES. J Ultrastruct Res 1965; 12: 92.
93. Mennemayer R, Hammar SP, Raisie JE, Tytus JS, Bockus D. Am J Surg Pathol 1979; 3: 3.
94. Spence AM, Rubenstein LJ, Conley FK et al. Acta Neuropathol (Berl) 1976; 35: 27.
95. Ghosh BC, Ghosh L, Huvos LC, Fortner JG. Cancer 1973; 31: 184.
96. Woodruff JM. Cancer 1976; 37: 2399.
97. McGavran MH. Ann Otol Rhinol Laryngol 1970; 79: 547.
98. Shanmugaratnam K, Sobin LH, eds. Upper respiratory tract tumours. Geneva: World Health Organization, 1978.
99. Bratton AB, Robinson SHG. J Pathol Bact 1945; 58: 643.
100. Smith KR, Schwartz HG, Luse SA, Ogura JH. J Neurosurg 1963; 20: 968.
101. Katz A, Lewis JS. Arch Otolaryngol 1971; 94: 351.
102. Hirsch LF, Stool SE, Langfitt TW, Schutt L. J Neurosurg 1977; 46: 85.
103. Deutsch H. Ann Otol Rhinol Laryngol 1965; 74: 637.
104. Love GL, Riehl PA. Arch Otolaryngol 1983; 109: 420.
105. Musser WA, Campbell R. Arch Otolaryngol 1961; 73: 732.
106. Mirra SS, Pearl GS, Hoffman JC, Campbell WG. Arch Pathol Lab Med 1981; 105: 540.
107. Blumenfeld R, Skolnik EM. Arch Otolaryngol 1965; 82: 527.
108. Berger L, Luc, Richard. Bull Assoc Fr Etude Cancer 1924; 13: 410.
109. Skolnik EM, Massari FS, Tenta LT. Arch Otolaryngol 1966; 84: 644.
110. Berger L, Coutard H. Bull Assoc Fr Etude Cancer 1926; 15: 404.
111. Lindstrom CG, Lindstrom DW. Acta Otolaryngol (Berl) 1975; 80: 447.
112. Kadish S, Goodman M, Wang CC. Cancer 1976; 37: 1571.
113. Friedmann I, Osborn DA. Minerva Otorinolaringol 1974; 24: 66.
114. Silva EG, Butler JJ, Mackay B, Goepfert H. Cancer 1982; 50: 2388.
115. Curtis JL, Rubinstein LJ. Cancer 1982; 49: 2136.
116. Osamura RY, Fine G. Cancer 1976; 38: 173.
117. Falck B. Acta Physiol Scand 1962; 56 (Suppl 197): 1.
118. Judge DM, McGavran MH, Trepukdi. Arch Otolaryngol 1976; 102: 97.
119. Dhillon AP, Rode J, Leatham A. Histopathology 1982; 6: 81.
120. Kameya T, Shimosato Y, Adachi I, Abe K, Ebihara S, Ono I. Cancer 1980; 45: 330.
121. Herrold KM. Cancer 1964; 17: 114.
122. Mendeloff J. Cancer 1957; 10: 944.
123. Fitz-Hugh GS, Allen MS, Rucker TN, Sprinkle PM. Arch Otolaryngol 1965; 81: 161.
124. Schenk NL, Ogura JH. Arch Otolaryngol 1972; 96: 322.
125. Joachims HZ, Altmann MM, Mayer SW. J Laryngol Otol 1975; 89: 335.
126. Fischer ER. Arch Pathol 1955; 60: 435.
127. Gerard-Marchant R, Micheau C. J Nat Cancer Inst 1965; 35: 75.
128. Hamilton AE, Rubenstein LJ, Poole GL. J Neurosurg 1973; 38: 548.
129. Bailey P, Barton S. Arch Otolaryngol 1975; 101: 1.
130. Singh W, Ramage C, Best P, Angus B. Cancer 1980; 45: 961.
131. Lewis JS, Hutter RVP, Tollefsen HR, Foote FW. Arch Otolaryngol 1963; 81: 169.
132. Rosalki SB, McGee LE. J Laryngol Otol 1962; 76: 133.
133. Saksela E, Holmstrom T, Grahne B. Acta Otolaryngol (Stockh) 1972; 74: 363.
134. Kjeldsberg CR, Minckler J. Cancer 1972; 29: 153.
135. Kang-loon Ho. Cancer 1980; 46: 1442.
136. Russell DS, Rubinstein LJ. Pathology of tumours of the nervous system. 4th ed. London: Edward Arnold, 1977; 73.
137. Godel V, Samuel Y, Shanon E et al. Arch Otolaryngol 1981; 107: 626.
138. Friedmann I, Osborn DA. Pathology of granulomas and neoplasms of the nose and paranasal sinuses. Edinburgh: Churchill Livingstone, 1982: 209.
139. Osborn DA. J Laryngol Otol 1959; 73: 174.
140. Fechner RE, Cooper PH, Mills SE. Arch Otolaryngol 1981; 107: 30.
141. Chelius MJ. A system of Surgery. Transl. by J.F. South. Vol. 2. London: H Renshaw, 1847: 726.
142. Chauveau C. Histoire des maladies du pharynx. Vol. 5. Paris: Baillière et fils, 1906: 562.
143. Acuna RT. Arch Otolaryngol 1973; 64: 451.
144. Handousa A, Farid H, Elwi LM. J Laryngol Otol 1954; 68: 647.
145. Harma RA. Acta Otolaryngol (Stockh) 1959; 49 (Suppl 146): 7.
146. Bhatia ML, Mishra SC, Prakash J. J Laryngol Otol 1967; 81: 99.
147. Osborn DA. J Laryngol 1959; 73: 295.
148. Munson FT. Ann Otol Rhinol Laryngol 1941; 50: 561.

149. Maniglia AJ, Mazzurella LA, Minkowitz S, Moskowitz H. Arch Otolaryngol 1969; 89: 527.
150. Gill G, Rice DH, Ritter FN, Kindt G, Russo HR. Arch Otolaryngol 1976; 102: 371.
151. Boles R, Dedo H. Laryngoscope 1976; 86: 364.
152. Schiff M. Laryngoscope 1959; 69: 981.
153. Zaynoun S, Juljulian HK, Kurban AK. Arch Derm 1974; 109: 689.
154. Chen KT, Bauer FW. Cancer 1982; 49: 369.
155. Fu Y, Perzin KH. Cancer 1974; 33: 1275.
156. Friedmann I, Osborn DA. Pathology of granulomas and neoplasms of the nose and paranasal sinuses. Edinburgh: Churchill Livingstone, 1982: 216.
157. Stout AP. Cancer 1949; 2: 1027.
158. Compagno J, Hyams VJ. Am J Clin Pathol 1976; 66: 672.
159. Babaris JG, Jacobs JB, Templeton AC. J Laryngol 1983; 97: 36.
160. Wick MR, Banks PM, McDonald TJ. Cancer 1981; 48: 2510.
161. Merino MJ, Berman M, Carter D. Am J Surg Pathol 1983; 7: 53.
162. Pantazoupulos PE. Arch Otolaryngol 1965; 81: 83.
163. Moran TE. Laryngoscope 1962; 72: 201.
164. Lack EE, Cubilla AL, Woodruff JM, Farr HW. Cancer 1977; 39: 397.
165. Byers PD, Norman Jones A. Br J Surg 1969; 56: 262.
166. Jaffe HL. Arch Pathol 1953; 15: 83.
167. Smith R. Br Med J 1977; 1: 365.
168. Friedmann I. Pathology of the ear. Oxford: Blackwell, 1974; 229.
169. Tubbax J. Acta Stomatol Belg 1974; 71: 293.
170. Schulz A, Delling G, Ringe JD, Ziegler R. Virchows Arch Path Anat 1977; 376: 309.
171. Rebel A, Malkani K, Basle M, Bregeon C. Calcif Tissue Res 1976; 20: 187.
172. Cooke SL, Powers WH. Arch Otolaryngol 1949; 50: 319.
173. Eversole LR, Sabes WR, Rovin S. J Oral Path 1972; 1: 189.
174. El Deeb M, Sedano HO, Waite ED, Int J Oral Surg 1980; 9: 301.
175. Jaffe HJ. Oral Surg 1953; 6: 159.
176. Lichtenstein L. Arch Pathol 1953; 56: 84.
177. Ochsner SF. Am J Roentgenol 1966; 97: 719.
178. Swain RE, Sessions DG, Ogura JH. Ann Otol Rhinol Laryngol 1974; 83: 439.
179. Windeyer B, Dische S, Mansfield CM. J Clin Radiol 1966; 17: 32.
180. Conley J, Stout AP, Healey WV. Am J Surg 1967; 114: 564.
181. Gane NFC, Rhona Lindup, Strickland P, Bennett MH. Br J Cancer 1970; 24: 705.
182. Soloway HB. Cancer 1966; 19: 1984.
183. Kauffman SL, Stout AP. Cancer 1961; 14: 469.
184. Blitzer A, Lawson W, Biller HF. Laryngoscope 1977; 89: 1497.
185. Townsend GL, Neel HB, Weiland LH, Devine KD, McBean JB. Arch Otolaryngol 1973; 98: 51.
186. Rice DH, Batsakis JG, Headlington JT, Boles R. Arch Otolaryngol 1974; 100: 398.
187. Wilmes E, Meister P. Laryngologie Rhinol Otol 1978; 57: 69.
188. Crissman JD, Henson SL. Arch Otolaryngol 1977; 104: 228.
189. Brookes GB, Rose PE. Malignant fibrous histiocytoma of the ethmoid sinus. J. Laryngol 1985; in press.
190. Bednar B. Cancer 1957; 10: 368.
191. Enzinger FM, Weiss SW. Soft tissue tumours. St Louis: Mosby, 1983: 170.
192. Leite L, Goodwin JW, Sinkovics JG, Baker LH, Benjamen D, Benjamen R. Cancer 1977; 40: 2010.
193. Fu Y, Perzin KH. Cancer 1974; 34: 453.
194. Miglets AW, Laura Rood, Lucas JG. Arch Otolaryngol 1983; 109: 417.
195. Gardner EJ. Am J Hum Genet 1951; 3: 167.
196. Mollison WM. Dental Record 1916; 36: 44.
197. Coates HL, Pearson BW, Devine KD, Unni KK. Trans Am Acad Ophthal Otolaryngol 1977; 84: 919.
198. Evans HL, Ayala AG, Romsdahl MM. Cancer 1977; 40: 818.
199. Dahlin DC. Bone tumours. 3rd ed. Springfield: Charles C Thomas, 1978: 226.
200. Sweetnam R. Br J Hosp Med 1982; 28: 112.
201. Dehner LP. Cancer 1973; 32: 112.
202. Livolsi VA. Arch Otolaryngol 1977; 103: 485.
203. Fu YS, Perzin KH. Cancer 1975; 35: 1300.
204. Fu YS, Perzin KH. Cancer 1976; 37: 364.
205. Dito WR, Batsakis JG. Arch Otolaryngol 1963; 77: 123.
206. Capell DF, Montgomery GL. J Pathol Bacteriol 1975; 44: 517.
207. Horvat BL, Caines M, Fisher ER. Am J Clin Path 1972; 53: 555.
208. Morales AR, Fine G, Horne RC. In: Sommers SC, ed. Pathology Annual 7. New York: Appleton Century Croft, 1972: 81.
209. Altmannsberger M, Osborn M, Treuner J, Holscher A, Weber K, Schauer A. Virchows Archiv (Cell Path) 1982; 39: 203.
210. Brooks JJ. Human Path 1982; 13: 969.
211. Heffner DK, Hyams VJ. Cancer 1984; 53: 2140.
212. Maurer H, Moon T, Donaldson M et al. Cancer 1977; 40: 2015.
213. Poole AG, Marchetta FC. Cancer 1968; 22: 14.
214. Touma YB. J Laryngol Otol 1971; 85: 125.
215. Booth JB, Cheesman AD, Vincenti NH. Ann Otol Rhinol Laryngol 1973; 82: 709.
216. Castro EB, Lewis JS, Strong EW. Arch Otolaryngol 1973; 97: 326.
217. Friedmann I, Osborn DA. Pathology of granulomas and neoplasms of the nose and paranasal sinuses. Edinburgh: Churchill Livingstone, 1982: 204.
218. Ringertz N. Acta Otolaryngol (Stockh) 1938; 27: 234.
219. Friedmann I. Proc R Soc Med 1961; 54: 1064.
220. Hellwig GA. Arch Pathol 1943; 35: 95.
221. Batsakis JG, Fries GT, Goldman RT, Karlsberg RC. Arch Otolaryngol 1964; 79: 613.
222. Batsakis JG. Tumours of the head and neck. 2nd ed. Baltimore: Williams & Wilkins, 1979: 472.
223. Gall EA, Mallory TB. J Pathol 1942; 18: 381.
224. Friedmann I, Osborn DA. Pathology of granulomas and neoplasms of the nose and paranasal sinuses. Edinburgh: Churchill Livingstone, 1982: 198.
225. Wang CC. Radiology 1971; 100: 151.
226. Lautz HA. Arch Otolaryngol 1958; 67: 78.
227. Eichel BS, Harrison EG, Devine KD, Scanlon PW, Brown HA. Am J Surg 1966; 112: 597.
228. Stewart IA, Stuart AE. J Laryngol Otol 1971; 85: 1069.

229. Tiwari RM. J Laryngol Otol 1973; 87: 85.
230. Henry K, Bennett MH, Farrer Brown G. In: Anthony PP, Woolf N, eds. Recent advances in histopathology 10. Edinburgh: Churchill Livingstone, 1978: 275.
231. Rappaport H. Atlas of tumour pathology. Section 3, Fascicle 8. Washington DC: Armed Forces Institute of Pathology, 1966.
232. Ishii Y, Yamanaka N, Ogawa K et al. Cancer 1982; 50: 2336.
233. Birt BD. J Laryngol Otol 1970; 84: 615.
233a. Fermont D, Bennett MH. Unpublished observations.
234. Varney DC. J Urology 1955; 73: 1081.
235. Johnson DE, Butler JJ. In: Johnson DE, ed. Testicular tumours. London: Lewis & Co, 1976: 234.
236. Duncan PR, Checa F, Gowing NFC, McElwain TJ, Peckham MJ. Cancer 1980; 45: 1578.
237. Aozasa K. J Clin Pathol 1982; 35: 599.
238. Aozasa K, Watanabe Y, Ikeda H. Path Res Pract 1981; 171: 314.
239. Aozasa K, Ikeda H, Watanabe Y. Path Res Pract 1981; 172: 161.
240. Aozasa K, Inoue A. J Path 1982; 138: 241.
241. Isaacson P, Wright DH. Human Pathol 1978; 9: 661.
242. Isaacson P, Wright DH. In: Wright DH, ed. Recent advances in gastrointestinal pathology. Philadelphia: WB Saunders, 1980: 193.
243. Bernstein JM. Laryngoscope 1966; 76: 621.
244. Jortay AM. Acta Chir Belg 1971; 70: 715.
245. Abrams HL, Spiro R, Goldstein N. Cancer 1950; 3: 74.
246. Castigliano SG, Rominger CJ. Am J Surg 1954; 87: 496.
247. Cash CD, Royer RQ, Dahlin DC. Oral Surg 1961; 14: 897.
248. McDaniel RK, Luna MA, Stimson PG. Oral Surg 1971; 31: 380.
249. Friedmann I, Osborn DA. Pathology of granulomas and neoplasms of the nose and paranasal sinuses. Edinburgh: Churchill Livingstone, 1982: 300.
250. Flocks RH, Boatman DL. Laryngoscope 1973; 83: 1527.
251. Schantz JC, Miller SH, Graham WP. J Surg Oncol 1976; 8: 183.
252. Friedmann I, Osborn DA. J Laryngol Otol 1965; 79: 576.
253. Eneroth CM, Martensson G, Thulin A. Acta Otolaryngol 1961; 53: 546.
254. Harrison MS, Doey WD, Osborn DA. J Laryngol Otol 1964; 78: 103.
255. Beckers JP, Morimont M, Van den Eeckhaut J. Acta Otorhinolaryngol Belg 1972; 26: 336.
256. Achar MVR. Arch Otolaryngol 1955; 62: 644.
257. Edwards WG. J Laryngol Otol 1964; 78: 96.
258. Garrett MJ. J Fac Radiol (London) 1959; 10: 151.
259. Myers EM. J Laryngol Otol 1968; 82: 485.
260. Shanmugham MS. J Laryngol Otol 1976; 90: 1061.
261. Bataille R, Schumann C, Rolland J. Rev Stomatol Chir Maxillofac 1971; 72: 129.
261a. Chang G, Weber A, Pappamkou A. Ann Otol Rhinol Laryngol 1983; 92: 309.
262. Subramanyam C, Lal M. Med J Malaysia 1970; 24: 306.
263. Salimi R. J Surg Oncol 1977; 9: 301.
264. Mukherjee DK. Ann Otol Rhinol Laryngol 1978; 87: 257.

PART TWO

I. Friedmann

The nasopharynx

5

Structure and function: Inflammatory diseases

STRUCTURAL AND FUNCTIONAL CONSIDERATIONS

The nasopharynx lies behind the nasal cavities and is the widest part of the pharynx. Anteriorly, it is continuous with these cavities through the posterior nares, or choanae, which are separated by the posterior edge of the nasal septum. The roof of the nasopharynx is formed by the thick layers of mucous membrane and periosteum on the undersurface of the basilar part of the occipital bone. The posterior wall of the cavity is formed by the mucous membrane that overlies the prevertebral muscles and fascia; the anterior arch of the atlas vertebra can be felt a little below the upper limit of the posterior pharyngeal wall. During swallowing, the nasopharynx is closed below by the soft palate: at other times there is free communication with the oropharynx.

The pharyngeal ostia of the auditory tubes (Eustachian tubes) are on the lateral walls of the nasopharynx, behind the inferior conchae; they are vertical clefts, bounded above and behind by the tori. These are expansions of the cartilage of the tubes, and behind them lie deep recesses, the pharyngeal recesses or fossae of Rosenmüller. The mucosa of this part of the nasopharynx contains much lymphoid tissue, sometimes known as the tubal tonsils. They form part of Waldeyer's ring of pharyngeal lymphoid tissue. A much more important part of Waldeyer's ring is the nasopharyngeal tonsil (Luschka's tonsil), a single mass of lymphadenoid tissue, the 'adenoid' or 'adenoids', situated in the area where the roof and posterior wall of the nasopharynx merge into one another.

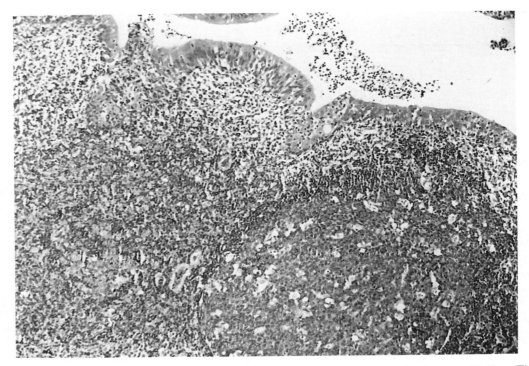

Fig. 5.1A Lymphoid tissue of nasopharyngeal tonsil ('adenoid') covered by pseudo-stratified columnar epithelium. There are large lymph follicles in the sub-epithelial cortical area.

Haematoxylin–eosin ×100

Histology

Because of its comparative inaccessibility, our knowledge both of the accurate dimensions and of the histology of the normal human nasopharyngeal mucosa is incomplete. Ali,[1] in an extensive study of 100 autopsy specimens, has described the histological features of the normal mucous membrane of the human nasopharynx in various age groups. He found that the area lined by stratified squamous epithelium is larger than the combined area occupied by the pseudostratified ciliated and intermediate epithelia (Fig. 5.1A).

Squamous metaplasia is common, particularly in adults; probably in consequence of chronic inflammation (Fig. 5.1B). Keratinization of the squamous area is, however, always pathological.

The intermediate epithelium forms a wavy junctional zone separating the nasopharynx from the oropharynx. There are numerous islands of intermediate epithelium all over the salpingopharyngeal fold, the pharyngeal recess, and the lining of the pharyngeal tonsils in the posterior wall. The intermediate epithelium resembles the transitional type urothelium. It is stratified, in contrast to the pseudostratified ciliated respiratory epithelium and appears to lack a full differentiation; its terminal maturation stage still resembles embryonic epithelium.[2]

The natural pathway taken by the secretions of the mucosal glands of the nose, including Bowman's glands in the olfactory area, is backward to the nasopharynx. The mucous blanket covering the epithelium of the nasal cavities and sinuses is constantly propelled in that direction by the action of the cilia (Fig. 5.1C and D), part of the stream passing above and part below the openings of the Eustachian tubes. This flow of mucus is wholly normal, and is part of the defences of the upper respiratory tract against infection.

Abnormal postnasal discharge

It is only when the quantity, odour and other characteristics of the nasal and postnasal secre-

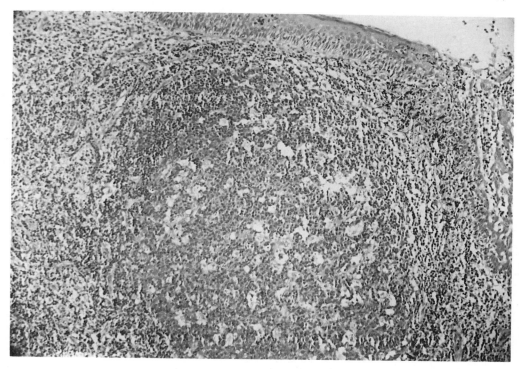

Fig. 5.1B Adenoid lymphoid tissue with large hyperplastic follicle containing large numbers of clear reticulocytes. The surface is covered by metaplastic squamous epithelium showing little or no keratinization.

Haematoxylin–eosin   × 100

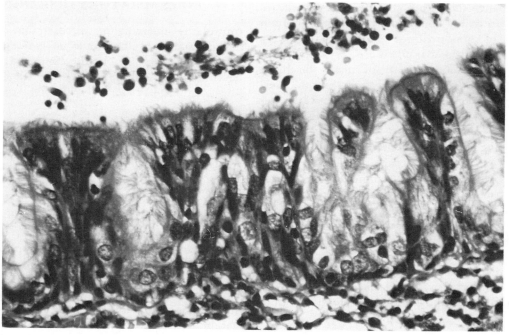

Fig. 5.1C Detail of ciliated respiratory epithelium of the nasopharynx covering the adenoid tissue.

Haematoxylin–eosin   × 500

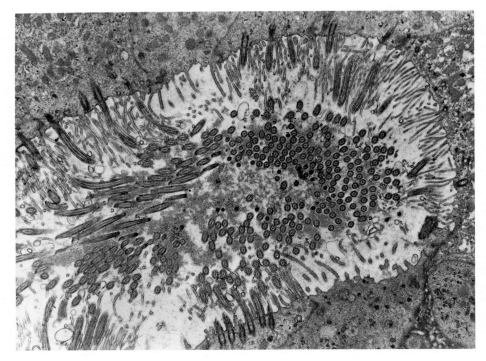

Fig. 5.1D Electron micrograph of the ciliated epithelium. There are large numbers of cilia protruding into the lumen. surrounded by long microvilli. The cilia are covered by some mucoid secretion.   × 7000

tions change that it becomes necessary to regard them as possibly abnormal. The most important causes of abnormalities are neoplasms, but chronic rhinitis and sinusitis are very much commoner. A blood-stained purulent discharge should always be regarded as suggesting the presence of a neoplasm until some other cause has been clearly demonstrated to be alone responsible.

Bleeding into the nasopharynx may result from trauma or disease. Fracture of the base of the skull is the commonest traumatic cause, apart from haemorrhage following adenoidectomy. Among the conditions in which bleeding is noteworthy are acute ulcerative forms of nasopharyngitis, infection complicating the presence of foreign bodies, spontaneous rupture of dilated superficial blood vessels in patients with arterial hypertension, and haemorrhagic states such as may accompany leukaemia and thrombocytopenia.

INFLAMMATORY DISEASES

Any of the inflammatory diseases that occur in the nose and nasal sinuses may affect the nasopharynx (see Chapter 2). Further comment here will be confined to a few points of particular local relevance.

Stenosis
Stenosis or narrowing of the nasopharyngeal lumen by scar tissue formation may occur not only after extensive surgery but also following tonsillectomy and adenoidectomy.[3]

Acute nasopharyngitis
The nasopharynx is commonly involved during the course of acute infections of the nose or of the oropharynx—for instance, acute tonsillitis, in which the causation organism is usually *Streptococcus pyogenes*. Rarely, the mucosal infection in diptheria is confined to the nasopharynx, a localization particularly prone to occur in children whose tonsils have been incompletely removed.

In acute nasopharyngitis, hyperaemia and oedema of the mucous membrane are accompanied by increasing secretion of mucus. Severer changes such as ulceration or membrane formation are sometimes found, their presence depending chiefly on the nature of the organism that is responsible and its pathogenic effects.

Chronic nasopharyngitis

Chronic inflammation of the nasopharynx occurs in association with certain nasal diseases, among them chronic sinusitis, obstruction of the airways by deviation of the nasal septum, and allergic rhinitis. It may be a troublesome consequence of working in a dusty atmosphere, the nasopharynx bearing the brunt of the irritation caused by the inhaled particles. The presence of residual adenoid tissue after incomplete excision predisposes to persistence of chronic nasopharyngitis.

Atrophic nasopharyngitis is a special form of chronic nasopharyngeal inflammation; it is usually associated with atrophic rhinitis, and its causes are the same (see p. 16).

Tuberculosis

Tuberculosis of the nasopharynx is rare, but its frequency in cases of chronic respiratory tuberculosis is appreciably greater than has generally been recognized.[4] Two types have been distinguished—the open ulcerative form and the closed type in which the mucosa is intact and the disease can be demonstrated only by microscopical examination. The lymphoid tissues are those most involved. Diagnosis is made by microscopic examination and culture of relevant material. Differential diagnosis from Wegener's granuloma may cause some difficulty.

Nasopharyngeal abscesses

Two varieties of nasopharyngeal abscesses have been described: both are very rare. *Tornwaldt's abscess* (first described in 1885)[5] is a chronic suppurative lesion in the midline of the adenoid, and is believed to result from infection in the remains of the median recess of the posterior nasopharynx (pharyngeal bursa).[6]

Internal Bezold abscess is the name given to a peculiar complication of acute suppurative otitis media in which pus tracks anteriorly along the outer aspect of the auditory tube until it reaches the pharynx, where a retropharyngeal abscess forms and eventually ruptures into the postnasal space. This lesion acquires its name from the supposed similarity between its pathogenesis and that of the traditional form of Bezold's abscess in which pus in the mastoid points into the soft tissues of the neck in the digastric fossa.

In osteomyelitis of the sphenoid bone, complicating sphenoidal sinusitis, the infection may extend through the mucoperiosteum and pus then discharges into the nasopharynx.

Enlargement of the pharyngeal tonsil

Although the term 'adenoids' has been used as a synonym for the pharyngeal tonsil, without implying the presence of any pathological state, it is generally used in clinical practice to denote an abnormal enlargement of this collection of lymphoid tissue. Adenoidal enlargement is common, especially in children from 5–10 years old. Its pathogenesis is still obscure. It may be part of a generalized hyperplasia of the lymphoid tissues throughout the body, or a purely local condition developing as a response to repeated infections of the adenoid tissue, possibly by viruses of the adenovirus group. Just as the adenoids are usually involved together with the faucial tonsils in acute inflammatory conditions of the throat, so chronic tonsillitis is likely to be accompanied by chronic inflammatory hyperplasia of the adenoids.

Histological examination of adenoids removed surgically shows a non-specific hyperplasia of the lymphoid tissues, often with many large, closely packed follicles with prominent germinal centres. It has been from fragments of such tissues that many of the adenoviruses have been cultured. There may be a narrow zone of hyaline fibrous tissue immediately deep to the epithelium, and also between the deep aspect of the adenoids and the tissues underlying them. Fibrosis of the lymphoid tissue itself is seldom conspicuous. Suppuration is much less frequent than in the faucial tonsils. The respiratory type of epithelium that normally covers the adenoids (Fig. 5.1A, C and D) is often replaced by squamous epithelium (Fig. 5.1B).

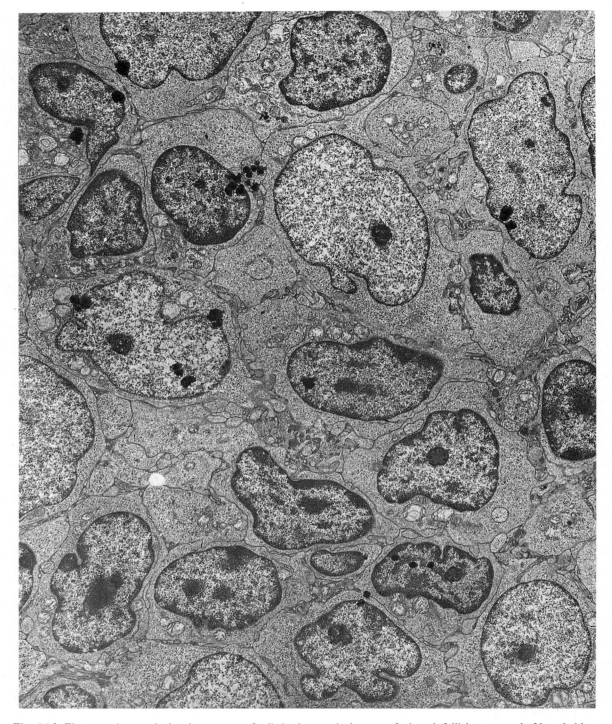

Fig. 5.2A Electron micrograph showing a group of cells in the germinal centre of a lymph follicle composed of lymphoblasts with pale nuclei and large nucleoli and dendritic reticulum cells with marked folding of the outer cell membrane.

× 7000

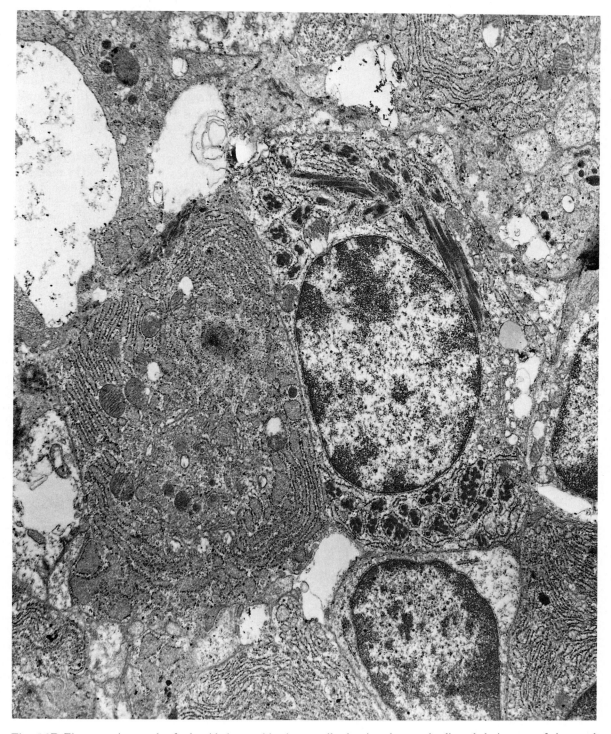

Fig. 5.2B Electron micrograph of adenoid tissue with plasma cells showing the greatly distended cisternae of the rough endoplasmic reticulum containing crystalline inclusions and secretory globules indicative of some immune activity.

× 12 500

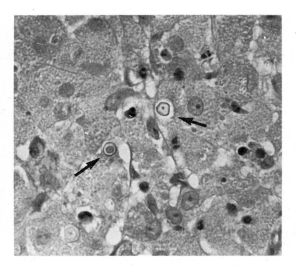

Fig. 5.2C Malakoplakia of the nasopharynx. Two inclusions are indicated.

Haematoxylin–eosin   × 120

(Provided by Dr A.H. Timme, Cape Town, and the Editor of the Journal of Laryngology.*)*

Electron microscopy of human adenoid tissue shows in addition to small and large lymphocytes dendritic reticulum cells with complex grossly folded outer cell membranes (Fig. 5.2A).[7] The presence of such cells and of active plasma cells with distended endoplasmic cisternae (Fig. 5.2B) indicates reaction of lymphoid tissue to an antigen, for example a viral antigen. The folds absorb and retain the antigen on their surfaces, activating antibody production by the cells.

Clinical findings
The typical symptoms are nasal obstruction, which leads to mouth breathing, especially at night, and a characteristic facies, with broadening and flattening of the nasal arch. Enlargement of the upper deep cervical lymph nodes is common. Children with enlarged adenoids suffer in general health; they tend to be nervous and irritable, backward at school and prone to colds and other infections of the upper respiratory tract. Hearing may be impaired as a result of obstruction of the Eustachian tubes, and such blockage also predisposes to infection of the middle ear and is accompanied by otitis media with effusion (the 'glue ear' syndrome).

Chronic sinusitis may be both the cause and the consequence of adenoidal hyperplasia. Allergic rhinitis may aggravate the local condition, for the added obstruction of the airways that is caused by the local swelling of the mucosa both increases the difficulty in breathing through the nose and helps to perpetuate the adenoidal enlargement by hindering the free drainage of discharges.

There are wide differences in the severity of the symptoms produced by adenoidal enlargement. It is possible that individual variations in the internal configuration of the nasopharynx may influence the effects of the enlargement on the airway, and help to determine the clinical significance of the condition in different cases.

Nasopharyngeal polyps
Polyps similar to those of the nose may be found in the nasopharynx. They usually arise in the maxillary antrum, whence they extend into the nasal cavity and eventually through the choana into the nasopharynx (choanal polyps). The so-called 'hairy polyps' are true neoplasms.

Malakoplakia
Malakoplakia, although rare, has been more widely recognized and its unique localization in the nasopharynx has recently been reported.[8] The lesion was composed of histiocytes containing the characteristic calcified inclusions (Michaelis–Gutman bodies) (Fig. 5.2C).

REFERENCES

1. Ali MY. J Anat 1965; 99: 657.
2. Batsakis JG, Solomon AR, Rice DH. Head Neck Surg 1981; 3: 511.
3. McDonald TY, Devine KD, Hayes AB. Arch Otolaryngol 1973; 98: 38.
4. Goodman RS, Mattel S, Kaufman D et al. Laryngoscope 1981; 91: 794.
5. Tornwaldt GL, Über die Bedeutung der Bursa pharyngea für die Erkennung und Behandlung gewisser Nasemachenraum-Krankheiten. Wiesbaden: JF Bergmann, 1985
6. Hollender AR, Szanto FB. Ann Otol 1945; 54: 575.
7. Friedmann I, Michaels L, Gerwat J, Bird ES. ORL 1972; 34: 195.
8. Timme AH. J Laryngol (in press).

6

Neoplasms of the nasopharynx

BENIGN TUMOURS AND TUMOUR-LIKE LESIONS

Most of the neoplasms of the nasopharynx are malignant; only about 10% are benign.

Epithelial tumours

Tumours arising from the surface epithelium are *squamous cell papilloma* and *transitional type papilloma*. The latter is identical with those that arise in the nose (see page 65); occasionally it may be confined to the nasopharynx.

Adenoma of the seromucous glands belongs to the least rare benign tumours of the nasopharynx. The commonest type is the *oncocytic* or *oxyphilic adenoma* which may be confused with an adenolymphoma. The lymphocytic element, however, surrounds the glandular structures whereas in the adenolymphoma it forms collections that invaginate and distort the lumen.

Pleomorphic adenoma ('mixed' tumour) may occur.

Connective tissue tumours

These include *fibroma*, *myxoma* (Fig. 6.1) and the *fibrous polyp*. Chondroma has only rarely been reported. Osseous tumours have not been reported in the nasopharynx.

Vascular tumours

Vascular tumours include the *cavernous haemangioma*. It is of some considerable clinical significance because surgical removal of the tumour can result in profuse and even fatal bleeding. *Lymphangioma* may also occur.

The *juvenile angiofibroma* is described on page 96.

139

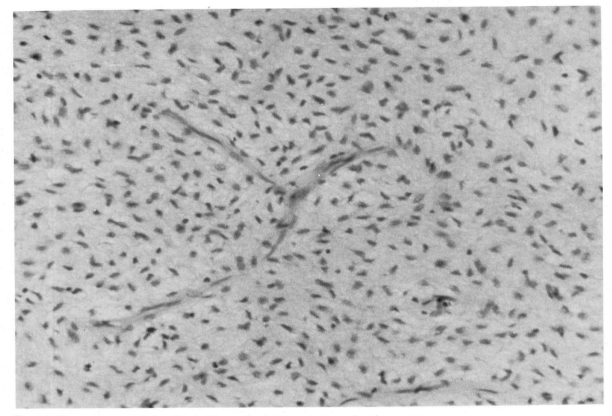

Fig. 6.1 Myxoma composed of uniform stellate cells with elongated cytoplasmic processes. Haematoxylin–eosin   × 250

Neurogenic tumours

Schwannoma and *neurofibroma* are rare and exhibit the same histological features as those seen elsewhere. Neurofibromas may produce bulky masses and may be confused with myxomas.

Tumour-like lesions

Hamartoma,[1, 2] dermoid and teratoma[3]
These tumour-like lesions are not true neoplasms but developmental malformations composed of two germinal layers, ectoderm and mesoderm. They can form pedunculated or sessile masses causing obstruction of the nasopharynx. They affect mainly children under 1 year of age; but a case occurring in a 71-year-old man has been reported.[1]

Microscopy shows various tissues e.g. skin, dermal appendages, hair follicles, fibrous and adipose tissue, muscle fibres, cartilage and bone.[4, 5] Nasopharyngeal dermoids have been called 'hairy polyps' because of their dermal contents.[6]

MALIGNANT EPITHELIAL TUMOURS

The nasopharynx has been described as a 'silent area' of cancer, for the primary malignant tumours that arise there may remain small and symptomless after widespread metastasis has occurred, whether to the regional lymph nodes or through the blood to the lungs or other viscera. Moreover, such tumours may easily be overlooked during clinical examination and they may be difficult to find at necropsy unless the region is dissected with special care. When the possibility of a small primary nasopharyngeal growth cannot be resolved by ordinary direct examination post mortem it is necessary to remove the whole of this region by the comparatively simple methods described by Graff[7] and Teo[8] which enables a detailed study to be carried out.

A special source of diagnostic difficulty is the almost inevitable presence of lymphoid tissue in specimens from the nasopharynx. As well as the problem of the so-called lymphoepithelioma (see below), this association leads to confusion because of the proneness of lymphocytes to become peculiarly altered by artefact, with consequent misinterpretation. Crushing or stretching the tissue during excision of a biopsy specimen may so distort lymphocytes that they come to resemble hyperchromatic tumour fibroblasts or anaplastic carcinoma cells of the small spindle-shaped type that characterizes, for example, the so-called 'oat-cell' carcinoma of the lower respiratory tract.

Again, delayed or otherwise insufficient fixation may result in confusing artefacts. For this reason, many of us whose work is in this field prefer the use of rapid fixatives, such as Zenker's fluid, to the more usual formol saline.

Many cancers of the nasopharynx have become ulcerated and infected by the time of biopsy. The secondary changes that result add to the difficulty of interpretation. They are not always avoided by taking material for histological examination from parts of the lesion that are not ulcerated, although such are generally preferable. In these cases it is, of course, important to remember that induration round a tumour may result from circulatory or inflammatory changes: a biopsy might thus be taken from tissue not directly involved by the nearby neoplasm, and an unwary report could delay the correct diagnosis when the latter might be made immediately by repeating the biopsy operation in another site.

Epidemiology of nasopharyngeal carcinoma

Carcinoma of the nasopharynx accounts for less than 1% of all carcinomas among Caucasians: the corresponding figure among the Chinese in the region of Canton exceeds 50%.[9] Inhabitants of Kwantung province show the highest incidence. The incidence of the disease among Chinese people born outside China is lower than in the Chinese born and living in the endemic areas of China. Nevertheless, it has remained higher also among the former than among Caucasians. The reluctance of immigrant Chinese to abandon their traditional way of life may be reflected in

Table 6.1 Tumours of the nasopharynx 1948–1971. Based on a survey, by the late Dr D. A. Osborn, of 154 nasopharyngeal tumours in the material of the Institute of Laryngology and Otology, London.

Carcinoma

Squamous keratinizing	21
Transitional type	15
Undifferentiated	51
Adenocarcinoma	5
Total	92

Malignant lymphoma

Non-Hodgkin's lymphoma	32
Hodgkin's lymphoma	1
Total	33

Sarcomas	8
Chordoma	3

Miscellaneous

Plasmacytoma	1
Transitional type papilloma	8
Duct adenoma	3
Haemangioma	2
Fibro-lipoma	1
Undetermined	3
Total	18

the relatively high incidence which is only slowly falling.

Incidence
In a series of 154 tumours of the nasopharynx we have studied (Table 6.1) there were 87 cases of squamous cell carcinoma and five cases of adenocarcinoma in a period from 1948–1971. A Canadian series listed 140 nasopharyngeal carcinomas in a period from 1970–1976.[10]

Age and sex
The age distribution shows a rise from the fourth to the seventh decade (Table 6.2). Males are more frequently affected (Fig. 6.2). The Child-

Table 6.2 Age incidence of carcinoma and malignant lymphoma of the nasopharynx and tonsillar region.

Decade	1	2	3	4	5	6	7	8	9	10
Nasopharynx										
Carcinoma	0	2	4	13	13	36	18	5	0	0
Lymphoma	0	0	2	0	4	12	8	6	0	1
Tonsil region										
Carcinoma	0	0	0	1	7	19	25	16	5	0
Lymphoma	4	2	0	10	11	19	16	12	3	0

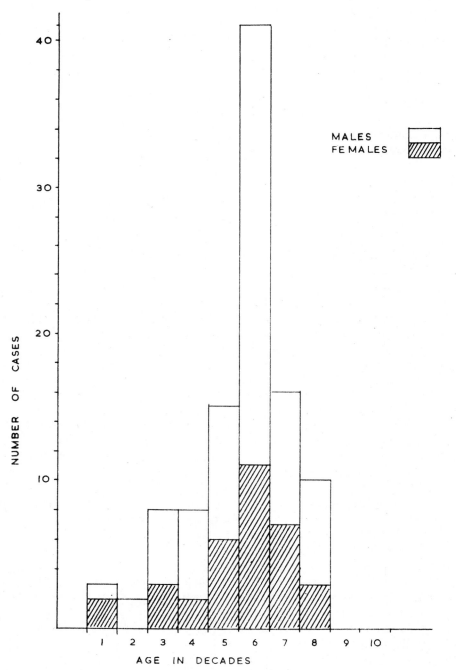

Fig. 6.2 Malignant tumours of the nasopharynx. Age and sex distribution.

ren's Tumour Registry in Manchester, UK, listed 12 cases of carcinoma of the nasopharynx in children up to 15 years of age, out of a total of 1482 cases of malignant disease of childhood from 1954–1980.

Clinical findings

The most frequent complaints of our patients included nasal obstruction (42%), nasal discharge (12%), loss of hearing (63%), epistaxis (19%), diplopia (16%) and tinnitus (6%).

The tissues of the nasopharynx are richly supplied with lymphatics: spread to the cervical lymph nodes is common (75–90% on presentation).[11] In our series there were palpable cervical lymph nodes in 45% of the patients when first seen. 20% of the patients presented with a recognizable swelling in the neck. The primary neoplasm could promptly be traced in the nasopharynx in the majority of the patients.

It is often difficult to define the side on which the tumour arose. Thus the distinction between homolateral and contralateral nodal involvement is often difficult to make. The retropharyngeal and upper jugular nodes tend to be involved.

Histological classification

The classification of nasopharyngeal neoplasms has remained debatable because of the varied histological features of these neoplasms. Technical difficulties in obtaining satisfactory biopsy specimens have contributed to the familiar difficulties encountered by the histopathologist.

The World Health Organization's Subcommittee for the Histological Typing of Upper Respiratory Tract Tumours divided nasopharyngeal carcinomas into the following groups according to their predominant pattern on light microscopy.[12]

Squamous cell carcinoma (keratinizing squamous cell carcinoma)

A nasopharyngeal carcinoma showing definite evidence of squamous differentiation with the presence of intercellular bridges or keratinization over most of its extent or both. It may be graded as well-, moderately- or poorly-differentiated.

Non-keratinizing carcinoma

The non-keratinizing squamous nasopharyngeal carcinoma is one that shows evidence of differ-

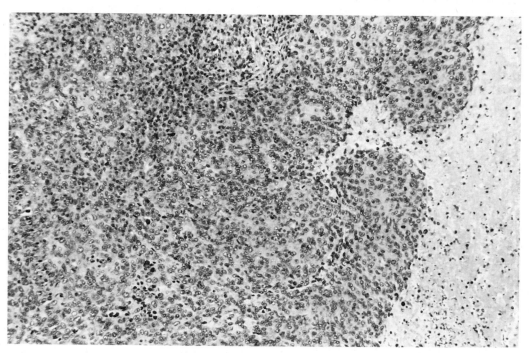

Fig. 6.3 Non-keratinizing poorly-differentiated squamous cell carcinoma. A plexiform pattern is recognizable and there is some tendency to stratification of the mainly irregularly distributed cells. . Haematoxylin–eosin   × 200

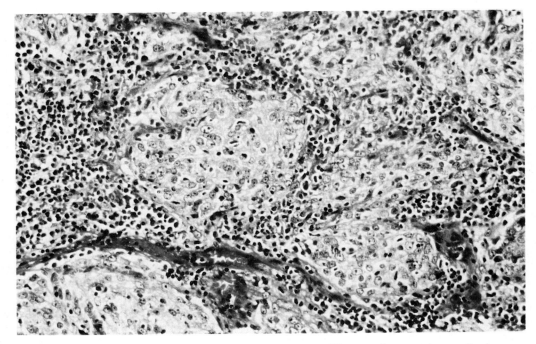

Fig. 6.4 Non-keratinizing squamous cell carcinoma of the nasopharynx. There are large aggregates of pale squamous-like epithelial cells in lymphoid tissue.   Haematoxylin–eosin   × 500

entiation with a maturation sequence that results in cells in which squamous differentiation is not evident on light microscopy. The tumour cells have fairly well-defined cell margins and show an arrangement that is stratified or pavemented and not syncytial. A plexiform pattern is common (Fig. 6.3). Some tumours may exhibit a clear-cell structure due to the presence of glycogen in the cytoplasm. There is no evidence of mucin production or of glandular differentiation.

In contrast to the keratinizing squamous cell carcinoma, which seldom poses diagnostic problems, the non-keratinizing carcinomas often cause difficulties (Fig. 6.4).[13–18] In an immuno-chemical analysis of 40 cases of nasopharyngeal neoplasms, utilizing an antibody against keratin, it was found that all the squamous cell carcinomas, whether regarded as keratinizing or non-keratinizing on examination of conventionally-stained sections, gave a positive immunochemical reaction for keratin.[14] The non-keratinizing tumours stained less extensively and more focally with the immunocytochemical methods than did the keratinizing neoplasms.[17]

Undifferentiated carcinoma (undifferentiated carcinoma of nasopharyngeal type)

The tumour cells have oval or round vesicular nuclei and prominent nucleoli. The cell margins are indistinct and the tumour exhibits an appearance that is syncytial rather than pavemented. Spheroidal tumour cells, some with hyperchromatic nuclei and prominent nucleoli, may be present. The tumour cells are arranged in irregular and moderately well defined masses or in strands of loosely-connected cells in a lymphoid stroma (Figs 6.5–6.8). The tumour cells do not produce mucin. These cytological and histological features are fairly characteristic and when present in metastatic tumours (Fig. 6.9), which are particularly common in the upper cervical lymph nodes, may enable a presumptive diagnosis of nasopharyngeal carcinoma to be made (Fig. 6.10). Localized amyloid may be deposited in the neoplastic tissue.[19]

Incidence

Among 423 cases of nasopharyngeal carcinoma in Singapore there were 73 cases of squamous car-

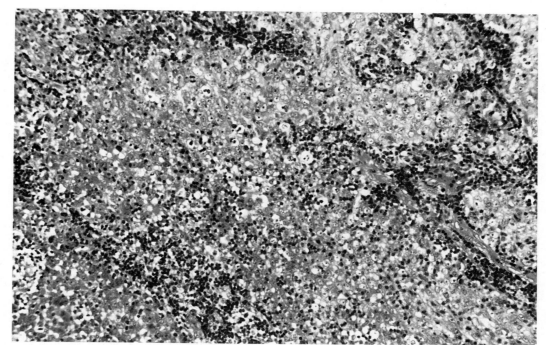

Fig. 6.5 Undifferentiated (non-keratinizing) carcinoma of nasopharyngeal type (anaplastic carcinoma). Note sheets of large pale carcinoma cells with prominent nuclei and nucleoli with an admixture of lymphocytes (of normal appearance).

Haematoxylin–eosin   × 125

Provided by Dr M.H. Bennett, Mount Vernon Hospital, Northwood, Middlesex, UK.

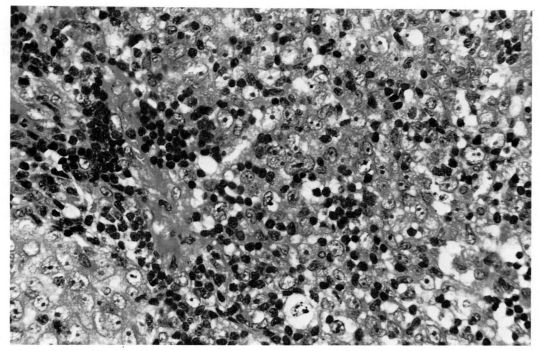

Fig. 6.6 As Figure 6.5.

Haematoxylin–eosin   × 500

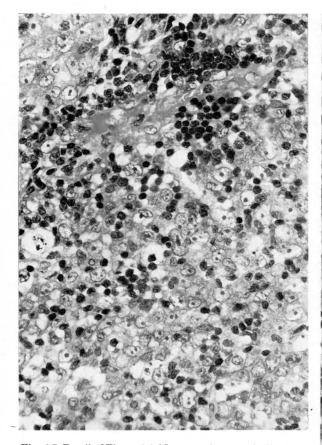

Fig. 6.7 Detail of Figure 6.6. Note prominent nucleoli.

Haematoxylin–eosin   × 250

Provided by Dr M.H. Bennett, Mount Vernon Hospital, Northwood, Middlesex, UK.

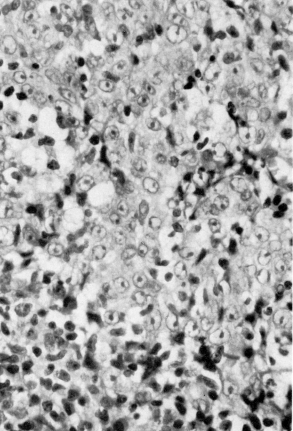

Fig. 6.8 Undifferentiated or anaplastic carcinoma of naso-pharyngeal type showing admixture of carcinomatous cells and lymphocytes. Caused secondary deposits in the brain (Fig. 6.7).

Haematoxylin–eosin   × 220

Provided by Professor P. Scheuer, Royal Free Hospital, London, UK.

Singapore there were 73 cases of squamous carcinoma, 178 cases of non-keratinizing squamous cell carcinoma, and 172 cases of undifferentiated carcinoma.[20] In our series of 92 carcinomas there were 51 cases of undifferentiated carcinoma (Table 6.1).

Undifferentiated carcinomas are not always easily distinguished from malignant lymphoma, for the tumour cells and the histological presentation are sometimes closely similar in the two forms of cancer in spite of their very different origins (p. 151). Moreover, the intimate association with the lymphoreticular tissue of the part tends to mask the identity of the malignant epithelium: the very frequent intermingling of cells of such different provenance and behaviour was the basis of the continuing controversy about the concept of 'lymphoepithelioma', which dates from the observations of Regaud in 1912[21] and of Schmincke in 1921,[22] both of whom regarded the lymphocytes and the epithelial cells as integral components of the neoplastic process. The already existing arguments over the functional relation between lymphoid tissue and its epithelial covering, seen particularly in Waldeyer's ring and in the intestines, provided a background to this concept of the tumours, which attracted more interest and support among clinicians than in the laboratory. Thus, a picture evolved of a

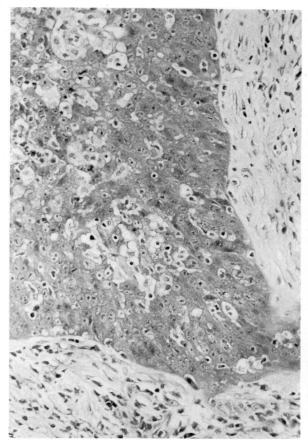

Fig. 6.9 Secondary deposit in the brain from primary carcinoma of the nasopharynx (in Fig. 6.5).

Haematoxylin–eosin × 130

Provided by Dr M.H. Bennett, Mount Vernon Hospital, Northwood, Middlesex, UK.

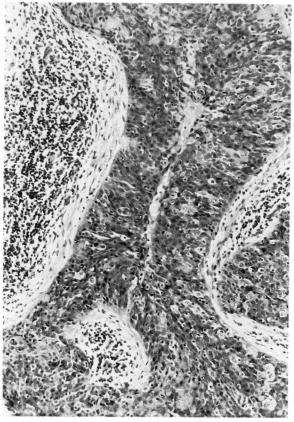

Fig. 6.10 Shows lymph node with metastatic squamous carcinoma, largely anaplastic and with some transitional appearing areas consistent with a nasopharyngeal primary.

Haematoxylin–eosin × 180

highly radiosensitive tumour that metastasized early and extensively to the lymph nodes on both sides of the neck.[23, 24]

Today, few pathologists accept that there is such an entity as the lymphoepithelioma. Some tumours that have been called 'lymphoepitheliomas' are not carcinomas but examples of histiocytic lymphoma. However, most are considered to be undifferentiated carcinomas with a conspicuous contribution of lymphocytes to the histological picture.[24, 25] The presence of the lymphocytes is explicable in two ways. It may merely reflect the carcinomatous invasion of the lymphoreticular tissues of the nasopharynx and,

of course, of the regional lymph nodes. Alternatively, it may represent active infiltration of the tumour by lymphocytes, possibly in the nature of an immunological defence, albeit an ineffectual one. The latter explanation accords better with the observation that distant metastatic deposits of these carcinomas, as in the liver, are often notably infiltrated by lymphocytes.

Recent investigations using antibodies against keratin protein from animal and human sources have confirmed that keratin is a major cytoplasmic element of squamous cells and that these antibodies can be employed in the study of human neoplasms and their differential diagnosis.[14, 15]

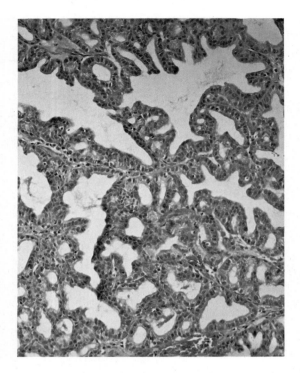

Fig. 6.11 Acinic-cell tumour of nasopharynx. Small, acinar type lumina are again present but general structure is papillary.

Haematoxylin–eosin   × 160

Immunocytochemical stains for three epithelial cell markers—keratin, epithelial membrane antigen (EMA), and carcino-embryonic antigen (CEA)—were used on paraffin-wax-embedded material from 14 patients with nasopharyngeal carcinoma in the course of a study to differentiate lymphomas from undifferentiated nasopharyngeal carcinoma.[16, 17] Tumour cells staining for keratin were found in all 14 cases and for EMA in 8; only 2 tumours were found to contain CEA-positive cells. 7 cases of Hodgkin's disease and 24 non-Hodgkin's lymphomas were uniformly negative. Keratin has proved to be the most reliable epithelial marker for identifying nasopharyngeal carcinoma and differentiating it from a lymphoma. The results of these investigations indicated that the regular finding of stainable keratin in non-keratinizing and undifferentiated nasopharyngeal carcinomas favours the view that nasopharyngeal carcinoma represents a homogeneous group with variable degrees of squamous differentiation.[16]

Prognosis

The survival rate of patients with undifferentiated carcinomas with a prominent lymphoid component has been considered to be higher than that of patients suffering from keratinizing squamous cell carcinoma of the nasopharynx.[26] A survey of 1555 consecutive cases of nasopharyngeal carcinoma in Taiwan, however, indicated that the histopathological classification of the tumours bears no relation to the survival rate of nasopharyngeal carcinoma.[27]

In the Singapore series[20] the 5-year survival rate for squamous cell carcinoma was lower than that for the combined group of non-keratinizing and undifferentiated carcinomas. The 3-year survival rate was higher for tumours with lymphocytic infiltrates but there was no difference in the 5-year survival rates. There was no significant correlation between the histopathological findings and the distribution of the tumours according to age, sex and/or the HLA (human leucocyte antigen) antigen profiles, or with the cell-mediated immune status of the patient. It was concluded that the three types of nasopharyngeal carcinoma as defined in the WHO classification are variants of a fairly homogeneous group of neoplasms in the population of Singapore.[19] In our series the 5-year survival rate for all types was only 10%.

Various systems have been employed in the clinical staging of nasopharyngeal carcinoma. A recent review of four widely-used staging systems has shown 'no statistically significant difference in predicting prognosis when the corresponding stages in each system are compared'.[28]

In a review of 99 patients with cancer of the nasopharynx[29] the only significant factor observed to influence survival was the age of the patient. It was best in the age group 0–20 years (44%) and poorest in patients over 60 years of age (14%). Longer treatment periods and higher dosage levels of radiotherapy offered, in some cases, a better prognosis.

Aetiology

In the aetiology of these tumours there are environmental and genetic factors that play an important role. The environmental factors may be external, such as carcinogenic chemicals, trace elements and viruses. Internal dietary deficiencies and endocrine disturbances may also be involved. There is some evidence that there are relatively high levels of oestrogens in the body among the people who belong to population groups with a particular liability to nasopharyngeal carcinoma. The inhalation of wood dust and coal tar products or snuff have been incriminated in the causation of the disease. High levels of arsenic, chromium and nickel have been found both in the environment and in the epidermal appendages of patients with nasopharyngeal carcinoma and in those of their relatives. Other portals of entry such as ingestion must also be considered because it is known that carcinogenic nitrosamines can be formed in vivo and dimethyl nitrosamine has been shown experimentally to have specificity for the upper respiratory tract. Nitrosamines were found in salted and pickled fish consumed by people in Hong Kong.

The sensitivity of the nasopharyngeal mucosa to various external factors may be enhanced by vitamin deficiencies such as the frequently occurring deficiencies of vitamins A and B in high incidence areas. Records show a male preponderance; this is highest among the Chinese, exceeding a ratio of 4:1, suggesting that hereditary factors play a part in the creation of the conditions together with the environmental factors which may be chemical or viral or both.

Epstein–Barr virus and nasopharyngeal carcinoma
The Epstein–Barr virus is present widely in human populations and following natural primary infection in childhood the virus presents throughout life, being harboured in circulating B-lymphocytes. It may be shed into the buccal fluid. The EB-virus is associated with two human malignancies: Burkitt's lymphoma and undifferentiated or poorly-differentiated carcinoma of the nasopharynx.[30]

The aetiological role of the Epstein–Barr virus in the causation of nasopharyngeal carcinoma cannot be doubted. Patients with nasopharyngeal cancer frequently have high titres of antibodies to the EB-virus (which has also been associated with infectious mononucleosis and Burkitt's lymphoma).[31] However, about 75% of adults contain antibodies in the serum to the EB-virus associated with infection that may remain latent throughout the lifetime of the individual. The virus has been identified in lymphoblast cell lines derived from biopsy specimens of nasopharyngeal carcinomas but also from normal or non-neoplastic nasopharyngeal biopsies.[8]

The question of the pathway of the EB-virus into the epithelial cells of the nasopharyngeal mucosa has attracted much attention. The only cells with receptors for the virus are a subpopulation of B lymphocytes. The EB-virus, like some other herpes viruses, is capable of fusing cells: the genome of the EB-virus could be introduced into an epithelial cell by fusion of the epithelial cell with an infected B-lymphocyte.[32] EB-virus in epithelium of nasopharyngeal carcinoma can be activated and is capable of replication in a cell type other than a primate B-lymphocyte.[33]

In an experiment in which tissue from two nasopharyngeal carcinomas was transplanted into nude mice (whose thymus is absent, rendering them unable to combat infections or alien tissues), herpes-virus-like particles were observed under the electron microscope in the transplanted tissue.[34] Similar viruses have been found in the biopsy specimens from these patients and were interpreted as latent murine oncorna viruses.[35] It is possible, theoretically, that a latent herpes virus, harboured in nasopharyngeal carcinomas, may be activated when transplanted into the nude mouse.[36]

Transitional-type carcinoma
The different types of nasopharyngeal carcinoma arise from the various cell types forming the normal or hyperplastic squamous epithelium of the nasopharyngeal mucosa. The intermediate epithelium at the junctional zone between the nasopharynx and the oropharynx[37] (also referred to as transitional epithelium) appears to lack full differentiation. In its terminal maturation stage it still resembles embryonic epithelium and may be more vulnerable than fully differentiated epithelia to carcinogenic agents. Transitional-type carcinomas and undifferentiated carcinomas arising from such cells are essentially of squamous

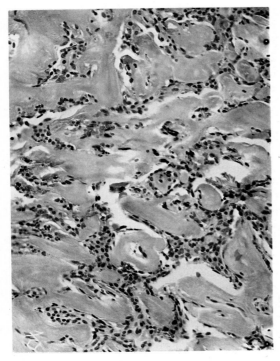

Fig. 6.12 Pleomorphic tumour of pharyngeal region. Hyalinized stroma in intimate relation with the epithelial component forming cylinders.

Haematoxylin–eosin × 200

epithelial origin as indicated by the presence of keratin when examined under the electron microscope or by immunochemical methods.

Formerly such carcinomas were usually diagnosed as lymphoepitheliomas; other have included transitional carcinomas in the classification of 'epidermoid carcinomas' of the nasopharynx.[38] We have found this diagnostic approach justified on both a morphological basis and as a helpful prognostic indicator.

Careful study of the tumours shows the characteristic tendency to retain the basal lamina noted in their counterparts in the nasal region (see p. 71). They have the same comparatively high survival rate as the latter.[39]

Verrucous carcinoma

Verrucous carcinoma has remained a controversial entity. There exists a great deal of confusion in the definition and interpretation of this unusual neoplasm. Many cases reported in the literature were, in fact, well-differentiated papillary invasive squamous cell carcinomas.[40] A doubtful verrucous carcinoma of the nasopharynx bearing all the characteristics of an invasive well differentiated squamous carcinoma was reported.[41]

Adenocarcinoma

Adenocarcinomas arising from mucosal glands are occasionally found in the nasopharynx. They show the microscopical features of the corresponding salivary gland tumours including well differentiated papillary tumours, acinic cell tumours (Fig. 6.11), pleomorphic (mixed) tumours (Fig. 6.12) and adenoid cystic (cribriform) adenocarcinomas (Fig. 6.13).

Adenoid cystic carcinoma[42]

The adenoid cystic carcinoma (cribriform adenocarcinoma, cylindroma) occurs at any age but is least rare in young adults. The prognosis is very poor: although initially radiosensitive recurrence is almost inevitable, mainly because the tumour has a special propensity for infiltrating alongside and within nerves. Haematogenous metastasis is common, especially to the lungs. The histogenesis of the adenoid cystic carcinoma is uncertain. Electron microscopy shows the regular presence of intracellular myofilaments supporting the concept that the tumours are derived from myoepithelial cells.[43, 44]

Blastoma

Embryomas or blastomas are very rare tumours of the respiratory tract. A blastomatous tumour of the nasopharynx was described in a 62-year-old man. Such tumours are considered to be malignant.[45]

MALIGNANT MESENCHYMATOUS TUMOURS

Sarcomas are uncommon in the nasopharynx but cases of fibrosarcoma, rhabdomyosarcoma and chondrosarcoma have been reported. Their

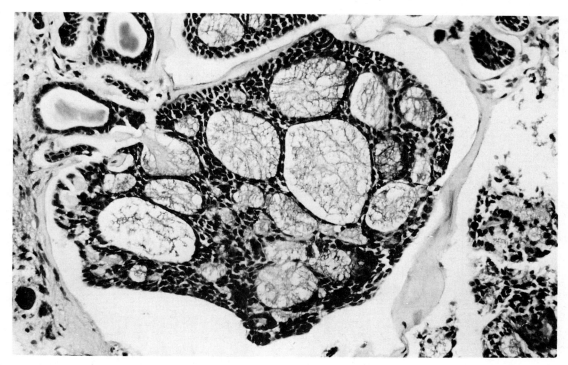

Fig. 6.13 Adenoid cystic carcinoma (cribriform adenocarcinoma) showing characteristic cribriform pattern made up of pseudocysts containing some mucoid secretion.   Haematoxylin–eosin   × 250

histological features do not differ from corresponding tumours in the nose and ear (pages 63 and 314). Here some of the presenting features in the nasopharynx will be briefly described.

Fibrosarcoma

Fibrosarcomas are least rare in adolescents and young adults but may be seen at any age. Extensive invasion of the skull may result in death well within a year of the first sign of the growth, or progress may be spread over many years, with or without recurrence after treatment. Often it is difficult to decide whether the histological picture is that of a sarcoma or of a benign lesion. In some cases there are associated angiomatoid features but these do not indicate any relation to the juvenile angiofibroma (p. 96), which is an altogether different condition, clinically as well as pathologically.[46]

Rhabdomyosarcoma (Fig. 6.14)

The lateral wall of the nasopharynx is one of the sites of election of this tumour. The patients are usually very young children and the tumour has been known to be congenital. Rapid extension into the nasal cavities and sinuses and into the base of the skull and the orbit is usual, with early death from haemorrhage, infection or widespread dissemination. The tumour is not usually very radiosensitive but multimodal chemotherapy has improved the prognosis of rhabdomyosarcoma of the head and neck in children.[47]

Chondrosarcoma

While chondrosarcomas occur in the nasopharynx they are less frequent than in other parts of the upper respiratory tract. They grow slowly and have little tendency to metastasize, although local recurrence after excision is not infrequent.

LYMPHOMA

Any variety of lymphoma may arise in the abundant lymphoreticular tissue of the nasopharynx.[48] The overall incidence, however, is not high.

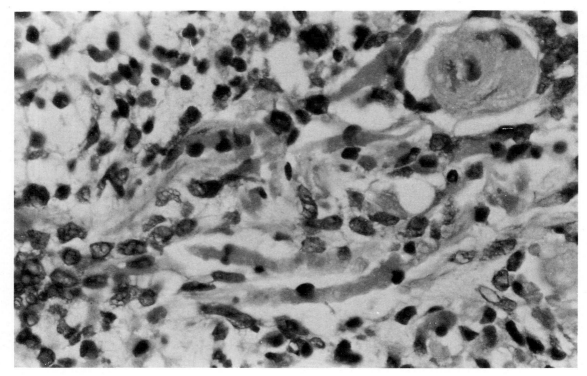

Fig. 6.14 Rhabdomyosarcoma of pleomorphic type in an 8-year-old girl to show round rhabdomyoblast and 'strap cells'. Haematoxylin–eosin × 720

Freeman et al reviewed 37 lymphomas reported in the nasopharynx.[49] In our series there were 33 malignant lymphomas among 154 neoplasms of the nasopharynx studied during the period of 1948–1971 at the Institute of Laryngology and Otology, London.

Clinical findings

The presenting symptoms in our series were nasal obstruction (54%), nasal discharge (18%), deafness (54%), epistaxis (6%), tinnitus (3%). Diplopia was not observed.

Swelling in the neck as early presenting sign was noted in 15% of the patients. There were palpable cervical lymph nodes present in 66% of the patients when first seen. The 5-year survival rate was higher (17%) than for carcinomas (10%).

Hodgkin's lymphoma

Comparatively infrequent in the nasopharynx, our series has included only one example of this tumour. The non-Hodgkin's lymphomas displayed widely different differentiation. Among the nasopharyngeal non-Hodgkin's lymphomas, large cell lymphomas predominated; formerly they were referred to as reticulum cell sarcomas.[50] There were 19 large cell lymphomas among 32 non-Hodgkin's lymphomas studied and 9 cases of diffuse lymphocytic lymphomas. 2 cases could be classified as immunoblastic lymphomas according to the classification proposed by the British National Lymphoma Investigation.[50]

PLASMACYTOMA

A plasmacytoma in the nasopharynx may be solitary or a manifestation of myelomatosis. Its occurrence in either circumstance is very much rarer than in the nose (see p. 118). As in the latter situation, electron microscopy may be helpful in the diagnosis of doubtful cases, the very characteristic and plentiful rough endoplasmic reticulum being readily demonstrated in the tumour cells.[51]

CHORDOMA

Virchow[52] described small tumours that he had found on the clivus (the sloping surface formed by the dorsum sellae and the contiguous upper surface of the basilar part of the occipital bone).[53] Because of their cartilage-like appearance he referred to these lesions as ecchondroses. He coined the word physaliphorous ('bubble-carrying') to describe the peculiar, bubble-like appearance of the cytoplasm of their constituent cells. Subsequently, Müller[54] recognized that these small lesions were derivatives of the notochord. He suggested that they should be called ecchordoses and that larger growths of comparable structure should be regarded as chordomas.

While a chordoma may arise at any site along the line of the notochord, from remnants of which it takes origin, the nasopharynx is one of the two sites most frequently involved clinically, the other being the sacrococcygeal region. Presentation in the nasopharynx is typical of chordoma arising in the base of the skull and can be associated with invasion of the cranial cavity and often of the sphenoidal sinuses and the orbits. The nasal cavity and paranasal sinuses may be involved. Compression of the brainstem and ulceration, infection and secondary haemorrhage are the outcome, the predominant manifestation being determined by the direction in which the tumour mainly extends.

Although slowly-growing tumours, chordomas cause widespread destruction of bone. They have been known to infiltrate between the dura and the bone, separating the two and extending quite widely between them. Extension alongside the petrous part of the temporal bone has been followed by penetration of the mastoid. Because of their invasiveness these cranial chordomas must be regarded as malignant tumours,[55]

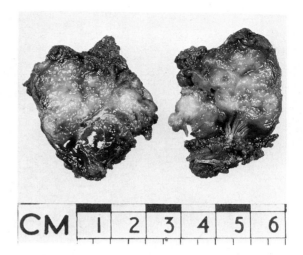

Fig. 6.15 Chordoma of the nasopharynx. Gross appearance to show lobular structure and gelatinous surface. Boy of 16.

although they seldom give rise to metastases, in contrast to their sacrococcygeal counterparts, which frequently metastasize.[56] It may be relevant that the duration of life is usually very considerably longer in the case of the latter, whereas the cranial chordomas are likely to prove fatal at a comparatively early stage as a result of their local effects and complications. A massive recurrent chordoma was described invading the intracranial cavity, the nasal cavity and the maxillary sinus.[57] A subgroup, the chondroid chordoma, has been associated with long survival.[58, 59]

Age and sex
Chordomas, whatever their site, may occur in either sex and at any age, though most of the patients are in the fourth decade.

Macroscopical appearances
Chordomas are lobulated or globular tumours, of whitish, translucent appearance, and firm or gelatinous in consistency (Fig. 6.15). Their cut surface may be loculated or solid, and there may be small or extensive foci of calcification. The bone adjoining the tumour is thinned and may be perforated, and it is unusual to find any evidence of the reactive formation of new bone.

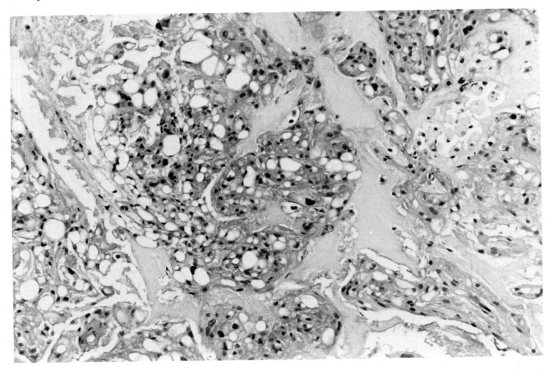

Fig. 6.16 Chordoma of the nasopharynx from a 72-year-old man. Microscopy shows groups of physaliphorous cells embedded in a mucinous matrix.   Haematoxylin–eosin   ×200

Provided by Dr J. Stewart, Essex County Hospital, Colchester, UK.

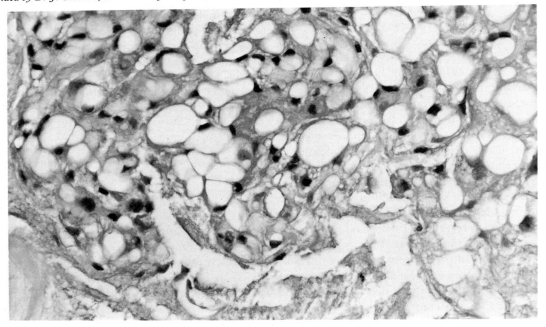

Fig. 6.17 Group of physaliphorous cells in a nasopharyngeal chordoma (as Fig. 6.16).   Haematoxylin–eosin   ×500

Provided by Dr J. Stewart, Essex County Hospital, Colchester, UK.

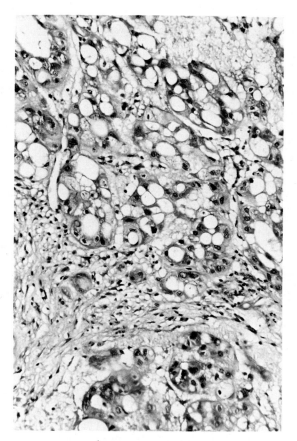

Fig. 6.18 Groups of physaliphorous cells separated by stellate cells (from another case of nasopharyngeal chordoma). Haematoxylin–eosin   × 130

These tumours can readily be mistaken macroscopically for chondromas or chondrosarcomas, craniopharyngiomas, or even secondary deposits of mucigenic or other carcinomas. The distinction between cartilaginous tumours, particularly the sarcomatous ones, and chordoma can also be difficult to establish on microscopical examination. Stewart and Cappell, in two classical papers,[60, 61] provided much of our knowledge of the light microscopy of the tumour.

Histopathology
The 'physaliphorous cells' are the characteristic feature of the histological picture. Their cytoplasm is riddled with clear vacuoles of different sizes, which are separated by fine strands of faintly eosinophilic cytoplasm (Figs 6.16–6.18). The vacuolation is often so striking that its appearance has been aptly described as frothy. The cells vary considerably in size, and may be very large, even as much as 70 μm in diameter. They are usually arranged in groups or cords, the general pattern being distinctly epithelial in character. The groups of cells are separated by a stromal matrix that has a frothy, vacuolated appearance similar to that of the cytoplasm of the chordoma cells. These vacuoles, both in the cells and in the matrix, are due to the presence of acid mucopolysaccharides, which can be demonstrated by the appropriate empirical staining methods and by histochemical studies. Another type of cell in chordomas has a stellate shape: there are usually no vacuoles in the granular cytoplasm of such cells—they may be the precursors of the physaliphorous cells.[62]

Sometimes the epithelial appearance of the tumour is accentuated by the formation of acinus-like structures that may even show papillary ingrowths. These are often formed of cuboidal cells that tend to be smaller and less vacuolated than the cells of the more characteristic areas.

In older parts of the tumour the cells are atrophic. The bulk of the tumour in these areas may consist of vacuolated ground substance. Biopsy of such an area presents considerable difficulty in interpretation, and is likely to lead to an erroneous diagnosis of chondrosarcoma. There is no staining method that is uniformly valuable for distinguishing between this type of chordomatous tissue and the ground substance of chondromas or chondrosarcomas and certain methods of silvering reticulin fibres have proved of doubtful value.[63]

In our experience chordoma can be recognized with certainty only by finding the characteristic physaliphorous cells in the mucoid matrix by light and/or electron microscopy.[62, 64] By electron microscopy intracellular tonofilaments and desmosomes have been noted in the cells of chordomas but not in chondrosarcomas.[59]

Immunocytochemical methods may prove of considerable assistance in the differential diagnosis of chordoma and chondrosarcoma by the use of specific antibodies against the intermediate filaments of the cells. Intermediate filaments form the major constituents of the cytoplasmic skeleton. It has been shown that chordomas are positive for keratin; in contrast chondrosarcomas are negative for keratin but positive for vimentin. These findings are indicative of the epithelial nature of chordoma.[65]

Chondroid chordoma[59]

This is a rare variety of chordoma and only about 30 cases of this tumour have been reported in the available literature. The differential diagnosis from chondroma of the classical type and chondrosarcoma can be difficult under the light microscope. Ultrastructural studies have discovered a helpful differential marker in the form of crystalline tubular structures within the rough endoplasmic reticulum of two chondroid chordomas.

Heterotopic pituitary adenoma

A case of heterotopic pharyngeal pituitary adenoma was described in a diabetic man in his late sixties. The tumour was easily removed from the roof of the nasopharynx.[66]

Paraganglioma

Paragangliomas form a prognostically intermediate group of neoplasms and nine cases of this rare tumour have been described in the nasopharynx.[67] Their origin is probably from paraganglionic tissue in the pterygopalatine fossa and their microscopical features are like those of paragangliomas in other sites.

REFERENCES

1. Bicknell MR. J Laryngol Otol 1967; 81: 1045.
2. Birt BD, Knight-Jones Eveline B. Br Med J 1969; iii: 281.
3. Hjertaas RJ, Morrison MD, Murray RB. J Otolaryngeal 1979; 8: 411.
4. Resta L, Santangelo A, Lastilla G. J Laryngol 1984; (in press).
5. Fu YS, Perzin KH. In: Principles and Practice of Surgical Pathology. New York. Wiley & Sons. 1983; 495.
6. Heffner D. Int J Pediat otorhinolaryngol 1983; 6: 1.
7. Robb-Smith AHTJ, Technic Meth 1937; 17: 66.
8. Teoh TB. J Path Bact 1957; 73: 451.
9. Clifford P. Int J Cancer 1970; 5: 287.
10. Payne DG. J Otolaryngol 1983; 12: 197.
11. Marsden HB. In: Duncan W, ed. Paediatric oncology. Berlin: Springer, 1983: 22.
12. Shanmaguratnam k, Sobin LH et al. Histological typing of upper resp tract tumours. Geneva: WHO, 1978: 19; 19.
13. Altmannsberger M, Osborn M, Schauer A, Weber K. Lab Invest 1981; 45: 427.
14. Madri JA, Barwick KW. Am J Surg Pathol 1982; 6: 143.
15. Nagle RB, McDaniel KM, Clark VA, Payne Claire M. Am J Clin Pathol 1983; 79: 458.
16. Gusterson BA, Mitchell DP, Warburton MJ, Carter RL. J Clin Pathol 1983; 36: 628.
17. Osborn M, Weber K. Lab Invest 1983; 48: 372.
18. Miettinen M, Lehto VP, Virtanen I. Virchows Arch (Cell Pathol) 1982; 40: 163.
19. Prathap K, Looi LM, Prasad U. Histopathology 1983; 8: 27.
20. Shanmuguratnam K, Chan SH, de-The G, Goh JEH, Kohr TH, Simons MJ, Tye CY. Cancer 1979; 44: 1029.
21. Regaud C, Crémieu R. C R Soc Biol (Paris) 1912; 72: 523.
22. Schmincke A. Beitr Pathol Anat 1921; 58: 161.
23. Cappell DF. J Pathol Bacteriol 1934; 39: 49.
24. Yeh S. Cancer 1962; 15: 895.
25. Friedmann I, Osborn DA. In: Systemic pathology. 2nd ed. Vol. 1. Edinburgh: Churchill Livingstone, 1974; 240.
26. Applebaum EL, Montravardi P, Haas R. Laryngoscope 1982; 92: 510.
27. Hsu MM, Huang SC, Lynn TC, Hsieh TI, Tu SM. Otolaryngol Head Neck Surg 1982; 90: 289.
28. Wei WI. Clin Oncol 1984; 10: 225.
29. Baker SR, Wolfe RA. Cancer 1982; 49: 163.
30. Epstein MA, North JR. In: McMichael AJ, Fabre JW, eds. Monoclonal Antibodies in Clinical Medicine. London: Academic Press, 1984; 278.
31. De Schryver A, Friberg S Jr, Klein G et al. Clin Exp Immunol 1969; 5: 443.
32. Costa J. Hum Pathol 1981; 12: 386.
33. Trumper PA, Epstein MA, Giovanella BC. J Cancer 1976; 17: 578.
34. Arnold W. Acta Otolaryngol (Stockh) 1983; 95: 447.
35. Achong BG, Trumper PA, Giovanella BC. Br J Cancer 1976; 34: 203.
36. Hirsch NS, Phillips SM, Solnik C, Black PH, Schwartz RS, Carpenter CB. Proc Natl Acad Sci USA 1972; 69: 1069.
37. Batsakis JG, Solomon AR, Rice DH. Head Neck Surg 1981; 3: 511.
38. Yeh S. Cancer 1962; 15: 895.
39. Osborn DA. Cancer (Philad) 1970; 25: 50.
40. McDonald JS, Crissman JD, Gluckman JL. Head Neck Surg 1982; 5: 22.
41. Jahn AF, Walter JB, Farkashidy J. J Otolaryngol 1980; 9: 84.
42. Conley J, Dingman DL. Arch Otolaryngol 1974; 100: 81.
43. Lawrence JB, Mazur MT. Hum Pathol 1982; 13: 916.
44. Batsakis JG, Kraemer B, Sciuba JJ. Head Neck Surg 1983; 5: 222.
45. Meinecke R, Bauer F, Skouras J, Mottu F. Cancer 1976; 38: 818.

46. Shanmugaratnam K, Sobin LH, et al. Histological Typing of upper res tract tumours. Geneva: WHO, 1978; 20.
47. Schuller DE, Lawrence TL, Newton WA Jr. Arch Otolaryngol 1979; 105: 689.
48. Wilder WH, Harner SG, Banks PM. Arch Otolaryngol 1983; 109: 310.
49. Freeman C, Berg JW, Cutler SJ. Cancer 1972; 29: 252.
50. Henry K. Clin Radiol 1981; 32: 481.
51. Booth JB, Cheesman AD, Vincenti NH. Annals Otol Rhinol Laryngol 1973, 82: 709.
52. Virchow R. Virchows Arch Pathol Anat 1857; 11: 79.
53. Horten BC, Montague SR. Virchows Arch [Pathol Anat] 1976; 371: 295.
54. Müller H. Z Rationelle Med 3rd series 1858; 2: 202.
55. Campbell WM, McDonald TJ, Unni KK, Laws ER. Laryngoscope 1980; 90: 4: 612.
56. Volpe R, Mazabraud A. Amer J Surg Pathol 1983; 7: 161.
57. Miller RH, Woodson GE, Neely JG, Murphy EC. Otolaryngol Head Neck Surg 1982; 90: 251.
58. Heffelfinger MJ, Dahlin DC, MacCarty CS et al. Cancer 1983; 32: 410.
59. Valderama E, Kahn LB. Am J Surg Pathol 1983; 7: 625.
60. Stewart MJ. J Pathol Bacteriol 1922; 25: 40.
61. Cappell DF. J Pathol Bacteriol 1928; 31: 797.
62. Friedmann I, Harrison DFN, Bird ES. J Clin Path 1962; 15: 116.
63. Crawford T. J Clin Path 1958; 11: 110.
64. Pardo-Mindan J, Guillen FJ, Villas C, Vazquez JJ. Cancer 1981; 47: 2611.
65. Miettinen M, Veli-Pekka Lehto, Dahl D, Virtanen I. Am J Pathol 1983; 112: 160.
66. Kopf PO, Kopf R, Nickol HJ. HNO 1983; 31: 28.
67. Schuller DE, Lucas JG. Arch Otolaryngol 1982; 108: 667.

PART THREE

I. Friedmann

The tonsils and oropharynx

7

Anatomy and histology
Inflammatory diseases

ANATOMICAL CONSIDERATIONS

The oropharynx varies greatly in shape and size owing to the movements of the tongue, which lies in front of it, and of the soft palate, which forms its upper limit. During swallowing the oropharynx is roofed by the soft palate. Its posterior wall is continuous with the posterior wall of the nasopharynx. The oropharynx becomes the hypopharynx at the level of the top of the epiglottis.

The paired tonsils (faucial tonsils) occupy the tonsillar fossae, which are triangular depressions of the lateral walls of the oropharynx, bounded in front by the palatoglossal arch and behind by the palatopharyngeal arch, and merging with the back of the tongue below. The fully grown tonsil is almond-shaped, 20–25 mm long, 15 mm wide and about 10 mm thick; its long axis is almost vertical. The upper pole may be partly embedded within the soft palate; the lower pole may be continuous with the lingual tonsil. The healthy tonsil does not project into the buccopharyngeal cavity beyond the plane of the faucial pillars. The medial aspect of the tonsil is covered by thin, firmly adherent stratified squamous epithelium which dips into the tonsillar crypts; there are between 10 and 20 of the latter and they penetrate the substance of the tonsil almost to its capsule. There is a distinct cleft in the upper part of many tonsils, and the part of the tonsil above the cleft may be covered by a mucosal fold, the plica semilunaris.

A similar fold, the plica triangularis, covers the lower anterior part of the tonsil in the fetus, the space between it and the tonsil being the tonsillar sinus. In most cases, this space is obliterated after birth, but it may persist and—in common with the other infoldings of epithelium described above—predispose to infection.

The lateral aspect of the tonsils is covered by a thin but distinct fibrous capsule, septa from which traverse the tonsillar tissue. The capsule is part of the pharyngeal aponeurosis but is separated from the muscle in the pharyngeal wall by loose areolar tissue, so that the whole tonsil can be moved quite freely on the underlying structures.

There are no afferent lymphatic vessels in the tonsil. Efferent lymphatic vessels can often be seen immediately under the surface epithelium. They pass to the upper deep cervical lymph nodes, and terminate particularly in a node situated immediately below and behind the angle of the mandible (the jugulodigastric or tonsillar lymph node).

Histological structure

The stratified squamous epithelium that covers the surface of the tonsils and lines their crypts is not keratinized. In the depths of the crypts, and particularly in the secondary crypts that open laterally from the main crypts, the epithelium is often very thin and may be obscured by the abundance of lymphocytes that is characteristic of the part. There is always some degree of lymphocytic infiltration of the tonsillar epithelium, even in 'healthy' tonsils.

In contrast to the lingual tonsil, the mucous glands in the vicinity of the faucial tonsils do not open into the tonsillar crypts, and consequently there is no adequate means of keeping the crypts clear of desquamated cell debris and food particles that may accumulate in them. Such emptying of the crypts as occurs is probably effected mainly by the massaging movements of the oropharyngeal muscles.

The lymphoid tissue of the tonsils generally lies immediately deep to the epithelium, although, particularly in adults, it may be separated from the latter by a narrow zone of fibrous tissue. It consists of well-formed lymphoid follicles, which may contain conspicuous germinal centres.[1, 2] The follicles may be closely packed, or they may be separated by varying amounts of looser-textured lymphoreticular

tissue. The lymphoid tissue of the tonsil, in contrast to that of lymph nodes, is devoid of lymph sinuses.

The B and T lymphocytes are distributed in a characteristic manner in the tonsil, as in the lymph nodes: the B cells are located in the lymph follicles and the T cells in the perifollicular tissue. The germinal centres may contain a small number of T lymphocytes.

The lymphocytes in the tonsils react to contact with antigens by the production of immunoglobulins which accumulate in the tonsil.[3] Polysaccharides and lipopolysaccharides derived from microbial membranes may cause abundant proliferation of the tonsillar lymphocytes.[4]

Involution of the palatine tonsils is a common feature of advancing age and can commence as early as 10 years.[5] The number of T lymphocytes increases with age and that of B lymphocytes decreases; this may be one of the underlying causes of chronic tonsillitis in the adult.

INFLAMMATORY DISEASES

Acute pharyngitis and tonsillitis

Aetiology

Acute tonsillitis is, essentially, a particular manifestation of an acute inflammation of the pharynx as a whole. The aggregation of lymphoreticular tissue that forms the tonsils and the tenuous epithelial lining of the depths of their crypts render the tonsils specially liable to be involved in infections that affect the throat. These infections are most frequently caused by beta-haemolytic streptococci, generally of Lancefield type A. Occasionally, *Streptococcus pneumoniae* and even *Staphylococcus aureus* may be responsible. In other cases, viruses of the adenovirus group may be implicated.[6, 7] In a study of samples from 204 tonsils and 186 adenoids, Israel[7] found that 26% of the former and 58% of the latter harboured adenoviruses of types 1, 2 or 5. Two strains of herpes simplex virus were also isolated, but influenza viruses, enteroviruses and salivary gland viruses were not encountered.[6]

In a microbial study of 248 children (1–10 years) who presented with acute tonsillitis, beta-haemolytic streptococci (mainly group A) were isolated from 129 (53%) of 244 cases and as the sole pathogen from 83 (47%) of 178 cases. Beta-haemolytic streptococci were especially common over the age of 6 years (68% of children) and relatively uncommon under the age of 4 years (18%). The potentially nephritogenic serotypes 4 and 12 were frequent and accounted for 42 (47%) of typable strains.[8]

Acute tonsillitis is a frequent complication of infectious mononucleosis and of agranulocytosis. In the latter condition, which can be caused by a wide range of myelotoxic drugs, the tonsillar region and surrounding pharyngeal wall may be covered by a grey, necrotic membrane, removal of which reveals severe ulceration of the mucous membrane. A similar picture is often seen in acute leukaemia. Diphtheria is considered below.

Clinical features
Intense hyperaemia of the mucosa develops, often with some swelling due to inflammatory ex-udate, and patchy ulceration of the pharynx may soon follow.

Although the whole of Waldeyer's ring, com-posed of the palatine, nasopharyngeal and lingual tonsils and the scattered laryngeal lymphoid tissue is affected, the involvement of the palatine tonsils is always prominent. The lesion takes one of two forms—acute follicular tonsillitis and acute parenchymatous tonsillitis. In both, the tonsils are enlarged and intensely hyperaemic, part of their surface may be covered by muco-purulent exudate and there may be small ero-sions. In acute follicular tonsillitis* the surface is studded with white or yellow spots that are, in fact, the crypts distended with collections of pus cells (Fig. 7.1), desquamated epithelium and other debris. In acute parenchymatous tonsillitis the entire lymphoid tissue of the tonsil is in-flamed and involvement of the crypts is often less striking.

Complications of streptococcal pharyngitis
Acute streptococcal pharyngitis occasionally

---

* It may be noted that the 'follicles' referred to in this traditional name are the tonsillar crypts (which used to be called follicles) and not the lymphoid follicles of the paren-chyma.

gives rise to a spreading cellulitis of the tissue of the neck, with very marked, brawny inflamma-tory oedema (Ludwig's angina*).[9, 10] In other cases, the infection spreads through the lymph-atics to the lymph nodes in front of the prever-tebral fascia, and a retropharyngeal abscess may then result. A retropharyngeal abscess may extend throughout the retropharyngeal space and cause necrotizing mediastinitis[10] or it may rup-ture into the pharynx, in which case aspiration of pus into the respiratory tract is likely to follow, causing streptococcal bronchopneumonia or, sometimes, a lung abscess. Streptococcal abscesses in the retropharyngeal space may be confused with cold abscesses that result from tuberculous osteomyelitis of the cervical verte-brae. The tuberculous cold abscess, however, is usually confined behind the prevertebral fascia, and tends therefore to track downward and later-ally in the plane of the muscles attached to the vertebrae.

Peritonsillar abscess, or quinsy, is a complica-tion of streptococcal tonsillitis, and presents a well-defined, fluctuant swelling above and to one side of the tonsil. Sometimes the condition is bi-lateral. Acute oedema of the glottis, which may gravely obstruct the airway, is another occasional complication.

In addition to these local effects of streptococ-cal infection, there are two important complica-tions of a systemic nature. The first, and less common, is streptococcal septicaemia; the other is the occurrence of allergic sensitization to the organism or its products, with the development some 1–2 weeks later of acute rheumatic fever or acute glomerulonephritis.

From the pathological standpoint, there is no difference between the local manifestations of the common form of streptococcal pharyngitis and those of the streptococcal pharyngitis of scarlet fever. Scarlet fever, with its typical rash,

---

* The old term angina is currently used both to describe the symptomatic pain of myocardial ischaemia associated with relative insufficiency of the coronary circulation ('angina pec-toris') and as the generic name for certain types of ulcerative pharyngitis (for example, Ludwig's angina, Vincent's angina, and the 'anginose form' of infectious mononucleosis). Its use in the second sense more nearly reflects the original meaning of the word, which implied choking by obstruction of the throat, and the associated sensation of compression.

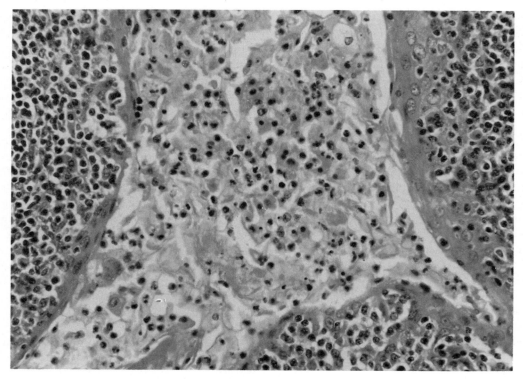

Fig. 7.1 Acute tonsillitis. Tonsillar crypt containing purulent exudate.
Haematoxylin–eosin   × 125

develops when the infecting strain of streptococcus is one that produces erythrogenic toxin (provided that the patient has not formed specific antitoxic antibodies as a result of previous infection).

Diphtheria

Formerly, faucial infection was the commonest clinical manifestation of diphtheria. The massive decline in the incidence of this disease during the present century in most prosperous countries has been one of the great triumphs of preventive medicine.

60 years ago, there were about 10 000 deaths yearly from diphtheria in England and Wales, whereas today, in most years, there are fewer than 10. This decline must be ascribed mainly to the widespread practice of active immunization during early childhood, although other changes, among them the greater prevalence of the less toxigenic varieties of *Corynebacterium diphtheriae* may also have played a part. There are many today who are unfamiliar with this disease, clinically and pathologically. Recent reports of outbreaks and accompanying fatalities demand a renewal of interest.[11]

In a typical case one or both tonsils and often some extent of the adjoining faucial and palatal mucosa are covered by a tough, whitish membrane. Removal of the membrane leaves bleeding points on a raw, necrotic surface. There is marked hyperaemia and oedema of the tissues and the breath has a characteristic smell that, once appreciated, may become of diagnostic value to the practitioner. There is always a marked enlargement of the regional lymph nodes, often with brawny oedema of the surrounding tissues.

Microscopically, the membrane consists mainly of fibrinous exudate that has formed on the necrotic surface of the infected tissue. The characteristic diphtheria bacilli are demonstrable in it. In the underlying lymphoid tissue there is often focal necrosis, particularly in the follicles. The bacilli remain confined to the infected mu-

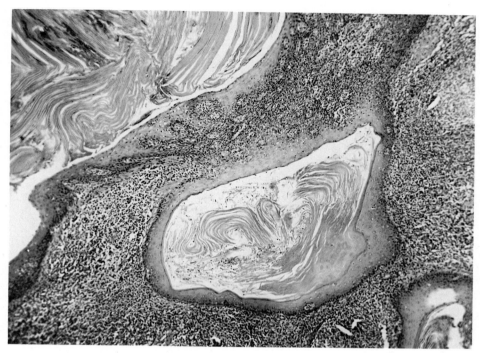

Fig. 7.2a Chronic tonsillitis. Dilated crypts filled with keratin.
Haematoxylin–eosin   × 50

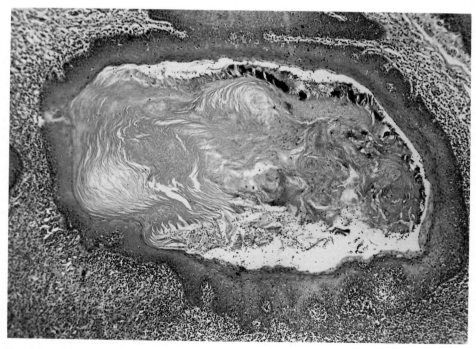

Fig. 7.2b Chronic tonsillitis Cross section of dilated crypt filled with keratin.
Haematoxylin–eosin   × 50

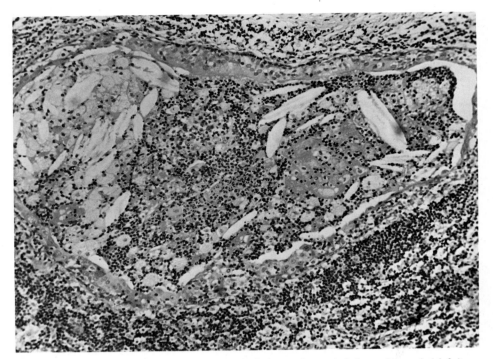

Fig. 7.3 Chronic tonsillitis. Distended crypt containing mixed cellular exudate and cholesterol crystals (clefts). Haematoxylin–eosin   × 140

cosal surface, the inflammatory reaction and necrosis in the underlying tissue and in the regional lymph nodes being a manifestation of the action of the absorbed exotoxin of the organisms, although in a few cases there may be a superimposed infection of the deeper tissues by beta-haemolytic streptococci.

The dangers of diphtheria are twofold. First, the effects of the bacillary toxin on the myocardium and nervous system may prove fatal. Second, extension of the infection to the larynx and trachea may be followed by obstruction of the airways by the membrane.

Nasal diphtheria is referred to in Chapter 2; cutaneous diphtheria may be mentioned here.[12, 13, 14] It is very much rarer in temperate climates than in the tropics. The typical lesion is an ulcer with a well-defined, irregular margin. The base of the ulcer is covered with a grey slough that is difficult to remove, and it is here that the diphtheria bacilli thrive. Absorption of their exotoxin as from other sites affected can produce peripheral neuropathy, paralysis of accommodation, and heart block. In some cases,

the patient is more concerned by symptoms due to the intoxication than by the ulcer. As in cases of fauciopharyngeal diphtheria, there may be severe lymphadenitis.

Chronic tonsillitis

Chronic non-specific tonsillitis is a controversial condition. Although its existence is denied by some authorities there can be no doubt that the clinicopathological state to which this name is commonly applied is not merely a manifestation of the physiological role of the tonsils in dealing with infected material. The principal features of these chronically inflamed tonsils are lymphoid hyperplasia, distension of the crypts and fibrosis of the parenchyma. The distended crypts contain keratin plugs, resulting from keratinization and desquamation of the lining epithelium (Fig. 7.2a, b); cholesterol esters may crystallize in the debris (Fig. 7.3) and neutrophils and lymphocytes accumulate. Large colonies of microorganisms may form, particularly in the deeper parts of the crypts. The organisms are usually cocci. Colonies of actinomycetes are by no means uncommon; in

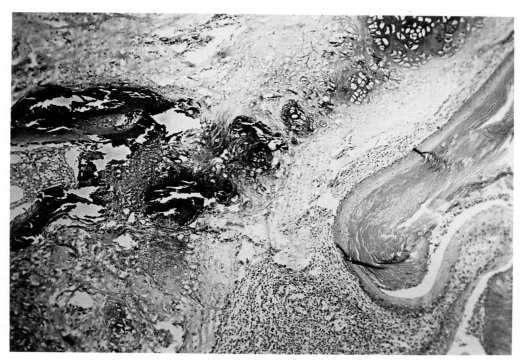

Fig. 7.4 Chronic tonsillitis. Metaplastic formation of cartilage and bone in the fibrotic tonsil. Haematoxylin–eosin × 75

some cases cultures have confirmed that these are *Actinomyces israelii*, but oftener they are non-pathogenic organisms such as *Leptothrix buccalis*. The significance of these actinomycetes in the tonsillar crypts is uncertain, but in the great majority of cases it seems likely that they are merely saprophytes. Careful microscopical examination of sections, however, may show unequivocal superficial invasion of the tonsillar parenchyma by the mycelium (tonsillomycosis).

Extensive fibrosis or focal scarring may be found in the tonsils as a sequel of attacks of acute tonsillitis, whether there had been abscess formation or not. The metaplastic formation of cartilage and bone has been observed in the scar tissue in such cases (Fig. 7.4).

Calcareous concretions (tonsilloliths) may form in the crypts in cases of chronic tonsillitis.[15] Such calculi may be single or multiple, and minute in size or up to 2–3 cm and more in diameter.

Chronic tonsillitis and the concept of 'focal sepsis'
Much less emphasis is nowadays placed upon focal infection as a cause of general disease than was formerly the custom. When considering the possibility that foci of chronic infection may be a contributory factor in the causation or persistence of any illness, it is imperative that all the evidence be weighed carefully before advising surgical procedures. Thus it must not be overlooked that a patient who has obviously diseased faucial tonsils may also have chronic infection of the nasal sinuses, the adenoid, the lingual tonsils or the teeth. There is no convincing evidence that wholesale surgical attack on multiple foci of chronic infection is specifically beneficial in cases of chronic diseases such as polyarthritis and psychoses.

It is noteworthy that chronic enlargement of the tonsils, with cheesy debris in the crypts, may be found in people who are clearly in good health otherwise. In fact, it is chronic inflammation of small, partly buried tonsils or of the foci of tonsillar tissue that remain after incomplete surgical removal that is most likely to cause symptoms. These symptoms include recurrent attacks of pharyngitis, persisting enlargement and possibly tenderness of the tonsillar lymph nodes, and discomfort in the throat. It is in such cases that tonsillectomy is likely to benefit the patient.

All tonsils excised ought to be submitted for histopathological investigation with modern methods employed in the study of lymphoreticular tissue in health and disease. Now that wholesale tonsillectomies are no longer performed no department of histopathology would be inundated by 'normal' tonsils.

CHRONIC SPECIFIC INFECTIONS

Tuberculosis

Tuberculosis of the tonsils may be primary, in which case the tonsillar lesion is almost always of microscopical extent only, the primary complex being represented clinically only by the involvement of the cervical lymph nodes.

Tonsillar tuberculosis is by far the commonest antecedent of tuberculous cervical lymphadenitis, and the picture is comparable to that of primary abdominal tuberculosis, in which the primary focus in the lymphoid tissue of the intestine is so unobstrusive that it is only rarely found, whereas the associated tuberculous mesenteric lymphadenitis is generally conspicuous. In many cases of primary tuberculosis the organism was *Mycobacterium bovis*: with eradication of tuberculosis in cattle and general pasteurization of milk this form of tonsillitis has become much rarer.

The tonsils frequently become infected in the course of chronic pulmonary tuberculosis. In one recorded series of 122 necropsies in cases of pulmonary tuberculosis, 91 presented tuberculous lesions in one or other tonsil and 76 had similar lesions in the corresponding upper cervical lymph nodes.[16] In those parts of the world where the great decline in mortality from tuberculosis has been manifest in recent decades, all these forms of the disease are much less common than formerly.

Syphilis

The tonsil is one of the rarer sites of a primary chancre. Although, like most syphilitic ulcers, the lesion may be painless, it is very liable to secondary infection, particularly by the organisms of Vincent's disease. The pain that then follows may be considerable, and by putting the doctor or dentist off guard, may expose him to a serious risk of infection. The presence of nonpathogenic oral treponemes that more or less closely resemble *Treponema pallidum* adds to the difficulty of diagnosing syphilitic lesions in the mouth, and may cause serious errors in the interpretation of the findings in films examined by dark-ground illumination.

The mucous patches and serpiginous ulcers typical of the secondary stage of syphilis may be seen on the tonsils. In the tertiary stage, gumma of the tonsil has been recorded: such lesions may be difficult to distinguish from carcinoma or other malignant tumours clinically, and from caseous tuberculosis microscopically.

Tularaemia

Tularaemia, an infectious disease caused by *Francisella tularensis*, is a rare cause of pharyngitis and tonsillitis. An 8-year-old boy was described with bilateral tonsillar enlargement and cervical lymphadenopathy.[17] Because of his long-standing febrile condition serological tests were carried out, resulting in an agglutinin titre of 1:5120 for tularaemia.

Mycoses

The condition that is conventionally referred to as tonsillomycosis has been mentioned (p. 167): the term 'tonsillomycosis' is best restricted to this usage.

Any of the deep mycoses may involve one or both tonsils, histoplasmosis (Fig. 7.5) (particularly African histoplasmosis, caused by *Histoplasma duboisii*) and rhinosporidiosis being perhaps likelier than others to be found in these sites.

Many patients with progressive disseminated histoplasmosis have oropharyngeal lesions. The predominant sites, in descending order of occurrence, are the tongue, palate, tonsil and buccal mucosa.[18] The painful lesions may be nodular, ulcerating or forming plaques. Most of the ulcers begin as small plaques or nodules which ultimately undergo central necrosis. The lesions are often accompanied by enlarged cervical lymphnodes.[18]

Microscopy shows an inflammatory tuberculoid granulation tissue with giant cells containing

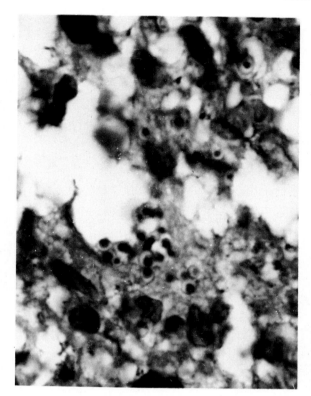

Fig. 7.5 Histoplasmosis. Note yeast form of *Histoplasma capsulatum* in a degenerated giant cell.

Periodic-acid/Schiff × 1200

the yeast form of the organism (Fig. 7.5). The organism stains distinctly with PAS and Grocott techniques. Necrosis and caseation is common, as well as pseudoepitheliomatous hyperplasia of the non-ulcerated surface epithelium. In common with other mycotic granulomas, this microscopical feature has been mistaken for carcinoma.

The diagnosis can be made by culturing the organism and biopsy or by the demonstration of the causative agent by indirect serologic methods.

Rhinosporidiosis of the tonsils may cause polypoid superficial lesions or a more uniform enlargement of the affected part; the characteristic sporangia are conspicuous in histological sections.

Leishmaniasis

Leishmaniasis of the tonsil is rare, although it may present as the primary manifestation of the disease.[19]

MALAKOPLAKIA

Malakoplakia (see pp. 138, 280) may occur in the upper respiratory tract and two cases have been described in the palatine tonsil.[20, 21] The lesion may be associated with various microbial and neoplastic conditions and in one of the tonsillar cases a soft tumour-like non-ulcerated mass was noted projecting from the surface of the right palatine tonsil. Microscopy revealed the presence of the characteristic Michaelis–Gutmann bodies and *Escherichia coli* was grown repeatedly from the tissues.

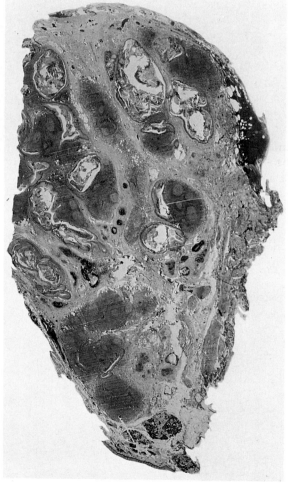

Fig. 7.6 Chronic tonsillitis. The enlarged tonsil contains many keratin cysts in a fibrous stroma. The lymphoid content appears to be reduced.

Haematoxylin–eosin × 6

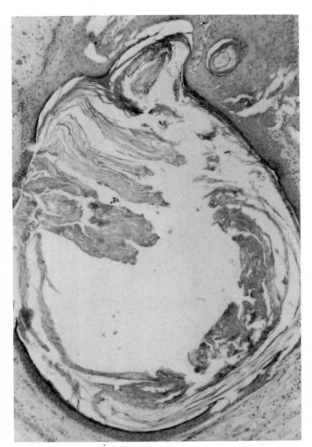

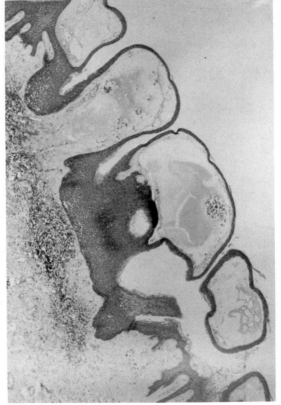

Fig. 7.7 Chronic tonsillitis. Detail of cyst lined by squamous epithelium and filled with laminated keratin.

Haematoxylin–eosin   × 30

Fig. 7.8 Bullous tonsillitis. The surface of the tonsil is covered by intraepithelial bullae filled with proteinaceous fluid.   Haematoxylin–eosin   × 35

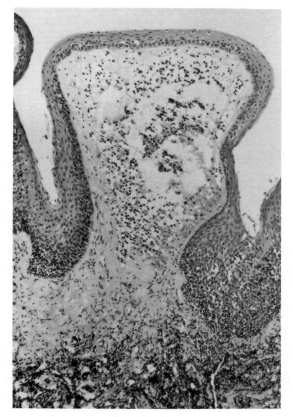

Fig. 7.9 Bullous tonsillitis. Detail of bulla in the squamous epithelium containing some proteinaceous fluid with few lymphocytes.

Haematoxylin-eosin   ×80

REFERENCES

1. Curran RC, Jones EL. Clin Exp Immunol 1978; 31: 251.
2. Crocker J. J Pathol 1981; 134: 81.
3. Curran RC, Jones EL. Clin Exp Immunol 1977; 28: 103.
4. Jannossy G, Greaves M. Transplant Rev 1975; 24: 177.
5. Siegel G. Int J Pediatr Otorhinolaryngol 1983; 6: 61.
6. Tyrrell DAJ, Balducci D, Zaiman TE. Lancet 1956; 2: 1326.
7. Israel MS. J Pathol Bacteriol 1962; 84: 169.
8. Douglas RM, Miles H, Hansman D, Fadejevs A, Moore B, Bollen MD. Pathology 1984; 16: 79.
9. Ludwig WF von. Med Corresp BL Württemb Ärztl Vereins 1836; 6: 21 (English translation in: Bull Hist Med 1939; 7: 1115).
10. Brondbo K et al. Otolaryngol Head Neck Surg 1983; 12: 50.
11. Anderson GS, Penfold JB. J Clin Pathol 1973; 26: 606.
12. Reiss F. Arch Derm Syph (Chic) 1947; 56: 216.
13. Robert P. Dermatologica 1947; 94: 334.
14. Haber H, Milne JA, Symmers WStC In: Systemic Pathology, 2nd ed. Vol. 6. Edinburgh: Churchill Livingstone, 1980; 2738.
15. Baumann J. HNO 1983; 31: 399.
16. Long ER, Faust R. Am J Pathol 1941; 17: 697.
17. Wills PI, Gedosh EA, Nichols DR, Smith F. Laryngoscope 1982; 92: 770.
18. Young L. Mycologia mycopathologia applicata 1972; 22: 65.
19. Laudadio P. J Laryngol Otol 1984; 98: 213.
20. Kalfayan B, Seager GM. Am J Clin Pathol 1982; 78: 390.
21. Destombes P, Loubière R, Fontanel A et al. Arch Opht 1975; 35: 427.

KERATOSIS

Keratosis is characterized by the appearance of whitish, horny projections on the surface of the tonsils or the formation of keratin cysts (Figs 7.6, 7.7). The condition is usually bilateral; it usually involves the lingual tonsil also, and often the wall of the pharynx. It is commoner in women, and most of the patients are aged between 15 and 40 years. The essential lesion is keratinization of the epithelial lining of the crypts of the tonsils, and of small areas of the pharyngeal mucosa. Intraepithelial bullous vesicles may form (Figs 7.8, 7.9).

8

Neoplasms of the tonsillar region

When considering tumours of the faucial tonsils it is necessary to take into account the growths that arise from the faucial pillars between which the tonsils lie. This reflects the impossibility in many cases of deciding whether a carcinoma has arisen from the epithelium covering the tonsil itself or from that of the adjacent pillars.

TUMOUR-LIKE LESIONS AND BENIGN TUMOURS

Aggressive fibromatosis

This tumour-like lesion occurs usually in the abdominal wall (desmoid tumour). It consists of bundles or whorls of fibrous tissue and may be difficult to differentiate from a fibrosarcoma (Figs 8.1–8.3). The aetiology is unknown but trauma and scar formation have been implicated in its development. Recurrence is common but metastasis does not occur.[1,2]

Squamous papilloma

The commonest benign tumour of this region is the squamous papilloma (Figs 8.4, 8.5)—it accounted for more than a third of a series of 278 benign and malignant tumours of the region studied at the Institute of Laryngology and Otology, London. The papilloma usually arises from a faucial pillar: fewer than a quarter develop on the tonsil itself. Keratinization of these lesions is uncommon. Although they occasionally recur after removal, malignant change is almost unknown.

Lymphangioma

Next in frequency, but much less common than the papilloma, is the lymphangioma, which

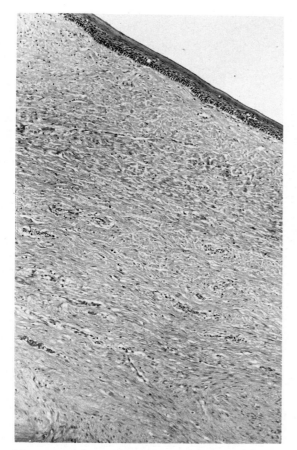

Fig. 8.1 Aggressive fibromatosis. Low-power picture of fi-bromatous lesion arising from the post-tonsillectomy bed. Its surface is covered by squamous epithelium. The specimen was from a young girl of 10 years who has developed a firm well defined tumour following tonsillectomy which recurred after excision. There was some central ulceration of the overlying mucosa. This case underlines the importance of submitting the tonsils for histopathological examination.

Haematoxylin–eosin   × 45

Provided by Dr A Stevens, University Hospital, Nottingham, UK.

generally presents as a pedunculate mass attached to the surface of the tonsil (Fig. 8.6). It consists of dilated and distorted lymphatics (Fig. 8.7a, b). Whether it is a hamartoma or an acquired lymph-angiectatic formation is debatable.

Rarer benign neoplasms
These include haemangiomas, fibromas, lipomas and Schwannomas (Fig. 8.8).

MALIGNANT NEOPLASMS

A survey of about 1900 tonsillar neoplasms re-corded in the otolaryngological registry of the Armed Forces Institute of Pathology, Washington, DC, over a period of 31 years (1945–1976) revealed 378 benign and 1535 malignant tumours of the tonsillar region.[3]

In the series of 278 benign and malignant tumours of the tonsillar region studied at the Institute of Laryngology and Otology, London, there were 73 carcinomas, 78 malignant lymphomas and one malignant melanoma. This study indicated no clinical features that enable the carcinomas and the lymphomas to be distinguished with certainty. Gross ulceration is common among tumours of each group, but rather less so in cases of lymphoma than in carcinoma. Bilateral disease is usual in lymphoma but may occur in carcinoma.

Lymph node enlargement in association with tonsillar lymphoma is usually due to the neoplastic disease itself but occasionally the enlargement may be inflammatory in nature and not caused by metastasis.

Carcinoma

Incidence
Carcinoma of the tonsil is one of the commonest cancers of the head and neck, comprising 10% of oral cancers and about 2% of all carcinomas in the region. In the USA there are approximately 12 000 new cases of carcinoma of the tonsil in a year.[4]

Age and sex
The greatest incidence of carcinoma is in the seventh decade and of lymphoma a decade earlier. There is a considerable overlap of the age incidence of the two groups and more cases have been occurring in younger persons than previously. Both groups of tumours affect males predominantly; the preponderance of males is much greater (about 5:1) in cases of carcinoma. A Canadian review[5] of 372 cases of tonsillar carcinoma noted a similar age distribution and a male:female ratio of about 2:1, which is lower than in other series.

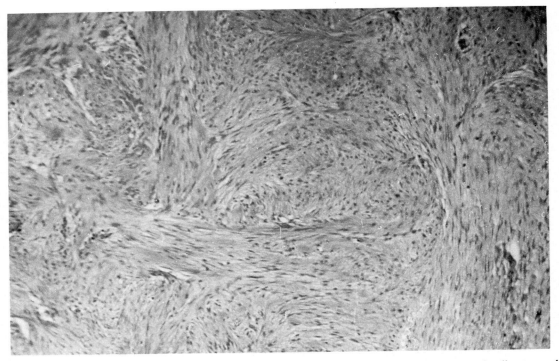

Fig. 8.2 Aggressive fibromatosis. Bundles of fibroblasts forming a storiform pattern of spindle-shaped cells arranged in cartwheel-like formation around narrow vessels (same specimen as Fig. 8.1).   Haematoxylin–eosin   × 160

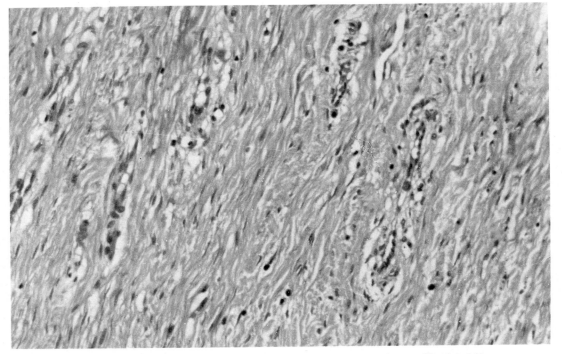

Fig. 8.3 Aggressive fibromatosis. A richly vascularized area of the tumour (same specimen as Figs 8.1, 8.2).
Haematoxylin–eosin   × 160

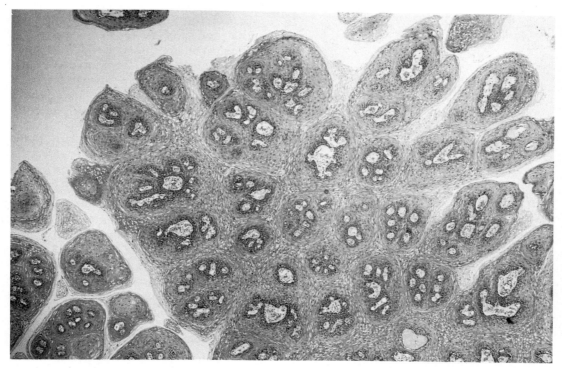

Fig. 8.4 Squamous cell papilloma of the tonsil showing the characteristic papillary pattern formed by proliferating squamous epithelium covering thin fibrovascular stalks.   Haematoxylin–eosin   × 50

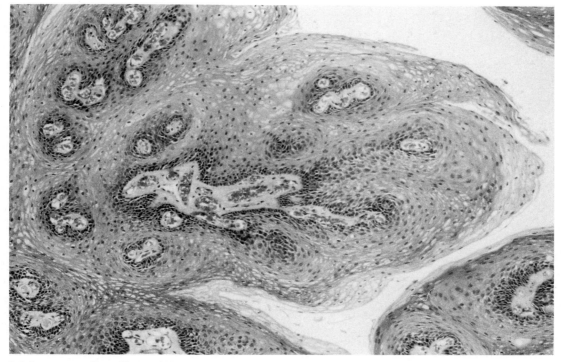

Fig. 8.5 Squamous cell papilloma of the tonsil. The squamous epithelium covering the central fibrovascular stalk displays uniform nuclei.   Haematoxylin–eosin   × 125

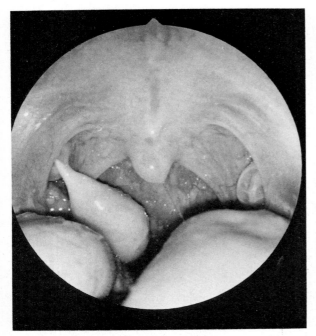

Fig. 8.6 Lymphangioma tonsil. Polypoid structure attached by a thin stalk to the soft palate.

Provided by Dr F. Hiraide, National Defense Medical College, Japan and the Editor, Journal of Laryngology.

An analysis of 142 clinically-diagnosed cases of tonsillar cancer at the Christian Medical College Hospital, Vellore, India, during 1968 to 1977 showed a male preponderance of 95%.[6] Most patients presented in an advanced stage, often with spread to the cervical lymph nodes. There were distant metastases in 8 cases, in bone in 5 cases (the skull in 3 and the pelvis in 2), in mediastinal lymph nodes in 2 cases, and in the subcutaneous tissues of the chest wall in 1 case.

Dysplasia and carcinoma in situ
The squamous epithelium covering the tonsils and the surrounding oropharyngeal mucosa displays morphological changes similar to those observed elsewhere (see larynx, p. 218). Hyperplasia, dysplasia and carcinoma in situ occurs and may, in inadequately removed biopsy specimens, disguise the true invasive nature of a tonsillar lesion.

Squamous carcinoma
Grossly, squamous carcinoma of the tonsil presents as an ulcer, as a tumour mass or as a mucosal discoloration. The ulcer appears crater-

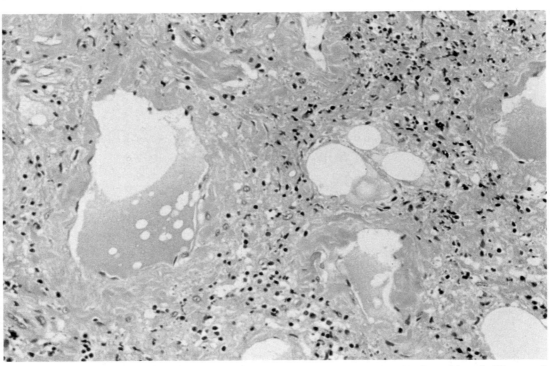

Fig. 8.7a The distended lymphatic vessels are filled with some white often moderately inspissated lymph. The vessels are lined by endothelial cells and hyalinized endothelial tissue. The surrounding tissue is oedematous and there are groups or scattered lymphocytes in it. Same specimen as Figure 8.6. Lymphangiomas have been considered to be congenital malformations of the lymphatic vessels.   Haematoxylin–eosin   × 120

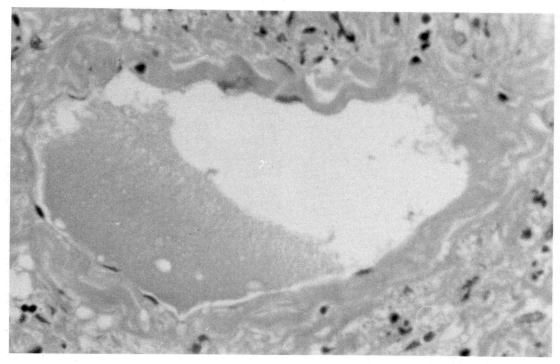

Fig. 8.7b Distended lymphatic vessels containing grey lymph. There are a few endothelial cells on the underlying hyalinized endothelial fibrous tissue lining the vessel.   Haematoxylin–eosin   × 360

like, with rolled elevated firm borders, infiltrated by the neoplastic tissue.

Histopathology (Figs 8.9, 8.10). Microscopy shows a proliferation of well-differentiated keratinizing neoplastic cells penetrating into the underlying lymphoid tissue, forming sheets, groups or strands (Figs 8.11, 8.12). In fact, the high proportion of differentiated carcinomas in the tonsillar region contrasts with the preponderance of anaplastic tumours in the nasopharynx. The prognosis is poor. The pattern of invasion and mitotic activity, rather than the degree of keratinization and irregularity of cellular and nuclear shape and size were found to be 'the most important histological variables predicting survival'. Infiltration of the host tissues by small groups of neoplastic cells or single cells—rather than along a broad front—appear to signify a poor prognosis.[7]

Transitional type carcinomas
These have a characteristic pattern of infolded ribbon-like swathes of epithelium bounded by an intact basement membrane. These tumours are often regarded as intraepithelial carcinomas, but they are liable to become invasive. Their prognosis appears to be somewhat better than that of the squamous carcinomas.

Undifferentiated carcinoma
These are often difficult to distinguish histologically from the large cell malignant lymphomas, a difficulty that is aggravated by the occasional association of pseudocarcinomatous hyperplasia of the epithelium overlying the latter.

Relative frequency
Squamous carcinoma accounts for about 75% of the carcinomas of the tonsillar region, the transitional type of carcinoma for about 10% and anaplastic carcinoma for about 15%.

Spread
Tonsillar carcinomas spread principally into the soft palate, tongue and anterior faucial pillar.

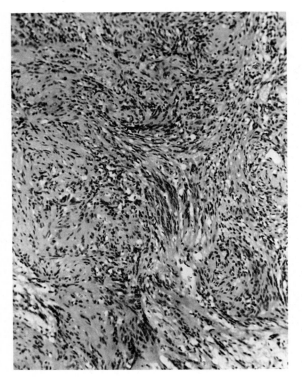

The retropharyngeal space, the medial compartment of the parapharyngeal space and the lateral wall of the pharynx may be invaded.

The parapharyngeal space is an ill-defined region, which may be divided into three parts: anterior or pre-styloid; medial or retro pharyngeal; and posterior or retrostyloid. It contains the internal carotid artery, internal jugular vein, the ninth, tenth and twelfth cranial nerves, the sympathetic chain and numerous lymph nodes and many glomus bodies. Various neurogenic tumours may occur in this space which can cause symptoms and signs due to direct involvement of the nerves, and can extend up to the base of the skull by perineural extension.[8, 9, 10, 11]

Lymph node involvement occurs in about three-quarters of the cases, and many cases present with metastasis to the cervical lymph nodes.[17] The tumour becomes disseminated through the blood stream in about 10% of cases.

Fig. 8.8 Schwannoma of tonsil. Showing characteristic palisading of the nuclei of the spindle-shaped cells and moderate nuclear irregularity.

Haematoxylin–eosin   × 80

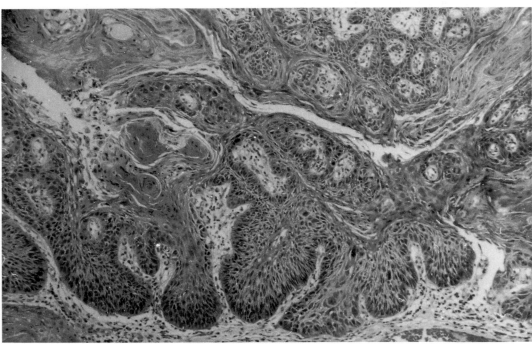

Fig. 8.9 Carcinoma in situ of the faucial tonsil. The hyperplastic and papillary squamous epithelium covering the faucial tonsil consists of irregularly-shaped cells with numerous hyperchromatic and atypical nuclei. There is loss of stratification and polarity and the diagnosis lies between severe dysplasia (TIN III) and carcinoma in situ (see also Fig. 8.10).

Haematoxylin–eosin   × 50

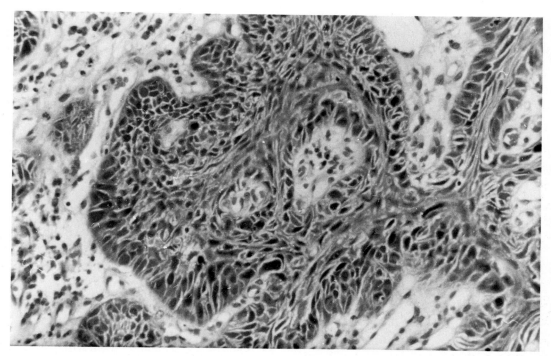

Fig. 8.10 Detail of an irregular papillary process growing down into the fibrous stroma containing an inflammatory reactive infiltrate. There is marked irregularity of the shape and size of the cells and their nuclei. Irregular down-growth is strongly suggestive of invasive activity.

Haematoxylin–eosin   × 170

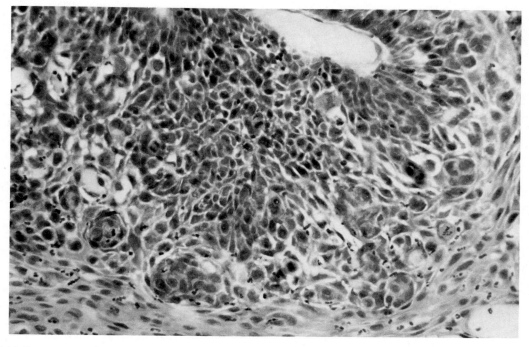

Fig. 8.11 Squamous carcinoma of the tonsil. Area of scattered foci of squamous cell carcinoma underneath the disorganized squamous epithelium.

Haematoxylin–eosin   × 320

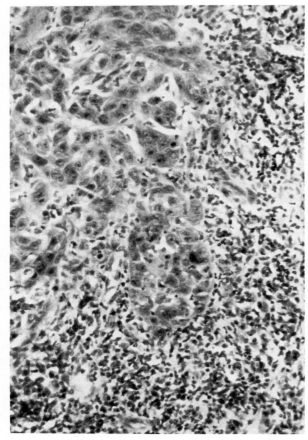

Fig. 8.12 Showing deeper invasion of lymphoid tissue by scattered groups of cells of a well differentiated squamous carcinoma (as Fig. 8.11).

Haematoxylin–eosin × 225

Fatal haemorrhage from the ulcerated area of the primary lesion occurs in about 5% of cases.

Prognostic staging
A system for staging carcinomas of the tonsil has been proposed:

Stage 1—Carcinoma confined to the tonsil.

Stage 2—Carcinoma that has spread to the soft palate, faucial pillars or tongue, but without palpable enlargement of lymph nodes.

Stage 3—Carcinoma with local extension beyond the area in Stage 2, or with palpable lymph nodes that are not fixed to adjacent structures.

Stage 4—Carcinoma with involvement of the skin, fixation of lymph nodes, or distant metastasis.

Radiation therapy has been recommended for Stage 1 and 2 disease and combination radiation therapy and composite resection for Stages 3 and 4.[4, 13]

The TNM staging system of the American Joint Committee on Cancer Staging and End Results Reporting has been widely used[14] and is as follows:

Cancer of the tonsil
T1 Tumour less than 2 cm in diameter.
T2 Tumour of 2–4 cm in diameter with no invasion of surrounding tissues.
T3 Tumour greater than 4 cm and/or limited extension to adjoining structures.
T4 Massive tumour or bone involvement.

Nodes
N0 No clinically palpable nodes.
N1 Clinically palpable homolateral cervical lymph nodes that are not fixed, metastasis suspected.
N2 Clinically palpable contralateral or bilateral lymph nodes that are not fixed, metastasis suspected.
N3 Clinically palpable lymph nodes that are fixed, metastasis suspected.

Glandular tumours
Occasionally a tumour of the seromucinous glands presents in the tonsillar region. Such tumours usually have the structure of the pleomorphic type of salivary adenoma, but other varieties occur, including adenoid cystic (cribriform) adenocarcinomas (Figs 8.13, 8.14). Their behaviour does not differ from that of comparable tumours elsewhere. They are sometimes known as 'ectopic salivary gland tumours', but this is misleading since they originate from glands that are normally present in the fauces.

Sarcomas[3, 6]
Sarcomas of the tonsil are very rare. There were only 12 sarcomas among 1535 malignant neoplasms of the tonsil.[3] These included three cases of embryonal rhabdomyosarcoma and synovial sarcoma each.

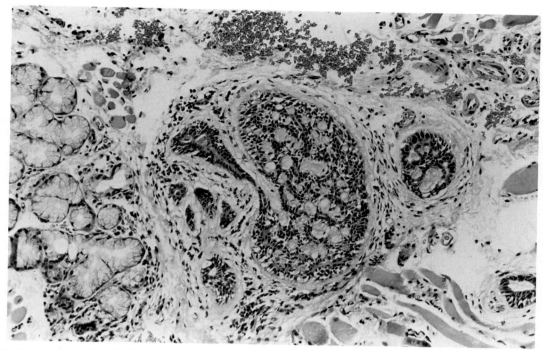

Fig. 8.13 Adenoid cystic (cribriform) adenocarcinoma near normal mucous glands. A small vessel is thrombosed by the tumour.   Haematoxylin–eosin   × 80

Lymphoma

Newer immunological concepts have influenced our views of lymphocytes and their neoplasms and have led to change in the nomenclature and classification of these neoplasms. There are several classifications: that offered by the British National Lymphoma Investigation[15, 16] has been favoured because it has the advantage that its terminology is more familiar to the practising clinician; the 'working formulation for clinical use' of the United States National Cancer Institute is essentially similar. Both classifications are closely related to prognosis.[13, 15, 16]

The large cell lymphoma (previously known as reticulum cell sarcoma) is the commonest of the lymphomas of the tonsillar region, forming about 60% of a series of 78 lymphomas of the tonsils studied at the Institute of Laryngology and Otology, London. Diffuse lymphocytic lymphoma accounted for 30% and Hodgkin's disease and follicular for about 5% each.

In a series of 1394 new patients treated between 1967 and 1978 at the Princess Margaret Hospital in Toronto, Canada for non-Hodgkin's lymphoma, there were 142 with involvement in the head and neck.[13] The tonsil was the primary site of lymphoma in 58 cases, the nasopharynx in 34 cases and the oropharynx in 4 cases; in the remainder various sites were affected such as the nose, nasal sinuses, tongue and salivary glands. Large cell lymphoma predominated and accounted for 63% of the 142 cases of non-Hodgkin's lymphoma of the head and neck; lymphocytic lymphoma accounted for 28%.[13]

Age

The large cell lymphoma occurs mainly in childhood whilst the fully-differentiated lymphocytic lymphoma is commoner in adults. Lymphomas, particularly differentiated ones, may not be distinguishable from non-neoplastic conditions when inadequate biopsy specimens, particularly 'punch biopsies', are provided: their recognition often depends on observation of the loss of the normal follicular pattern.

As in the nasopharynx, the histological distinction between large cell lymphoma and the anaplastic carcinoma is often debatable: in the

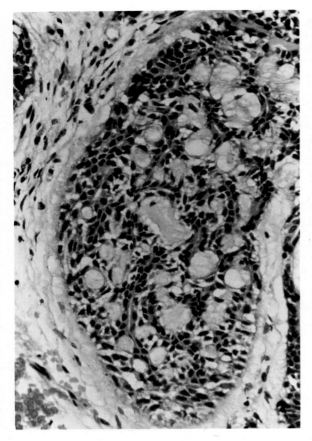

Fig. 8.14 Adenoid cystic (cribriform) adenocarcinoma of the tonsil (same specimen as Fig. 8.13). Detail of neoplastic tissue showing the characteristic cribriform pattern of the glandular tumour. The pseudocysts are surrounded by myoepithelial cells.

Haematoxylin–eosin   × 135

tonsillar region the lymphoma is much the commoner of the two tumours.

Spread

Lymphomas of the tonsil tend not to spread locally beyond the palate and the lateral pharyngeal wall. Generalization of the disease is the natural outcome, and even in treated cases is a frequent terminal manifestation.

Some patients with lymphoma of Waldeyer's ring develop a gastrointestinal lymphoma.[17] In the absence of direct lymphatic connection between the two sites, the association of these tumours has prompted several hypotheses: that the gastrointestinal lymphoma is a concomitant primary tumour, or that it is related to the swallowing and implantation of tumour cells, or that it represents the 'homing tendency' of the gut-associated lymphoid tissue.

The reverse pattern of involvement (that is, a lymphoma in Waldeyer's ring following gastrointestinal lymphoma) provides evidence against the concomitant primary theory and the swallowing theory. The homing tendencies of gut-associated lymphoid tissue may offer some explanations for this interesting observation. Five cases were described in which lymphoma of Waldeyer's ring developed after an initial diagnosis of gastrointestinal lymphoma had been made;[18] the interval ranged from 10 months to 5½ years.

Comparative prognosis

Distinction between lymphoma and carcinoma in this region is particularly important because of the difference in prognosis, which largely reflects the better response of the former to therapy. The crude 5-year survival rate of the lymphomas is about 39% while that of the carcinomas is about 19%.

PLASMACYTOMA

The upper respiratory tract is the most frequent site of extramedullary plasmacytomas. It is a rare, usually solitary tumour of the tonsillar region.

Microscopically they are composed of closely packed cells with a fine vascular connective tissue stroma which may impart a packeted appearance to groups of cells, more easily appreciated with reticulin stains.

The tumour cells may be so well differentiated that they closely resemble normal plasma cells or they may be so primitive that they may be confused with malignant lymphoma or anaplastic carcinoma though they usually have eccentric nuclei and a pale paranuclear 'hof'. There is usually an element of pleomorphism and cells with two and three nuclei are common (Fig. 8.15). Amyloid may be present in the stroma in about 15% of cases (Fig. 8.16).

Extramedullary plasmacytoma must be re-

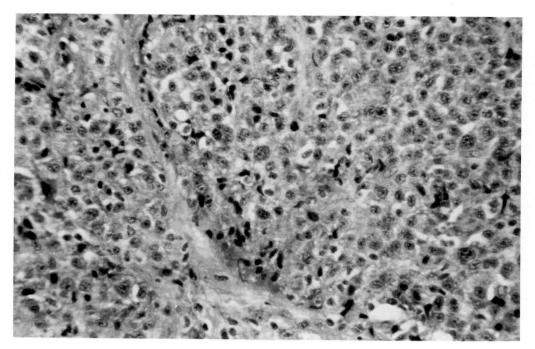

Fig. 8.15 Plasmacytoma of the oropharynx. The lobulated tumour is composed of mainly mature plasma cells some of which contain two nuclei. The characteristic hyperchromatic nuclei have prominent nucleoli.   Haematoxylin–eosin   × 195

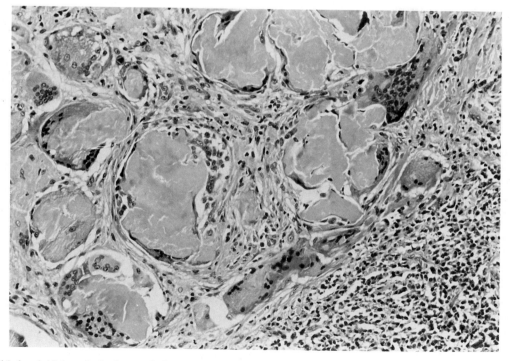

Fig. 8.16 Amyloid deposits in the tonsil. There are clumps of amyloid surrounded by foreign-body giant cells in the lymphoid tissue.   Haematoxylin–eosin   × 225

garded as a malignant tumour. In a small proportion of cases it is a manifestation of myelomatosis, usually antedating the symptoms of the latter. This means that in every case of extramedullary plasmacytoma, biochemical, radiological and bone marrow investigation must be done.

Secondary neoplasms

Secondary neoplasms of the tonsils are rare. A metastatic malignant melanoma in the tonsils was described in a 49-year-old man following the excision of a primary malignant melanoma from the wall of his chest about 5 years previously.[19]

A comparatively more frequent source of secondary deposits in the tonsil are renal carcinomas. In five out of 13 reported cases the tonsillar metastasis was the first manifestation of the renal carcinoma.[20]

REFERENCES

1. Masson JK, Soule EH. Am J Surg 1966; 112: 609.
2. Schwartz HE, Ward PH. Ann Otol 1979; 88: 12.
3. Hyams VJ. Clin Otolaryngol 1978; 3: 117.
4. Givens CD, Johns ME, Cantrell RW. Arch Otolaryngol 1981; 107: 730.
5. Garrett PG, Beale FA. J Otolaryngol 1983; 12: 2.
6. Kuruvilla A. J Laryngol Otol 1983; 97: 735.
7. Crissman JD, Liu WJ, Gluckman JL et al. Cancer 1984; 54: 2995
8. Maran AGD, Mackenzie IJ, Murray JAM. J Laryngol Otol 1984; 98: 371.
9. Rouviere H. Anatomie humaine. 2nd ed. Paris: Masson et Cie, 1927.
10. Shumrick DA, Gluckman JL. In: Suen JY, Myers EN, eds. Cancer of the Head and Neck. New York: Churchill Livingstone, 1981; 345, 346.
11. Ferlito A, Pesavento G, Recher G, Nicolai P, Narne S, Polidoro F. Head & Neck Surg 1984, 7: 32.
12. Shaw HJ. J Laryngol 1970; 84: 249
13. Clark RM Fitzpatrick PJ, Mary K. Gospodarowicz. J Otolaryngol 1983; 12: 4.
14. Nofal F. J Laryngol 1984; 98: 161.
15. Bennett MH, Ferrer-Brown G, Henry K, Jelliffe AM. Lancet 1974; ii: 405.
16. Henry K. Clin Radiol 1981; 32: 499.
17. Banfi A, Bonadonna G, Carnevali G et al. Cancer 1970; 26: 346.
18. Ree HJ, Knisely RE et al. Cancer 1980; 46: 1528.
19. Myer CH M III, Wood MD, Donegan OJ. Ear Nose Throat J 1983; 62: 538.
20. Bom JWA, Baarsma EA, Hacette PE. Bull Med Surg 1981; 14: 1159.

PART FOUR

I. Friedmann and J. Piris

The larynx

9

Anatomy
Malformation

ANATOMICAL CONSIDERATIONS

For descriptive purposes, the larynx may be divided into three regions: 1) the superior or supra-glottic region, which includes the epiglottis, the aryepiglottic folds, the arytenoid cartilages and the interarytenoid fold, the vestibular folds (false vocal cords), and the laryngeal sinuses (ventricles); 2) the middle or 'glottic region, which includes the vocal cords (true vocal cords), and the anterior commissure; and 3) the inferior or subglottic region, which is that part of the larynx which lies below the level of the vocal cords.

The hypopharynx is the part of the pharynx behind the larynx, and it extends, therefore, from the level of the top of the epiglottis to the beginning of the oesophagus at the level of the lower margin of the cricoid cartilage. Its named regions are: 1) the piriform fossae, which lie one on each side of the lower half of the laryngeal opening, between the aryepiglottic folds medially and the lamina of the thyroid cartilage and thyrohyoid membrane laterally; and 2) the postcricoid region, behind the cricoid cartilage.

Attention to the anatomical situation of the lesions is important in diseases of the larynx, and particularly in relation to cancer, for therapeutic measures and prognosis depend to a large extent on the part of the larynx which is affected.

Thus, the abundance and extent of the anastomoses between the lymphatics of the extrinsic parts of the larynx and those of the adjoining parts of the throat and mouth account for the early and extensive spread of carcinomas arising in this region of the larynx: in contrast, there is relatively little communication between the lymphatics of the glottis and those of the adjacent structures, and this is one of the factors that

187

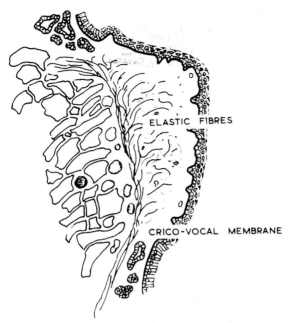

Fig. 9.1 Diagram of normal vocal cord.

account for the very much better prognosis of glottic cancers.

Histology of the normal larynx

Much of the epithelium covering the supraglottic and subglottic regions of the larynx is pseudo stratified columnar ('respiratory') epithelium with interspersed goblet cells, although scattered metaplastic patches of stratified squamous epithelium are found in approximately 50% of normal adult larynges. Recent studies using macroscopic staining methods, which enable the identification of both squamous and respiratory epithelium have shown small islands of squamous epithelium in the subglottic area in 40% of normal larynges and may be present at birth.[1, 2, 2a] Similar results were also found in the supraglottis; only 50% of all the specimens show the vestibular folds to be covered entirely by respiratory epithelium. It is believed that this represents a metaplastic change. The vocal folds are covered by non-keratinizing stratified squamous epithelium (Fig. 9.1).

The elastic fibres in the lateral part of the conus elasticus (cricovocal membrane) become attenuated as they approach its free border, which forms the edge of the vocal cord. Although the mucosa is attached firmly to each aspect of the edge of the membrane over which it is stretched, there is a potential space between the lines of attachment: separation of the mucosa in the plane of this potential space is important in the pathogenesis of polyps of the vocal cords.

Seromucous glands are present in the submucosa of various parts of the larynx. Their distribution is variable, but they are generally most numerous (and best developed) in the laryngeal sinuses, in the region of the ventricular folds and on the epiglottis. They are also numerous in the subglottic region but absent from the vocal cords and their immediate vicinity.

Metaplastic fibroelastic cartilage was found in the vestibular folds of 43 out of 111 unselected human larynges.[3] Metaplasia is the transformation of one differentiated tissue into another as a response to injury. Since the term 'injury' is applicable to a wide range of insults, it is quite consistent for metaplastic cartilage to be formed from connective tissue which has undergone degeneration.

The lymphatic system of the larynx

The lymphatic system of the interior of the larynx is poorly developed and is subdivided by the vocal cords into supraglottic and subglottic regions. The vocal cord itself has a sparse lymphatic supply. The supraglottic region is drained through lymphatics running alongside the superior laryngeal veins directly to the deep cervical lymph nodes. The subglottic region is drained through the anterior laryngeal nodes (along the lower margin of the thyroid cartilage) to the deep cervical lymph nodes.

MALFORMATION AND ACQUIRED DEFORMITIES

There are a number of congenital abnormalities affecting the cartilaginous skeleton of the larynx, the most common of which are seen in the supraglottic area where they give rise to laryngeal stridor; these might be due to a generally floppy laryngeal superstructure or an abnormality resulting in an omega-shaped epiglottis and short aryepiglottic folds. Complete atresia at the glottic

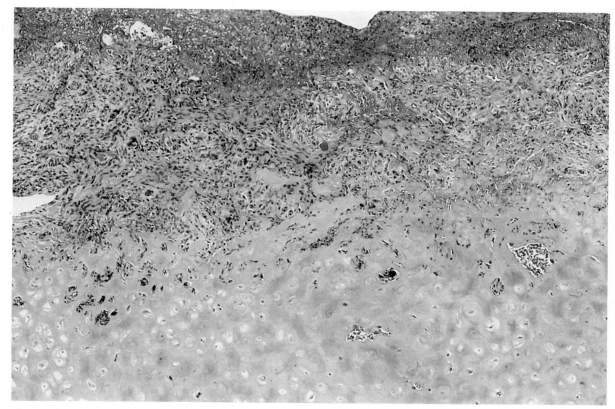

Fig. 9.2 Laryngeal cartilage showing perichondritis. The peripheral area is replaced with granulation tissue and the chronic inflammatory cells are seen infiltrating the matrix. Some revascularization is seen.   Haematoxylin–eosin   × 80

level is incompatible with life; partial atresia is very rare. Subglottic stenosis may also be encountered at birth with a frequency of 1 in 1000 live births. These conditions may lead to long-term complications often due to repeated upper respiratory tract infections.

Laryngeal web

The so-called laryngeal web is the most common congenital malformation of the larynx. The web may be a thin and translucent membrane, made up of epithelium with some connective tissue joining the anterior portion of both vocal cords. In some cases, however, the web is thicker: adequate surgical excision of its insertions is then necessary. There may be adhesions in the supra-glottic and subglottic regions.

Stenosis

This may be congenital or acquired. Congenital stenosis may be due to compression of the larynx or to cysts or webs. Acquired stenosis of the larynx is due to scar formation or destruction of the cartilaginous part of the larynx, and may be traumatic in origin (including surgical measures) or, more frequently, due to burns or caustic substances. Stenosis may also result from tertiary syphilis, tuberculosis, scleroma, typhoid, diphtheria, measles and other infections.

Perichondritis

Accompanying or following irradiation of neoplasms of the larynx, perichondritis may lead to destruction of the cartilaginous skeleton of the larynx and so give rise to stenosis or severe deformities (Fig. 9.2). Relapsing perichondritis is described below.

Laryngocele

A laryngocele is an enlargement of the laryngeal

ventricle and saccule. It is of congenital origin and regarded as an atavistic structure, homologous with the air sacs of monkeys. Its enlargement is further increased by intralaryngeal pressure due to coughing and, perhaps, the playing of wind instruments. It may become infected, resulting in the condition of laryngopyocele which, if untreated, may prove fatal.

Relapsing perichondritis

Relapsing perichondritis is a rare disorder of cartilage that may affect the larynx, the auricle and other organs.[4] Microscopy shows loss of metachromasia, necrosis and calcification of the cartilage and acute and chronic inflammatory granulation tissue. The cause of the disorder is obscure but it may be associated with rheumatic disease, autoimmune diseases, sinusitis, diabetes mellitus and non-specific granulomas. Death may be due to respiratory tract obstruction. Emergency tracheotomy is often indicated. Laryngeal biopsy in patients with relapsing perichondritis may enhance the respiratory difficulties.[5]

REFERENCES

1. Stell P M, Gregory I, Watt J. Clin Otolaryngol 1980; 5: 389.
2. Stell P M, Watt J, Stell I M. Clin Otolaryngol 1982; 7: 335.
2a. Yung M W, Barr G, Stell P M. Clin Otolaryngol 1984; 9: 145.
3. Hill M J, Taylor C L, Scott G B D. Histopathology 1982; 4: 205.
4. McAdam L P, O'Hanlan M A, Bluestone R et al. Medicine 1976; 55: 193.
5. Moloney J R. J Laryngol Otol 1978; 92: 9.

10

Non-neoplastic diseases of the larynx

INFLAMMATORY DISEASES

Misuse of the term 'laryngitis'
In many textbooks of laryngology various non-inflammatory conditions are included under the term 'laryngitis'. It has, indeed, become a clinical convention to describe as laryngitis any laryngeal disturbance that presents with a history of hoarseness and is not the result of paralysis of the vocal cords or of cancer. The more important conditions that are thus mistakenly described as laryngitis are the various polyps and polypoid lesions of the vocal cords, and keratosis. This carelessness in terminology is regrettable because it contributes to a confusion already existing in the nomenclature of many of these lesions.

Acute laryngitis
Various infections, both bacterial and viral, may cause acute laryngitis. The bacteria most commonly concerned are *Streptococcus pyogenes*, *Haemophilus influenzae* and, possibly, *Strep. pneumoniae*. In diphtheria, and exceptionally in typhoid fever, the larynx may be acutely inflamed and ulcerated. It seems likely that the importance of viruses as causes of laryngitis has been much underestimated in the past. Apart from influenza virus, the adenoviruses are now well recognized causes. Chickenpox may cause pustular laryngitis as was also found in some cases of smallpox. Exposure to dust or to irritant fumes can be the direct cause of acute laryngitis. Chronic laryngitis may ensue.

In acute laryngitis, the mucosa is hyperaemic and infiltrated by neutrophils; ulceration may result from epithelial necrosis with a fibrinopurulent exudate covering the ulcers. Acute oedema

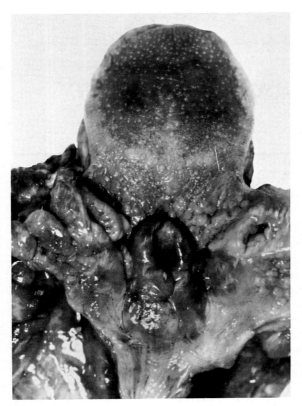

Fig. 10.1 Acute epiglottis to show grossly swollen oedematous aryepiglottic folds. The causative organism was *Haemophilus influenzae*. The patient, a 3½-year-old boy, died within 12 hours of the onset of the disease.

of the glottis is a rare complication, except after exposure to irritant chemical vapours.

Acute epiglottitis

Acute epiglottitis is a serious disease occurring mainly in early childhood (2–7 years) which has been recognized more frequently in recent years.[1–4] It is caused by *Haemophilus influenzae* type B. Frequently a previously healthy child develops a sore throat and, within a few hours of the onset, becomes severely ill.

On examination of the respiratory tract, pharyngitis and laryngitis with supraglottic oedema is found. The most important clinical feature which may be missed unless the tongue is depressed or pulled forward is a swollen, red epiglottis that bears a strong resemblance to a bright red cherry, obstructing the pharynx on the base of the tongue.[5] The epiglottis is grossly swollen, brawny and red (Fig. 10.1). No obvious ulceration can be seen with the naked eye, and generally no other part of the larynx or of the mouth or pharynx is involved. No lesions are found elsewhere in the body, apart from the non-specific effects of the overwhelming toxaemia, which—often with septicaemia—accompanies the infection. Microscopically, there may be superficial ulceration of the epiglottis, but the changes are essentially those of an acute, histologically non-specific inflammation.

Blood culture is an important investigation because it may provide unequivocal retrospective evidence about the nature of the infection. Isolation of an untyped *H. influenzae* strain from the throat or epiglottis is of no significance, because non-capsulated strains of this species can be recovered from such sites in 50% or more of healthy children. The isolation of a type B strain is diagnostic since this organism is carried by only a few members of healthy communities but has been found responsible for nearly all cases of epiglottitis in which careful bacteriological investigations have been carried out.[2]

Acute epiglottitis in the adult

Acute epiglottitis is less likely to occur in adults because the adult larynx is wider and larger. Nevertheless, it is important to be aware that the disease may also develop rapidly in adults.[6, 7] A review of 64 cases seen in Sydney Hospital, showed that acute epiglottitis occurred at any age from infancy to adulthood and 'never recurred'.[3] The pathological changes, oedema and acute inflammation involve only the supraglottic structures: the ventricular folds, arytenoids, aryepiglottic folds and epiglottis. The pharynx, vocal cord, subglottic area and trachea are not affected.

An unusual case of acute necrotizing epiglottitis caused by *Aspergillus flavus* was described in a 21-year-old woman dying of acute lymphocytic leukaemia.[8] A herpetic lesion of the epiglottis that was mistaken for a carcinoma has been described.[9]

Chronic laryngitis

Non-specific, chronic inflammatory changes are commonly found in the larynx, particularly in

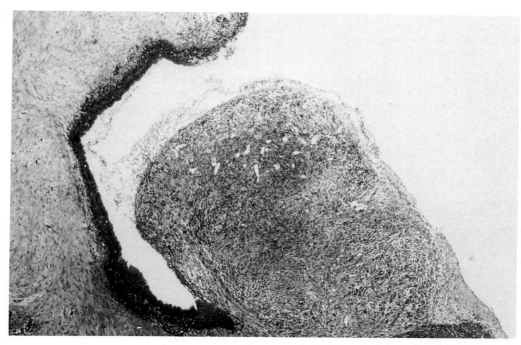

Fig. 10.2a Low-power view of a polypoid non-specific granuloma composed of vascular granulation tissue from the larynx of a 57-year-old woman. The repeatedly recurrent lesion was of unknown aetiology.

Haematoxylin–eosin   × 40

smokers, town-dwellers and those who persistently overuse their voices. In some cases thinning of the covering epithelium with subepithelial fibrosis and atrophy of seromucinous glands results (atrophic laryngitis). Non-specific inflammatory changes are frequently seen near other chronic laryngeal lesions, such as the various polyps and tumours and as part of chronic inflammatory conditions of the upper respiratory tract (sinusitis, rhinitis) and in some cases of chronic bronchitis. Attention has been drawn to a variety of chronic laryngitis in the posterior third of the larynx which may be caused by gastric reflux; mainly in patients with a hiatus hernia.[9a]

GRANULOMAS

Pyogenic granuloma
Attention has been drawn to a common condition which may involve the larynx, the so-called pyogenic granuloma.[10] It is well known that the distinction between pyogenic granuloma—an exuberant formation of vascular granulation as a consequence of trauma—and the benign capillary haemangioma is sometimes impossible. A careful study[10] of 639 vascular lesions of the oral cavity, larynx and trachea revealed that all laryngeal lesions followed some traumatic episode, biopsy procedure, intubation, crush injury etc. and no cases of lobulated capillary haemangioma were encountered; this contrasted with the spontaneously-occurring lesions on the lips or tongue, or elsewhere in the oral cavity, or in the nasal mucosa which presented in young patients, particularly in pregnancy, of whom less than 10% refer to a history of trauma. Histologically, the post-traumatic pyogenic granuloma has a uniform structure whereas the capillary haemangioma is usually lobulated.

Non-specific recurrent granulomas may cause considerable discomfort and diagnostic difficulties (Fig. 10.2a,b).

Nodular fasciitis
Nodular fasciitis (also called pseudosarcomatous fasciitis) is a proliferative process of soft tissues.

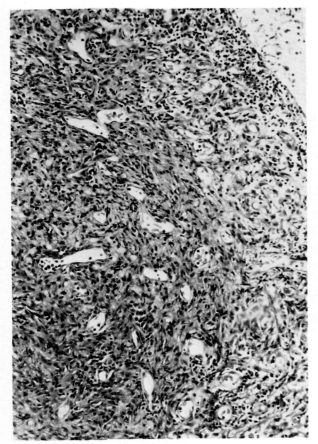

Fig. 10.2b Detail of Figure 10.2a.
Haematoxylin–eosin   × 170

Microscopy shows plump bizarre fibroblasts intermingled with proliferating endothelial cells and supported by a mucinous matrix. The vascular lesion displays considerable mitotic activity and the tumour may be mistaken for a sarcoma. Myxomatous areas and lymphocytic infiltrates with occasional foreign body giant cells are present. The lesion may recur after excision but it is benign.

Nodular fasciitis has been described in a 61-year-old man forming a firm submucosal tumour of the vocal cord which was excised. There was no recurrence for at least 7 years after the operation. Histological interpretation may cause considerable difficulties.[11]

Plasma cell granuloma[12]

The upper respiratory tract, and in particular the supraglottic region of the larynx, may be densely infiltrated by plasma cells. The clinical symptoms and signs may be suggestive of a neoplasm and the lesion can recur after excision. Microscopy shows essentially mature plasma cells of polyclonal type. This argues against a plasmacytoma and for the diagnosis of a reactive plasma cell granuloma of unknown aetiology.

Intubation granuloma

Intubation granuloma is a complication of endotracheal anaesthesia. It is a condition, however, which is becoming more frequent due to the increasing role of intubation in modern surgery. An understanding of the pathogenesis of intubation granuloma is of value not only in the prophylaxis but also in the treatment of this lesion. In a series of 99 cases in adults who came to post mortem, intubation had been maintained for periods that ranged from 15 minutes to 176 hours during the 30 days preceding death.[13] All the recorded cases have been in adults. Women are four times likelier to be affected than men. The difference in the sex incidence may be due to the smaller size of the larynx in women. Intubation granulomas are invariably on the vocal processes of the arytenoids. They are bilateral in approximately half the cases.

The effects of nasogastric tubes on the larynx of anaesthetized dogs have been studied histologically, comparing those resulting when the tube is in the midline with those resulting when the tube is in a lateral position.[14] The histological study confirmed that tubes cause severe inflammation in the postcricoid region. Various theories have been postulated to explain this complication; it is evident from analysis of the literature that no single factor can be exclusively incriminated. The structure of the intubation granuloma is simply that of non-specific granulation tissue partially covered by squamous epithelium (Fig. 10.3). There is no justification for referring to this condition by the histologically ill-defined term 'granuloma pyogenicum'.

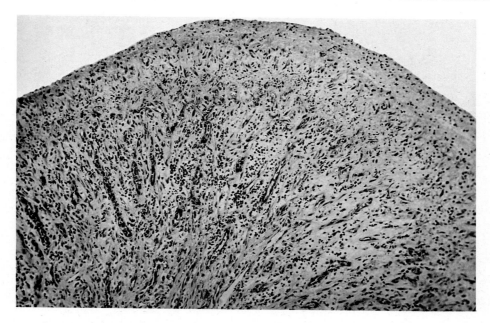

Fig. 10.3 Intubation granuloma composed of non-specific inflammatory granulation tissue covered by squamous epithelium. Haematoxylin–eosin × 120

The larynx in 'cot death'

The larynx was examined in an unselected series of 209 necropsies on young children (91 'cot deaths', 11 stillbirths and 107 deaths from recognized diseases). There were lesions affecting the vocal cords which ranged from focal or generalized hyalinization of the basal lamina and subepithelial or deeper deposits of fibrin, to necrotic purulent foci and ulceration of the mucosa. Although these lesions were not confined to the 'cot death' situation, they seem to indicate the existence of an unknown laryngeal disorder causing reflex apnoea.[15]

In some cases inflammatory infiltration of the upper respiratory passages may be present, suggesting infection by a virus or other microorganism.[15a]

Teflon granuloma

Laryngeal injection of Teflon has been widely used for the treatment of vocal cord paralysis. This technique has proved successful and innocuous but occasional complications have been reported. The extrusion of the substance between the thyroid and cricoid cartilage can form a localized mass simulating a thyroid tumour.[16] A foreign-body granuloma was found at the site of injection in the case of a patient who died 14 months after treatment.[17] A similar foreign-body reaction (Fig. 10.4) has been described with particular reference to the absence of any evidence of malignant change caused by the injected material.[18]

In studies by light and electron microscopy of tissue from 12 vocal cords which had been injected with Teflon from 4 weeks to 16 years earlier, it was found that Teflon had produced only a minimal histological response.[19]

Primary eosinophilic granuloma

Eosinophilic granuloma is a benign non-neoplastic histiocytic proliferation which may or may not be linked with the group of *histiocytosis X*. The disease is usually confined to the bones in which the lesions may be solitary or multiple. Extraosseous involvement has been observed in various organs, as in cases of primary eosinophilic granuloma of the larynx.[20-23] The subepithelial tissue is infiltrated by large numbers of histiocytes with pale vacuolated cytoplasm and a large round nucleus containing a small centrally placed nucleolus; large numbers of eosinophils are also

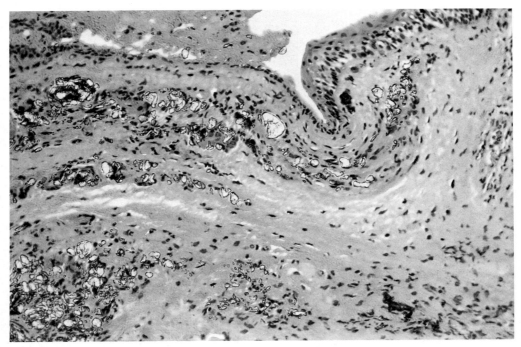

Fig. 10.4 Teflon granuloma—refractile crystalline 'Teflon' is seen in the subepithelial tissues of the vocal cord and ventricle. Haematoxylin–eosin × 250

present. No cells in mitosis and no atypical nuclei are seen. Occasional multinucleated giant cells are present and the granulomatous tissue is partly surrounded by lymphocytes and plasma cells. The surface epithelium shows marked pseudocarcinomatous hyperplasia, keratinizing squamous cells forming 'epithelial pearls'.

The diagnosis may be difficult if only small samples of tissue are available because the eosinophils may be so unevenly distributed that they are absent in some areas and abundant in others. Larger representative specimens present no difficulty in recognizing eosinophilic granuloma by light microscopy.

Lesions in bones have not been found. Electron microscopy may assist in confirming the diagnosis. The absence of Langerhans granules suggests that the condition is not related to histiocytosis X. The Langerhans granules, an ultrastructural component of the immunologically-active Langerhans cell, are rod-shaped and possess an internal lamellar structure. A vesicular dilatation at its tip may give the granule a tennis-racquet-like appearance. They

may occur in histiocytosis X and some other lesions: Langerhans cells containing the granules have been described in invasive squamous cell carcinoma of the larynx.[23]

SPECIFIC INFECTIOUS DISEASES OF THE LARYNX

Tuberculous laryngitis

Tuberculous infection of the larynx was frequent in cases of advanced pulmonary tuberculosis before drug treatment became effective. Nowadays, tuberculous laryngitis is less common, not simply because of the great fall in the incidence of all forms of tuberculosis, but also because treatment of chronic pulmonary tuberculosis, even when it fails to cure the disease in the lungs, is still likely to reduce the number of viable tubercle bacilli in the sputum and thus to hinder the establishment of infection in the mucosa of the upper air passages. Nevertheless, tuberculous laryngitis continues to demand clinical consideration because it may be confused with other chronic infections

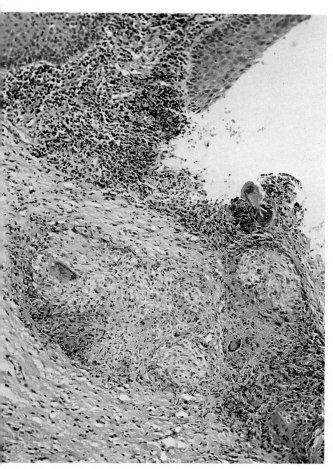

Fig. 10.5 Tuberculous laryngitis of a 62-year-old man. Note ulcerated vocal cord infiltrated by giant-cellular tuberculous nodules. The lesion was clinically suspected for a carcinoma.

Haematoxylin-eosin   ×110

and with carcinoma of the larynx. Biopsy shows characteristic tuberculous tissue beneath the surface epithelium. There is little or no pulmonary disease associated with the laryngeal condition in such cases, and this may indicate the decrease in the incidence of tuberculosis in this portion of the upper respiratory tract as has been observed in the similar cases of tuberculosis of the nose and ear. The disease in the larynx usually takes the form of multiple, small superficial ulcers (Fig. 10.5), with a tendency for the interarytenoid fold, the ventricular and vocal cord and the epiglottis to be involved in that order. Often the underlying cartilage becomes exposed and under-

goes necrosis. The infected mucosa may be swollen and reddened, as in any form of acute inflammation, even when histological examination shows only tuberculous granulation tissue. Clinically this condition may mimic keratosis or carcinoma[24] (Fig. 10.6a,b). Tuberculous laryngitis can heal with the formation of much scar tissue and eventual stenosis of the larynx.

Other forms of mycobacteria have been found to give rise to laryngitis.

Syphilis

A primary chancre of the larynx is a rarity. Secondary syphilis causes diffuse erythema, which may be mistaken for diffuse acute non-specific laryngitis.

The gumma of tertiary syphilis, which may appear as a well-defined 'tumour' or as a diffuse infiltration of the larynx leads sooner or later to the formation of a characteristic punched-out ulcer. Secondary infection results in perichon-

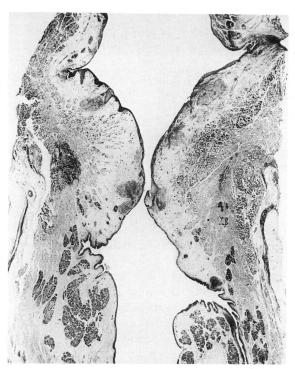

Fig. 10.6a Whole vocal cord removed by laryngofissure. The lesion was clinically mistaken for a carcinoma. Note widely dispersed tubercular foci.

Haematoxylin-eosin   ×7

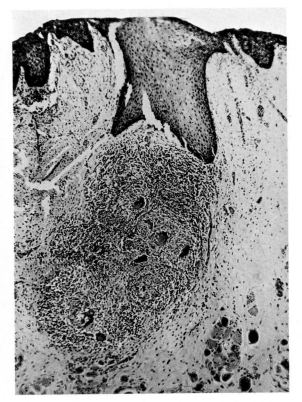

Fig. 10.6b Detail of Figure 10.6a to show isolated tuberculous nodule covered by thickened squamous epithelium.
Haematoxylin–eosin   × 45

dritis and then necrosis of the adjacent cartilage. Subsequently, the formation of scar tissue causes stenosis or other distortions of the upper air passages. The healing of congenital syphilitic lesions may also lead to stricture of the larynx.

Mycoses
When confronted with a clinical picture of chronic hoarseness and granulomatous laryngeal lesions, which on biopsy and culture are negative for acid-fast bacilli, one must consider the diagnosis of mycotic laryngeal disease.

Some of the deep-seated fungal infections may cause fungating and ulcerative, granulomatous lesions of the larynx, for example in *histoplasmosis*[26] (Fig. 10.7) and in *rhinosporidiosis*.[27] Superficial infections of the laryngeal mucosa by *Candida* may complicate severe thrush in the mouth and throat and occasionally produce a reactive

epithelial hyperplasia which may be mistaken for keratosis or carcinoma.[28]

Aspergillosis
Aspergillosis of the larynx (Fig. 10.8a,b) has been described.[29] Aspergillus epiglottitis has been seen as a complication of acute lymphocytic leukaemia.[8]

Blastomycosis
Blastomycosis a mycotic infection endemic in the mid-western and southern United States, may affect the larynx.[30, 31] The microscopic findings resemble those of tuberculosis; the epithelium shows pseudoepitheliomatous hyperplasia, a reactive proliferation of the squamous cell epithelium mimicking carcinoma.

MISCELLANEOUS DISEASES

Sarcoidosis
Involvement of the larynx in sarcoidosis is a rare occurrence. In a study of 2319 patients at the Mayo Clinic between 1950 and 1981 the region of the head and neck was affected in 220 (9%).[25] The larynx was involved in 13 of the 220 patients; in 7 of these cases there were manifestations of the disease elsewhere in the body but in 6 the larynx was the only known site. The most common presenting feature was an oedematous, pale, diffuse enlargement of the supraglottic structures. The diagnosis is made by clinical, and laboratory tests and confirmed by the microscopical finding of non-caseating granuloma.

Wegener's granulomatosis
Laryngeal lesions of Wegener's granulomatosis may be striking in their presentation. In one case[32] in which the histological findings were compatible with Stewart type midfacial granuloma there was early involvement of the uvula and the supraglottic and glottic parts of the larynx. Subglottic stenosis has been observed in a patient with Wegener's granulomatosis during remission induced by azathioprine.[33] The increase in the number of surviving patients that has resulted from advances in the treatment of

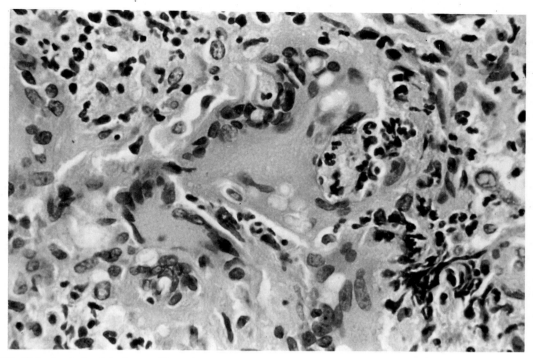

Fig. 10.7 Histoplasmosis of the larynx. Note giant cells containing the organism. The patient, a young black man, responded well to treatment.   Periodic-acid Schiff   × 800

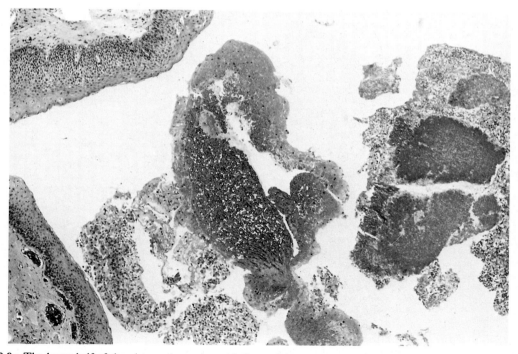

Fig. 10.8a The lower half of the picture shows the epithelium of the vocal cords and on the luminal surface a mycetoma of aspergillus.   Haematoxylin–eosin   × 80

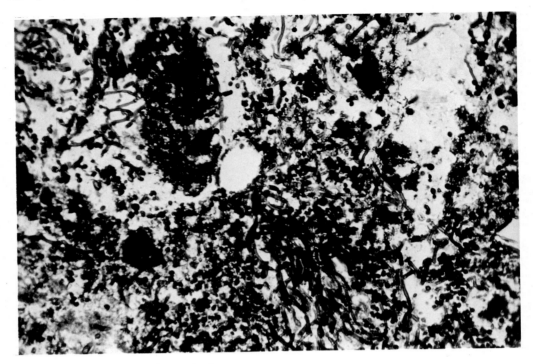

Fig. 10.8b Detail of the aspergillus colony stained.

Grocott   × 500

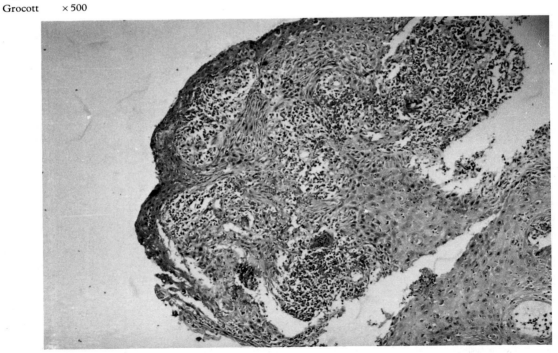

Fig. 10.9a Wegener's granulomatosis. Biopsy of the vocal cord shows the characteristic giant cellular granulation tissue infiltrating the stroma. The patient a 16-year-old girl at the time of this, the third biopsy, died 4 years later of cerebral failure.

Haematoxylin–eosin   × 100

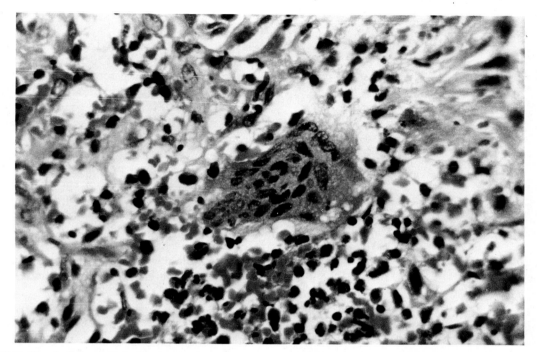

Fig. 10.9b Detail of Figure 10.9a. To show characteristic 'Wegener-type' giant cell packed with nuclei. Haematoxylin–eosin × 540

Wegener's granulomatosis is likely to be accompanied by an increase in the number of cases of laryngeal stenosis resulting from this disease.

Differential diagnosis
The histological appearances of Wegener's granulomatosis are all too often mistaken for those of tuberculosis (Fig. 10.9a,b). Such incorrect diagnoses may delay proper treatment.

Scleroma
This condition may also involve the larynx (see page 30). A case is illustrated in Figure 10.10.

Schistosomiasis
A granulomatous reaction to the presence of schistosome ova with extensive fibrosis has been noted in a case presenting with ankylosis of both cricoarytenoid joints.

Rheumatoid disease
The cricoarytenoid joints are overtly inflamed in about a quarter of all patients with rheumatoid arthritis. It has been accepted by most observers

as the cause of laryngeal stridor that may develop at a late stage of this disease. During remission, the mucous membrane over the cartilage becomes thickened and movement is limited or the joints become fixed.

Rheumatoid arthritis is believed to impair laryngeal function both by involving the cricoarytenoid joints and by direct injury to the adjacent muscles.[35]

Rheumatoid nodules have been observed in the larynx. Micro-laryngoscopical studies indicate that they are by no means uncommon.

The newly formed rheumatoid nodule of the vocal cord[36] consists of a central focus of granulation tissue with peripheral fibrinoid necrosis (Fig. 10.11). Further sections may disclose the characteristic peripheral histiocytic palisading if this is not apparent in those examined initially.

Gout
An uncommon cause of hoarseness is the deposition of sodium urate in the vocal cords or in the subglottic region. This occurs only in the presence of longstanding gout. The deposits may

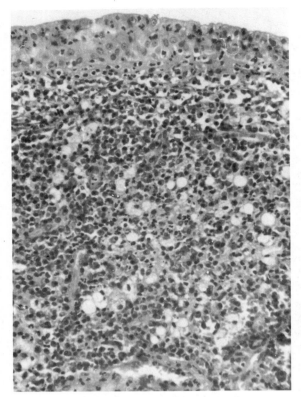

Fig. 10.10 Scleroma in the larynx. Note many clear Mikulicz cells in the mainly plasma cellular infiltrate covered by pseudostratified columnar epithelium infiltrated by polymorphs. Haematoxylin–eosin   × 49

form nodules up to several millimetres in diameter. There may be an accompanying giant cell granulomatous reaction, as in gouty deposits in other parts of the body[37] (Fig. 10.12).

Asbestos-body content of the larynx

Asbestos bodies were demonstrated at necropsy in two out of five asbestos workers but in none of ten control patients who had no known exposure to asbestos.[38] No dysplastic changes were found in the mucosal epithelium in the two cases in which the asbestos bodies were present.

The occurrence of laryngeal tumours in two patients who had been exposed to asbestos have been reported.[39] Extracts from the laryngeal tissues yielded large numbers of uncoated asbestos fibres in both cases but no asbestos bodies.

OEDEMA

The larynx may be affected in cases of cardiac, renal or other generalized forms of oedema. In such cases, the swelling of the laryngeal tissues seldom causes respiratory embarrassment. However, if the oedema is due to obstruction to the venous return from the head and neck—as happens, for instance, if there is thrombosis of the superior vena cava—the laryngeal swelling may be acute and extensive, with correspondingly greater risk of impeding respiration. 'Angioneurotic oedema' sometimes involves the soft tissues of the larynx as a manifestation of allergic hypersensitivity to a particular food or drug. Wasp and bee stings may prove fatal from the same cause, but the commonest of the dangerous causes of laryngeal oedema are diphtheria and streptococ-

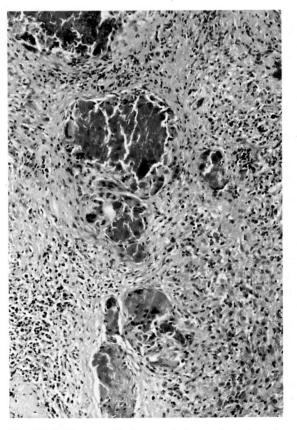

Fig. 10.11 Rheumatoid disease of the vocal cord to show submucosal necrotizing nodular foci and giant cells. Haematoxylin–eosin   × 252

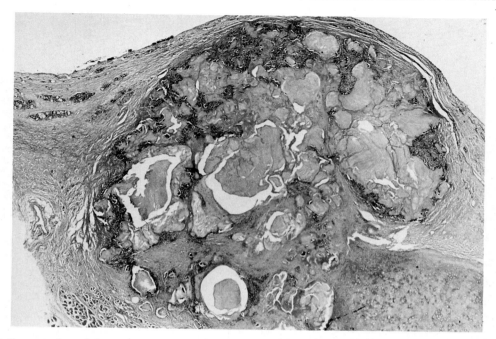

Fig. 10.12 Gouty tophus of the larynx from a 64-year-old man suffering from gout for over 20 years. Note tumour-like deposit covered by the intact mucosa.

Haematoxylin–eosin   × 75

Provided by Professor Alfio Ferlito, University ENT Department, Padua, Italy.

cal infection (including Ludwig's angina) and the acute inflammation that results from exposure to steam or the accidental inhalation of irritant gases such as ammonia or sulphur dioxide.[40]

Fluid can collect in the soft alveolar tissues of certain parts of the larynx. Its spread in some directions is limited by the firm adherence of the mucosa to the underlying tissue—the resulting swelling is, therefore, characteristically seen first over the arytenoid cartilages and in the aryepiglottic folds, spreading thence into the epiglottis and the vestibular folds; it does not, however, extend into the vocal cords or past the pharyngoepiglottic folds. It is mainly the swelling of the posterior ends of the aryepiglottic folds that obstructs the passage of air.

AMYLOID DISEASE

The larynx may be involved in primary and secondary generalized amyloidosis. The deposition of amyloid in the laryngeal tissues as part of generalized amyloidosis is unlikely to cause any functional disturbance.

There is also a form of amyloidosis which is confined to the larynx. It may be noted that the respiratory tract is by far the commonest part of the body to be the site of localized amyloid disease which may occur in the nose and nasal sinuses, the nasopharynx, the trachea and the bronchi.

Localized amyloidosis of the larynx

Amyloid disease limited to the larynx may present either as tumour-like deposits, which may be solitary or multiple and reach a centimetre or even more in diameter, or as a diffuse thickening of parts of the mucosa. The surface of the deposits is smooth or nodular. Either form may eventually obstruct the laryngeal airways, necessitating tracheostomy and surgical excision. In most cases the disease does not progress after initial diagnosis; in a few, slow progression does take place. Surgical excision of the amyloid deposit is usually effective in treating the symptoms

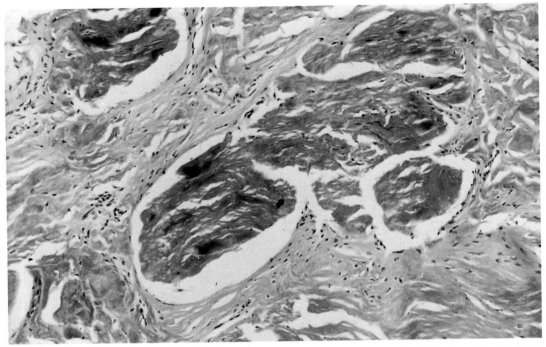

Fig. 10.13 Amyloid deposit in the vocal cord positive with Congo red. There is nodular infiltration of vessels and of the inflamed laryngeal tissue.

Congo red   × 180

produced by it. Primary amyloidosis of the larynx is rarely followed by generalized amyloidosis. In every case care must be taken to exclude the possibility that amyloid deposition in the larynx is a manifestation of generalized amyloidosis.

Histopathology

In haematoxylin–eosin preparations amyloid appears as a pale pink, homogeneous substance. In some cases there is a well marked foreign-body type of giant cell reaction round the amyloid deposits.[41]

The β-pleated sheet structure of the amyloid fibrils, gives them strong affinity for Congo red (Fig. 10.13), negative birefringence when seen in polarized light, and dichroism when stained with Congo red. Amyloid also shows strong secondary fluorescence in ultraviolet light when stained with thioflavine T. It also has a high degree of resistance to extraction with proteolytic enzymes, such as pepsin. These reactions usually establish the sometimes difficult distinction between amyl-

oid and the hyaline material which is found in some laryngeal polyps.[42]

The presence of amyloid can also be confirmed by electron microscopy, which shows the amyloid fibre to be composed of two filamentous elements, mainly fibrils, composed of one to four laterally-aligned filaments (75 nm in diameter). The amyloid fibrils form parallel bundles or criss-cross at random, resembling 'chopped straw', accounting for the phenomenon of birefringence.

Aetiology and pathogenesis

The nature of amyloidosis is obscure. Most evidence suggests that immune mechanisms are involved in the pathogenesis of human and experimental amyloidosis. There is an apparent contradiction in the observations that amyloidosis can not only complicate immune deficiency states but also that its production in experimental animals can be accelerated by steroids, immuno-suppressive agents and ionizing irradiation, all of which may compromise the immune response.

It is interesting that localized amyloidosis is occasionally a complication of the rare, primary extra-skeletal plasmacytoma, one of the most frequent sites of which is the larynx. In fact, the topographical distribution of primary localized amyloidosis of the respiratory tract is essentially the same as that of amyloid deposition complicating extra-skeletal solitary myeloma.[43] However, these neoplasms are rare. The fact that the deposition of amyloid occurs in the same sites is likely to be a result of the propensity of the mucosa of the respiratory tract to chronic infection which stimulates the local accumulation of plasma cells and much local production of immunoglobulin. This view is supported by the fact that the secondary type of generalized amyloidosis is usually associated with chronic infections characterized by prolonged production of antibodies, or with other conditions, such as myelomatosis, in which immunoglobulin production is very much increased.

POLYPS OF THE VOCAL CORD

The study of polyps of the vocal cords has been complicated unnecessarily by a confusing nomenclature which is largely due to discrepancies between clinical impressions and histological findings. Some clinicians freely describe simple nodules by such pathological terms as myxoma, fibroma and angioma, without microscopical confirmation and merely because of a superficial resemblance between the lesion and these tumours. The term chorditis tuberosa is commonly used in some clinics, although the implication of an inflammatory process is not strictly correct. The least objectionable clinical terminology is that based on occupation and has the merit of indicating that polyps occur predominantly in those whose work involves much strain on the voice. Such terms are singer's, hawker's, teacher's, preacher's, lawyer's, politician's, heckler's, ranter's and chairman's nodes or nodules.

It must be emphasized, before describing the lesions more fully, that the nature of such polyps can be determined only by microscopical examination, and that this should never be omitted. Failure to take this precaution may allow the oc-

casional early carcinoma that presents as a polypoid nodule to pass undetected at a stage when the chance of cure is greatest.

Aetiology and pathogenesis

Conflicting statements about the incidence of polyps of the vocal cords are to be found in different textbooks of laryngology. Experience at the Royal National Throat, Nose and Ear Hospital in London has been that they occur twice as often in men as in women.[44] However, there were 307 females out of 591 patients presenting with vocal cord polyps in a recent study.[45] No age is exempt; to some extent, the patient's occupation may determine the age at which polyps appear.

The polyps result from mechanical injury to the connective tissue of the vocal cords. This injury is incurred mainly through persistent misuse when there is an incidental laryngitis, or after symptoms of polyp formation have already appeared. Faulty voice production is as important a cause as overuse, and the commonest fault is forcing the voice after most of the available air has been exhaled, in an effort to compensate for the sharp fall in the air flow. This leads to the vocal cords being pressed unduly firmly together at a time when their rapid vibration is liable to cause injury. Altering the pitch of the voice in order to make it better heard in noisy surroundings, a means commonly adopted to avoid shouting, is another frequent source of 'voice strain', a colloquial expression that aptly describes the effect on the vocal cords. Straining the voice in such ways can bring about immediate changes in the vocal cords as has been shown by indirect laryngoscopy after conversation for a few minutes in a noisy London underground railway carriage; efforts, even by experienced speakers, to converse under such conditions may be followed by hyperaemia and increased secretion of mucus, and occasionally by slight swelling of the vocal cords.

The polyps that develop as a consequence of vocal stress are believed to be the result of vascular engorgement, oedema and focal haemorrhage in the subepithelial tissue. The distortion is usually localized, and the commonest site for polyps is the medial aspect of the vocal cord at about the junction of the anterior and middle thirds. In many cases the lesion is bilateral, but

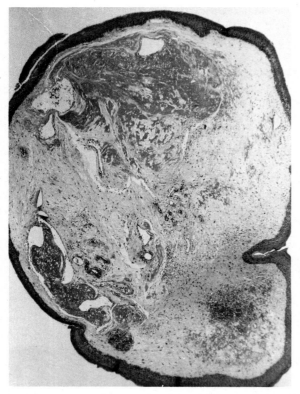

Fig. 10.14a Vocal cord polyp—recurrent. Survey picture of a polyp removed from the vocal cord covered by squamous epithelium. The structure is composed of vascular fibrous tissue containing varicose distended vessels partly filled with fibrinoid material—some of it appears in the stroma. Man of 45.

Haematoxylin-eosin   × 25

often the polyps of the two sides differ in size. In some cases, the changes are more extensive, and in extreme instances there is polypoid degeneration of the entire membranous part of the vocal cord—that is, its anterior two-thirds.

Histopathology

The subepithelial structure of the polyp seems to depend upon the fate of the initial exudate. Ingrowth of blood vessels from the deep aspect of the upper part of the cricothyroid membrane may produce a predominantly vascular tissue which can be mistaken for an angioma (Fig. 10.14a,b,c). By contrast, if proliferation of simple connective tissue predominates, a fibrous nodule simulating a fibroma may be formed. Myxomatous degeneration in such fibrous tissue has sometimes led to the misdiagnosis of myxoma. Careful histological examination will reveal the non-neoplastic nature of these lesions.

Enhanced permeability of the blood vessels may contribute to the polypoid swelling.[46] Bleeding into the stroma is common, especially in angiomatoid polyps, and occasionally the resulting haematoma may interfere with respiration. Organization of the clot leads to fibrosis, and the resulting scar tissue is often heavily pigmented with haemosiderin.

Hyaline change is found in many polyps, either through hyalinization of the collagen, or through some alteration in the proteins of the exudate in the interstitial tissue. Hyaline material may even occupy most of the polyp but usually it forms small, discrete deposits. These may be found in three situations: 1) as rings round blood vessels; 2) within blood vessels, as a result of hyalinization of thrombi, the affected vessels appearing as plexiform, distended, thin-walled channels, occluded by the hyaline mass; and 3) in the stroma, usually in the form of fine, thread-like deposits. It may be difficult to distinguish amyloid deposits from hyalinized polyps, since the characteristic staining reaction with Congo red may be elicited by some varieties of connective tissue hyaline, resulting in erroneous diagnosis. In contrast with amyloid, hyaline deposits show no metachromasia, low affinity for Congo red, weak birefringence in an unstained state, no birefringence if stained with Congo red, weak or negative fluorescence with thioflavine T, low resistance to pepsin digestion, areas that stain with phosphotungstic acid haematoxylin, and a high affinity for the picric acid component of Van Gieson's stain.[42] Hyalinized collagen closely resembles amyloid in appearance in haematoxylin and eosin preparations but can be distinguished from the latter by its fuchsinophilia with Van Gieson's stain.

The covering squamous epithelium may show hyperplasia, with an increase in the thickness of the basal layer and keratinization; not uncommonly it appears thin and atrophic. Atypical features are seen only rarely.[45]

It must be stressed again that all polypoid lesions of the vocal cords should be examined microscopically in order to arrive at the precise

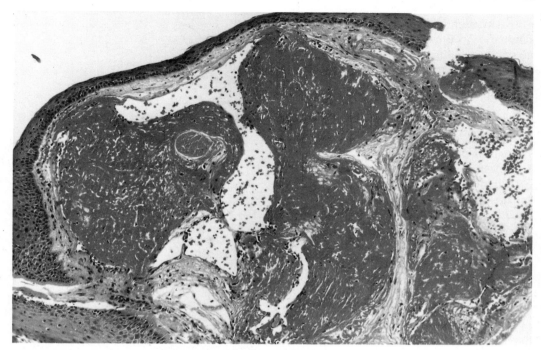

Fig. 10.14b Vocal cord polyp—recurrent. Detail of varicose dilation of vessels.
Haematoxylin–eosin   × 250

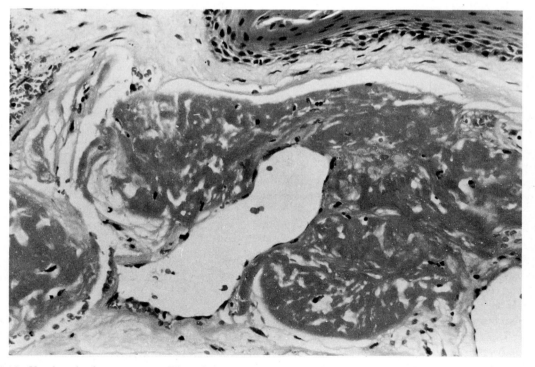

Fig. 10.14c Vocal cord polyp—recurrent. Distended vessel surrounded by fibrinoid matter in the stroma.
Haematoxylin–eosin   × 240

diagnosis. Although in most cases the microscopical examination confirms the clinical impression that the polyp is benign, such lesions may prove to be amyloid foci, squamous papillomas, keratotic nodules or even early squamous carcinomas.

Plasma cell polyps (plasma cell granulomas)[12]

Some laryngeal polyps consist of dense accumulations of plasma cells throughout an oedematous stroma. Small numbers of lymphocytes and macrophages are also present. These infiltrates may be severe forms of the chronic inflammatory reactions often seen in laryngeal polyps. Two unusual features are sometimes seen: first the presence of small, faintly haematoxyphilic, globular clumps of material that histochemically can be identified as precipitates containing ribonucleic acid, and second, fine deposits of amyloid. The only practical significance of these peculiar lesions, as far as is yet known, is that the precipitates may be mistaken for fungi or parasites. Myelomas (plasmacytomas) may also occur in the form of polypoid lesions.

CYSTS

Most laryngeal cysts result from obstruction of the ducts of mucous glands, due either to inflammation nearby or to contraction of scar tissue after healing of a local ulcer. These retention cysts are found on the lingual aspect of the epiglottis or in the aryepiglottic folds, and only occasionally at other sites, such as the vocal cords.[47] They are smooth-surfaced, tense, translucent structures, ranging from 5-15 mm in diameter and filled with thick, very glairy mucus. They are liable to become infected and they may occasionally cause death through suffocation.

Rarely, excision of what had seemed to be a simple retention cyst is followed by recurrence of the lesion. This may be merely the result of incomplete removal of the wall of a benign cyst, which formed again from the remains. Sometimes, however, such a recurrence discloses the neoplastic nature of the original lesion.

Some cysts of the epiglottis appear to arise

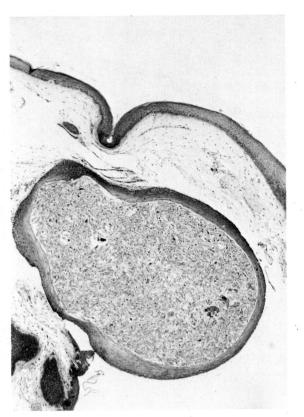

Fig. 10.15 Epidermoid cyst in the vocal cord. The cyst lies deeply in the stroma but appears to be protruding into the ventricle. Note keratinized content of the cyst.

Haematoxylin-eosin   × 50

within the substance of the cartilage as a degenerative change in its matrix.

In children, the larynx may be involved in the form of a generalized lymphangioma, with cystic dilatation of lymphatics. As the larynx grows the size and effect of these cysts become proportionally less.

Occasionally epidermoid cysts may be formed (Fig. 10.15).

REFERENCES

1. Cherry JD. Arch Otolaryngol 1981; 107: 19.
2. Addy MG, Ellis PD, Turck DC. Br Med J 1972; 1: 40.
3. Benjamin B, O'Reilly B. Ann Otol Rhinol Laryngol 1976; 85: 565.
4. Baugh R, Baker SR. Otolaryngol Head Neck Surg 1982; 90: 157.
5. Barenberg W, Kevy S. N Engl J Med 1958; 258: 870.

6. Hawkins DB, Miller AH, Sachs GB, Bone RT. Laryngoscope 1973; 83: 1211.
7. Johnstone JM, Lawy HS. Lancet 1967; ii: 134.
8. Bolivar R, Gomez LG, Luna M, Hopfer R, Bodey GP. Cancer 1983; 51: 367.
9. Schwenzfeier CW, Fechner RE. Arch Otolaryngol 1976; 102: 374.
9a. Lancet 1983; i: 512.
10. Fechner RE, Cooper PH, Mills SE. Arch Otolaryngol 1981; 107: 30.
11. Jones SR, Myers EN, Barnes L. Otolaryngol Clin North Am 1984; 17: 170.
12. Fu YS, Perzin KH. In: Silverberg SG ed. Practice and principles of surgical pathology. Vol. 1. New York: Wiley, 1983; 479.
13. Donnelly WH. Arch Pathol 1969; 88: 511.
14. Friedman M, Baim H, Shelton V, Stobnicki M. et al. Ann Otol 1981; 90: 469.
15. Cullity GJ, Emery JL. J Pathol 1975; 115: 27.
15a. Forfar RO, Arneil GC. Textbook of paediatrics. 2nd ed. Edinburgh: Churchill Livingstone, 1978: 1520.
16. Sanfilippo F, Shelburne J, Ingram P. Ultrastruct Pathol 1980; 1: 471.
17. Lewy RB. Arch Otolaryngol 1966; 83: 355.
18. Stephens CB, Arnold GE, Stone JW. Arch Otolaryngol 1976; 102: 432.
19. Dedo H, Carlsoo B. Acta Otolaryngol (Stock) 1982; 93: 475.
20. Friedmann I, Ferlito A. J Laryngol Otol 1981; 95: 1249.
21. Booth JB, Thomas RS. J Laryngol 1970; 84: 1123.
22. Lhotak J, Dvorackova I. J Laryngol 1975; 89: 771.
23. Schenk P. Laryngol Rhinol Otol (Stuttg) 1980; 59: 232.
24. Yarnal JR, Golish JA, van der Kuyp F. Arch Otolaryngol 1981; 107: 503.
25. Neel H, McDonald TJ. Ann Otol Rhinol Laryngol 1982; 91: 359.
26. Amat C, Amat D, Demaldent JE, Camilleri JP. Arch Cytol Pathol 1979; 27: 45.
27. Pillai OS. J Laryngol Otol 1974; 88: 277.
28. Hicks JN, Peters GE. Laryngoscope 1982; 92: 644.
29. Ferlito A. J Laryngol Otol 1974; 88: 1257.
30. McLean WC, Fitz-Hugh GH. South Med J 1959; 52: 667.
31. Blair PA, Gnepp DR, Riley RS, Sprinkle PM. South Med J 1981; 74: 880.
32. McKinnon DM. J Laryngol Otol 1970; 84: 1193.
33. Lampman JH, Querubin R, Kendapalli P. Chest 1981; 79: 230.
34. Manni HJ, Lema PN, van Raalte JA, Westerbeek GF. J Laryngol Otol 1983; 97: 1177.
35. Wolman L, Darke CS, Young A. J Laryngol Otol 1965; 79: 403.
36. Abadir WF, Forster PM. J Laryngol Otol 1974; 88: 473.
37. Di Bonito L, Ferlito A. Clin Otolaryngol 1971; 23: 94.
38. Roggli VL, Greenberg SD, McLarty JL, Hurst GA, Spivey GG, Heiger LR. Arch Otolaryngol 1980; 106: 533.
39. Hirsch A, Bignon J, Sebastien P, Gaudichet A. Chest 1979; 76: 679.
40. Salmon LFW. In: Scott Brown's Diseases of the ear, nose and throat. 4th ed. Vol. 4. London: Butterworths, 1979: 375.
41. McAlpine JC, Fuller AP. J Laryngol Otol 1964; 78: 296.
42. Michaels L, Hyams VJ. J Pathol 1979; 128: 29.
43. Symmers W St C. J Clin Pathol 1956; 9: 187.
44. Epstein SS, Winston P, Friedmann I, Ormerod FC. J Laryngol Otol 1957; 71: 673.
45. Kambic V, Radsel Z, Zargi M, Acko M. J Laryngol Otol 1981; 95: 609.
46. Frenzel H, Kleinsasser D, Hort W. Virchows Arch (Pathol Anat) 1980; 389: 189.
47. Asherson N. J Laryngol Otol 1957; 71: 750.

11

Neoplasms of the larynx

Benign epithelial tumours
    Papillomas
    Keratosis
Malignant tumours
    Carcinoma in situ
   Squamous cell carcinoma
    Invasive squamous cell carcinoma
    Prognosis of laryngeal squamous carcinoma
    Verrucous carcinoma
    Spindle-cell squamous carcinoma
Tumours of the seromucous glands
    Adenomas
    Malignant tumours of the seromucous glands
    Other rare carcinomas
    Giant cell carcinoma
    Clear cell carcinoma
Neuroendocrine tumours
    Paraganglioma (chemodectoma)
    Carcinoid tumours
    Small cell anaplastic carcinoma ('oat cell' carcinoma)
Secondary tumours
Multiple primary malignant tumours
    Tumours of identical histological type
    Tumours of different histological types
Mesenchymatous tissue tumours
    Fibrosarcoma
    Cartilaginous tumours
    Tumours of adipose tissue
    Osteosarcoma (osteogenic sarcoma)
Tumours of muscle derivation
    Tumours of smooth muscle
    Rhabdomyoma
    Rhabdomyosarcoma
    Malignant fibrous histiocytoma
Vascular tumours
    Benign haemangioma
    Haemangiopericytoma
    Angiosarcoma
Lymphoma
    Mycosis fungoides
    Leukaemia
    Plasmacytoma
Peripheral nerve tumours
    Granular-cell tumour (granular-cell myoblastoma)
    Schwannomas (neurilemmomas) and neurofibromas
    Other neural tumours and tumour-like conditions

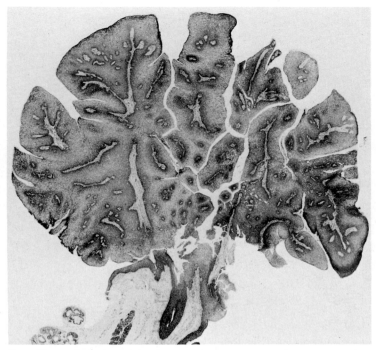

Fig. 11.1 Squamous cell papilloma of the larynx is a common lesion. This figure shows a juvenile type. Note branching fibrovascular stalks covered by a hyperplastic layer of parakeratotic squamous epithelium.

Haematoxylin–eosin   × 20

BENIGN EPITHELIAL TUMOURS

Papillomas

Papillomas are well-circumscribed, benign neoplasms of the lining squamous epithelium. They are the most common benign laryngeal tumours and there are two main varieties, the juvenile and the adult.

Juvenile laryngeal papilloma (juvenile papillomatosis; multiple papillomas of the larynx in childhood)

As indicated by some of its synonyms the tumour is commonly multiple; the lesions tend to spread, recur after surgery and eventually regress or disappear spontaneously, usually at puberty. In 1923 Ullmann[1] demonstrated the presence of viral particles by injecting cell-free extracts of papillomatous tissue into his own forearm, and observing the appearance of warty lesions after 90 days. Electron microscopy has demonstrated the presence of virus-like particles in a small proportion (20%) of specimens.[2] Recently, success

in identifying viral antigenic material in tissue sections of papillomas has been achieved by using anti-human-papilloma-virus antibodies (by an immunoperoxidase technique). In 48% of 102 laryngeal papillomas from 35 patients, positive staining within the nucleus of squamous cells in the superficial third of the epithelium was seen.[3] These observations and the realization that a substantial proportion of mothers of children with laryngeal papillomatosis had genital condylomas at the time of delivery, which may represent a source of infective virus,[4] are strong evidence of the viral aetiology of this condition.

The papillomas are soft, mobile, pale pink, finely lobulated and usually 2–5 mm in diameter. Histologically (Fig. 11.1), the lesion consists of multiple, small, papillary processes, the bulk of which is made up by a thickened prickle-cell layer containing cells of normal size with minimal production of keratohyaline granules and nuclei which often display more than one nucleolus; full keratinization is characteristically absent and there is no cellular atypia. In spite of the high

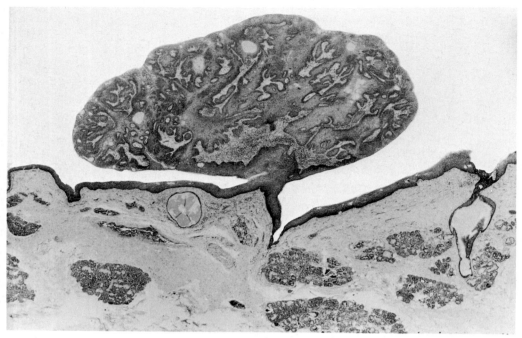

Fig. 11.2 Shows an adult type papilloma of larynx. Note a greater degree of disarray in the epithelium. Required complete laryngofissure.   Haematoxylin–eosin   × 20

recurrence rate, the microscopical appearances remain constant in the great majority of the cases. Malignant degeneration is sometimes observed, especially after irradiation; a number of cases of squamous carcinoma in children with laryngeal papillomatosis who had not had radiation therapy have recently been reported.[5, 6]

Papilloma of the larynx in adults
The commonest benign neoplasm of the larynx is almost invariably a single lesion and occurs on the vocal cords (Fig. 11.2); it also differs from the juvenile form in that it shows keratinization. Its distinction from a well-differentiated keratinizing squamous carcinoma is not always obvious and requires careful histological examination of the completely excised lesion, which may show considerable dysplasia. Many of these lesions proved to be benign in follow-up studies, but malignant transformation occurs with a frequency which is reported as between 2 and 3% (Fig. 11.3).[7]

Two examples of a variety of squamous papilloma displaying features similar to those of the verruca vulgaris of skin have been described.[8]

Human papilloma virus antigenic material was demonstrated with an appropriate antibody in tissue sections of one of the tumours. The authors remarked on the similarity of these lesions to verrucous carcinoma and the possibility of confusion with the latter.

Keratosis
The squamous epithelium of the vocal cord is prone to undergo some moderate to severe morphological changes which may be difficult to interpret. Comparative studies have been hampered by both inherent difficulties and also by terminological inexactitudes. Gynaecological pathologists have contributed to the better understanding and practical classification of the pre-cancerous squamous epithelial changes that figure prominently in the early diagnosis and treatment of squamous cell carcinoma of any site.

None of the classifications, whether on clinical or histological grounds, is entirely satisfactory or reliable. The interpretation of borderline patterns has been fraught with considerable difficulty, often affected by the perhaps unavoidably subjective approach of the diagnostician.

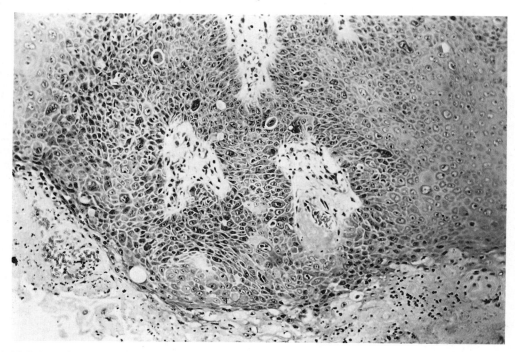

Fig. 11.3 Malignant change in recurrent squamous papilloma of the larynx. Note in-situ-type lesion with large numbers of bizarre cells and nuclei. The patient was a middle-aged woman. Haematoxylin–eosin × 160

The terms keratosis, hyperkeratosis, leucoplakia and pachydermia have been applied to a form of hyperplasia of the laryngeal epithelium. These conditions have their counterparts in the mucosa of the mouth and pharynx and of the vulva, vagina and uterine cervix. In fact, such changes are common to all mucous membranes with epithelium that normally is of non-keratinized, stratified, squamous type. They are often the outcome of chronic irritation, which stimulates keratin formation in non-keratinized squamous cells. Although much effort has been expended in seeking to define the supposed differences between keratosis, hyperkeratosis, leucoplakia and pachydermia, it now seems apparent that they are merely variants of a single type of reactive change and that little is to be gained by trying to distinguish between them. In this chapter they are considered inclusively under the term keratosis.

Crissman[9] used the term 'keratosis', which we favour, because excess keratin formation is a common feature of the changes observed; he divided it into three groups, or grades, according to its severity. Various histological categories have been suggested;[10] we follow a classification based on the predominant microscopical changes in the squamous epithelium of the larynx (see below):

Keratosis—hyperplasia, hyperkeratosis
Dysplasia—low-grade (mild, moderate)
Dysplasia—high-grade (severe).

Histopathology
The thickness of the involved epithelium is usually increased (acanthosis) as a result of hyperplasia of the basal or, more often, the prickle cell layer (Fig. 11.4). In addition, the cells of the superficial layers of the epithelium show production of keratohyaline granules, and form squames (keratinization). Two forms of keratinization are seen: in one of these—orthokeratosis—the keratinized cells have shed their nuclei; in the other—parakeratosis—the nuclei are retained as a small, flat, pyknotic central 'spot' in the cell (Fig. 10.19). The relative proportions of acanthosis and keratinization vary greatly. Fre-

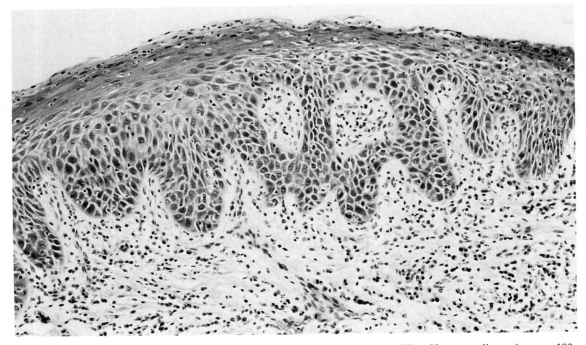

Fig. 11.4 Keratosis of the vocal cord in an elderly man to show severe dysplasia (LIN III).   Haematoxylin–eosin   × 180

quently, the basal layer shows downgrowth into the subepithelial tissue but retains an intact basal lamina. An important additional feature which may or may not be present in laryngeal keratosis is faulty maturation (dysplasia); it is manifested by various degrees of disarray in the orientation and layering of the cells—loss of polarity—and morphological abnormalities of the individual cells such as increased nucleo-cytoplasmic ratio, nuclear pleomorphism, individual-cell keratinization and increased mitotic activity. The features of dysplasia vary in degree and it is usual to grade them—rather arbitrarily—into mild, moderate and severe; severe dysplasia, however, is difficult to separate from the so-called carcinoma in situ in which the changes are seen throughout the whole thickness of the epithelium (Figs 11.5, 11.6a,b). For practical purposes this distinction may be of limited interest only since the treatment of both conditions should be the complete surgical removal by local excision. Malignant change, whether of the in situ or frankly invasive type, however, may be very localized, and this greatly increases the difficulties of diagnosis (see below).

Further biopsies are often necessary, because the finding of equivocal appearances requires examination of other parts of the lesions before the presence of carcinoma can be excluded. Keratosis is an uncommon precursor of laryngeal carcinoma and most critical reviews agree that the incidence of carcinoma following keratosis is below 5%. However, some well-documented cases have been reported[11] and the need for careful follow-up of cases should be emphasized, particularly of those in which dysplasia is a feature.

Microscopical differential diagnosis
The conditions to be considered in the differential diagnosis of keratosis of the larynx are carcinoma in situ and well-differentiated squamous carcinoma. Carcinoma in situ has to be considered particularly when there is conspicuous variation in the size, shape and intensity of staining of the nuclei and irregularity in the arrange-

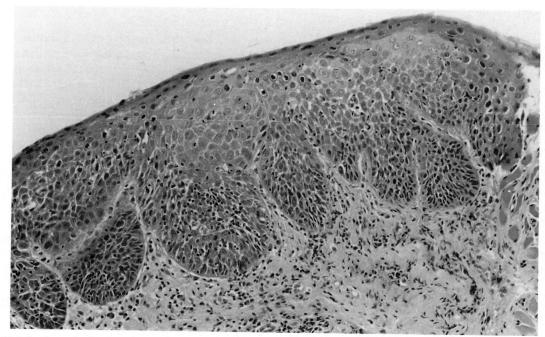

Fig. 11.5 In situ and microinvasive carcinoma of vocal cord of an elderly man. Haematoxylin–eosin × 190

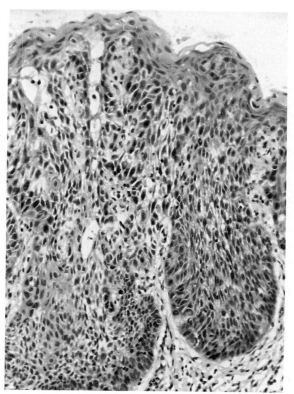

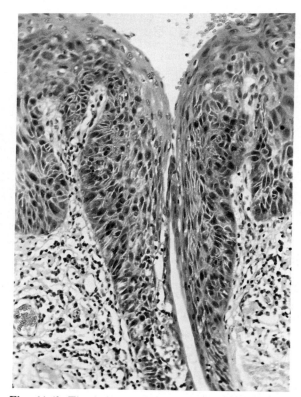

Fig. 11.6a Carcinoma in situ or severe dysplasia of the vocal cord (LIN III). Note characteristic loss of polarity nuclear irregularity of size and shape and nuclear hyper-chromasia. The basal lamina appears to be intact.

Haematoxylin–eosin × 165

Fig. 11.6b The lesion extended into the opening of the underlying gland.

Haematoxylin–eosin × 165

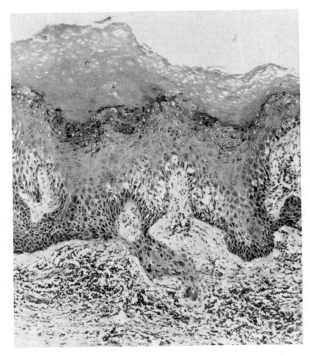

Fig. 11.7a Keratotic vocal cord with dysplastic basal layer and limited microinvasive break in the basal lamina. Female of 50. Heavy smoker for many years.

Haematoxylin–eosin   × 80

ment of the cells throughout most of the lesion. Malignant change, whether of the in situ or frankly invasive type, however, may be localized (Fig. 11.7a) and this greatly increases the difficulties of diagnosis. Electron microscopy shows the weakened basal lamina penetrated by the cytoplasm forming protrusions (Fig. 11.7b). In practice, it is often harder to distinguish confidently between a well-differentiated squamous carcinoma and keratosis than between keratosis and carcinoma in situ, because the haphazard nuclear arrangement and variations in nuclear shape and size are much more distinct in carcinoma in situ.

MALIGNANT TUMOURS

Carcinoma in situ (intraepithelial carcinoma)

This term was introduced in 1932 by Broders[12]

who also described the first case in the larynx; it can be defined as a proliferative disorder of the epithelium displaying all the cytological and structural changes seen in overt malignant tumours but with no evidence of invasion below the basal lamina. Conceptually the name 'carcinoma' infers that the lesion is malignant, but on the other hand malignancy implies that it invades the adjacent tissues and this criterion is not met by the definition of carcinoma in situ given above: this is perhaps why so much controversy still exists with regard to the nomenclature applied to lesions of this type. The problem, of course, is not confined to the larynx but is common to all mucocutaneous epithelia such as those of the oral cavity and the lower female genital tract, particularly in the uterine cervix. It must be said, however, that it is not agreed generally that the laryngeal carcinoma in situ is biologically identical to the same lesion in the cervix. This, to a great extent, may be due to the considerable variation in the criteria of in situ lesions used by different authors, to the necessarily subjective application of such criteria (known to vary even when one pathologist assesses the same case on different occasions) and to the inability to indicate on the basis of morphological features when—or even if—a given lesion will invade. In addition, the often reported observation that many invasive tumours do not pass through a stage of carcinoma in situ, but are invasive from the start, gives rise to questions as to the usefulness of the concept. It is for these reasons that there has recently been a proposal for the adoption of a simplified system of classification which distinguishes between those abnormalities of the squamous epithelium in which there is a significant risk of progression into an invasive carcinoma and those in which this potential is minimal or non-existent:[13] the second group includes such changes as basal cell hyperplasia, simple keratinization, hyperplasia of the prickle-cell layer and acanthosis. The first group, lesions of potential invasive malignancy, is made up of abnormalities traditionally categorized as dysplasia and carcinoma in situ, which are now encompassed in a single diagnostic category of intraepithelial neoplasia (for example, cervical intraepithelial neoplasia and laryngeal intra-

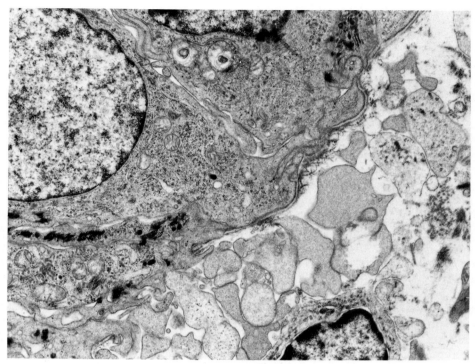

Fig. 11.7b Electron photomicrograph to show the weakened basal lamina of the squamous epithelium of the vocal cord with multiple invaginations or extrusions of the cytoplasm of the basal cells. A characteristic process in malignant change at the epithelial–mesenchymatous junction.   × 14 200

epithelial neoplasia). Three grades of morphological (histological) abnormalities are recognized:

—Laryngeal intraepithelial neoplasia Grade I— LIN I: morphologically equivalent to mild epithelial dysplasia.
—Laryngeal intraepithelial neoplasia Grade II— LIN II: morphologically equivalent to moderate epithelial dysplasia.
—Laryngeal intraepithelial neoplasia Grade III—LIN III: includes both severe dysplasia and carcinoma in situ (see Figs 11.5, 11.6a, 11.7).

The implications of such an approach are significant; the changes of laryngeal intraepithelial neoplasia are considered to be a morphological manifestation of a *neoplastic process* not a *precancerous lesion*. Laryngeal intraepithelial neoplasia presents a continuous spectrum of histological abnormalities. These abnormalities can be subdivided, for descriptive and epidemiological purposes only, into three grades. It is recognized

that lesions classified as intraepithelial neoplasia Grade III are more likely to progress to invasive carcinoma than those of Grade I, but there is no substantial evidence to indicate that invasion occurs only when a Grade I lesion has progressed to a Grade III lesion. Such progression is seen in some cases but there should remain little doubt that occasionally a carcinoma is found in a site where previous biopsy specimens have revealed mild dysplastic features only.

It could be argued that the relatively minor histological abnormality both under the light- and electron microscope (see Fig. 11.7a) associated with Grade I intraepithelial neoplasia does not warrant the 'alarming' connotation of potential malignancy, which may lead to excessive treatment. We believe that these objections cannot be seriously entertained. On the one hand, this system of nomenclature encourages the pathologist to be precise and unequivocally to separate unrelated (reactive) changes (such as basal-cell hyperplasia or simple keratinization of the epithelium) from truly neoplastic lesions; it also spares the pathologist the sometimes impossible and always fruitless task of differentiating between severe dysplasia and carcinoma in situ. On the other hand, the understanding of laryngeal intraepithelial neoplasia as a single process, regardless of the grade, will allow the necessary therapeutic approach to be adopted in all cases, thus avoiding neglect of individual cases on the basis that only mild or moderate dysplasia was seen and, perhaps, ensuring against unnecessarily intensive or radical treatment in cases of carcinoma in situ wrongly interpreted as showing imminent malignant transformation.

Histological appearances of laryngeal intraepithelial neoplasia

Grade I (mild dysplasia). The general tendency of the squamous epithelium to show stratification is preserved and the superficial layers show cytoplasmic differentiation (maturation) with easily seen intracellular bridges and keratinization. The orientation of the cells in the lower layers is not maintained and 'nuclear crowding' is conspicuous, with some pleomorphism and increased nuclear–cytoplasmic ratio. Nucleoli are prominent but mitotic figures are not common.

Grade II (moderate dysplasia). The histological changes are similar to those of Grade I but the undifferentiated (immature) cells extend to two-thirds of the thickness of the epithelium; differentiation and stratification are still seen in the superficial third of the epithelium. Mitotic figures are more numerous.

Grade III (severe dysplasia and carcinoma in situ). The non-stratified, undifferentiated cells occupy more than two-thirds of the epithelium up to its full thickness; this is usually accompanied by a more obvious degree of nuclear pleomorphism which may include the presence of bizarre large nuclei. Mitotic figures are seen with increasing frequency and in all layers; not uncommonly they are of abnormal appearance. There is no keratinization in the great majority of cases but occasionally a thin layer of keratin is seen at the surface with complete lack of orientation of the cells below.

Incidence

Published reports of cases of carcinoma in situ indicate that there are considerable discrepancies regarding its incidence. In one study, five to six times as many patients with invasive carcinoma were seen during the period of 28 years in which 300 patients were seen with carcinoma in situ.[14] In a series of 193 patients seen during a period of 14 years 39 had severe dysplasia or carcinoma in situ.[15] The rates range from nil to 15% of the total number of carcinomas of the larynx collected from the literature.[16] Two possible factors explain the discrepancies:[16] 1) carcinoma in situ may accompany an undiagnosed invasive lesion; and 2) carcinoma in situ may be incorrectly diagnosed by pathologists.

Some authors believe that the finding of severe atypia in a laryngeal biopsy is only rarely followed by the development of carcinoma, and that a conservative approach to the interpretation of keratosis is indicated.[11]

The degree of atypia has been considered to be the most important histological criterion. It has the advantage of permitting objective evaluation by photometry.[17]

A study of 942 larynges at post mortem examination showed cells with atypical nuclei somewhere within the larynx in 84%.[18] 'With a frequency of epithelial atypia as high as this in a population effectively healthy so far as concerned the larynx, the histologist should be wary of over-diagnosis with biopsies from patients whose larynx is not healthy or at least has demanded biopsy.'[19]

While there is general agreement that morphological assessment is fairly reliable, continued attempts are being made to develop quantitative methods derived from growth kinetic and histometric measurements.[17]

Prognosis

The difficulties already mentioned with regard to the diagnosis and incidence of carcinoma in situ of the larynx make assessment of its behaviour and prognosis uncertain since it is quite obvious that a number of different clinicopathological entities are sometimes described under this name. The figure emerging from long-term studies[14] suggest that in a significant number of cases (about 15%) the condition will progress to invasive carcinoma even after what is thought to be adequate treatment. In one study,[14] the greatest rate of invasion occurred after irradiation treatment: only one of 60 patients treated by laryngofissure and cordectomy developed invasive cancer. In a series,[15] 9 out of 39 (23%) patients in Group III (severe dysplasia and carcinoma in situ) developed invasive carcinoma. The interval before invasion occurs varies quite considerably; it can be from 2 months to 8 years after the initial diagnosis and treatment.[14]

The observations referred to above lead to a number of important considerations: 1) the recognition of the abnormal morphological features of the laryngeal epithelium classified here as intraepithelial neoplasia (keratosis with atypia, epithelial dysplasia, carcinoma in situ) should alert the clinician to search for the existence of an invasive lesion nearby; 2) it should be treated by local excision initially; and 3) there should be a long-term follow-up, and recurrences should be dealt with appropriately to minimize the chances of invasion.

SQUAMOUS CELL CARCINOMA

Invasive squamous cell carcinoma

Squamous cell carcinoma represents approximately 90% of all malignant tumours of the larynx and accounts for 1–2% of all human cancers. World Health Organization statistics for 1961, covering 35 countries, disclosed an average of 1.2 cases of laryngeal cancer per 100 000 inhabitants.[20] Epidemiological studies show a very strong association between carcinoma of the larynx and cigarette and pipe-tobacco smoking; its effect in the laryngeal epithelium is also closely related to the overall amount of exposure to cigarette smoke and a recent study of the larynx in 148 men at autopsy[21] showed a normal squamous epithelium covering the vocal cords in 83% of the non-smokers but in only 30.6% of the heavy smokers. Intraepithelial neoplasia or invasive carcinoma was found in 4.2% of the non-

smokers and in 47.2% of the heavy smokers. In those men who had given up smoking for a number of years before death the findings were similar to those in the other non-smokers.[21] These findings are supported by experimental work on Syrian hamsters which demonstrated a linear dose–response effect of tobacco smoking, a promoting influence of alcohol consumption, and induced progression to invasive carcinoma of non-invasive intraepithelial neoplastic changes. The role of alcohol consumption in the aetiology of laryngeal carcinoma, particularly if associated with cigarette smoking, has been emphasized in a recent study.[22] In both Britain and Australia there has been a recent increase in the number of cases of laryngeal carcinoma in parallel with the increase in consumption of alcohol and cigarettes since the second world war; it is of interest that a relatively greater increase of this malignancy in women (particularly in the younger age group), has occurred in line with the fact that in the past 30 years women smoke and drink alcoholic beverages more than before, while cigarette smoking amongst men has remained more or less stable.

The carcinogenic effect of irradiation on the larynx has been well-documented.[23] 10 patients out of 266 initially treated with radiotherapy for carcinoma of the larynx developed a second cancer within the head and neck area. Radiation for benign conditions, such as thyrotoxicosis, tuberculous lymphadenitis or juvenile laryngeal papillomatosis, has occasionally been followed by the appearance of a carcinoma of the larynx after an interval of 20–30 years.[24–26]

Age and sex

Carcinoma of the larynx is predominantly a disease of middle-aged men; approximately 95% of all patients are men aged from 40–70 years with a peak incidence between 55 and 65. As mentioned above, the increase in the number of women who smoke appears to account for the small rise in the occurrence of this cancer amongst them. Younger people are not exempt. A recent publication recorded 33 patients under the age of 35 years.[27] A 12-year-old boy developed an invasive squamous carcinoma following the surgical removal of a papilloma on the right vocal cord at the age of 8 years: the malignant tumour, also on the right vocal cord, was histologically similar to the type commonly found in adults.[28] There was no known history of smoking or of exposure to unusual fumes. The literature since 1868 includes references to 54 other cases of laryngeal carcinoma in children under 15 years old; it is of interest that 40% of these children were girls although the histological type of tumours was similar to that found in adults.[28] Attention must be drawn to the possibility that laryngeal cancer in children may present with persistent hoarseness.

Among 600 laryngeal neoplasms treated at the London Institute of Otolaryngology between 1960 and 1981 there were 18 patients with carcinoma of the larynx under the age of 35.[29] Histologically 17 were squamous cell carcinomas and one a cribriform (adenoid-cystic) adenocarcinoma. The male to female ratio was 2:1, in contrast to the much higher incidence in adult men.[30]

Classification

It is important, in assessing the factors which influence the prognosis of laryngeal carcinoma, to establish the precise location of the tumour and the extension within and outside the larynx, as well as the histological features of individual lesions (Figs 11.8, 11.9). For practical purposes, tumours of the larynx are classified topographically according to their origin in the three main anatomical compartments:

1. Supraglottic (vestibular) tumours. They arise from the posterior surface of the suprahyoid glottis (the tip of the epiglottis, the aryepiglottic folds and the arytenoids) or the infrahyoid level of the epiglottis, the vestibular folds and the ventricles.

2. Glottic tumours. They arise from the vocal cords and the anterior and posterior commissures.

3. Subglottic tumours. These are the tumours arising below the vocal cords and above the first tracheal ring.

This topographical classification excludes tumours arising from the piriform fossae and

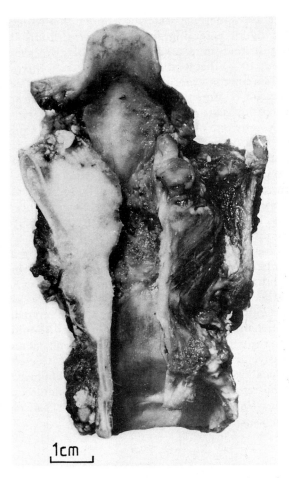

Fig. 11.8 Coronal section of a laryngectomy specimen showing deep invasion not clinically obvious.

the postcricoid area: these are now classified as laryngopharyngeal carcinoma. Recently, a novel technique of examination has been used to prepare transverse sections through the whole extent of the larynx by cutting it on a slicing machine. This method enabled 11 examples of ventriculosaccular carcinoma to be detected among a total of 76 laryngeal carcinomas.[31] Follow-up studies of up to 12 years showed no evidence of lymph node involvement or of local recurrence of the tumour in any of the 11 cases: this suggests that lesions in this location may be associated with a better prognosis than that of cancer arising elsewhere in the larynx. Some of the features that suggest the diagnosis of ventriculosaccular carcinoma are: 1) the presence of a ventricular

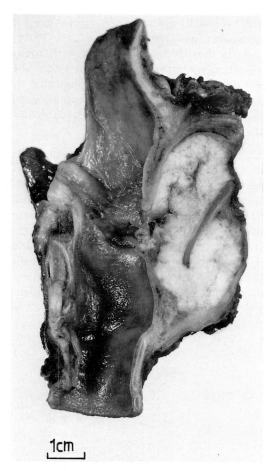

Fig. 11.9 Carcinoma of the larynx. The larynx has been divided sagittally through the midpoint of the right vocal fold, where there was a barely visible ulcer with everted edges. It is seen that the tumour has extended in an exuberant manner from this point anteroinferiorly, through the cricothyroid membrane, to invest the lamina of the thyroid cartilage, apparently without invading the perichondrium. The tumour has also extended anterosuperiorly, through the thyro-epiglottic ligament and into the pre-epiglottic space. The specimen illustrates the extent to which a superficially small carcinoma may have spread into the more deeply situated structures of the larynx and its vicinity.

tumour; 2) a supraglottic bulge above it; 3) a paraglottic swelling on CT scan, covered by a smooth laryngeal mucosa; and 4) the histological features of well-differentiated carcinoma.[31]

Pathological considerations
1. Supraglottic carcinomas. These usually involve the epiglottis and vestibular folds and do not extend to the supporting cartilaginous frame of the larynx; they stop at the level of the anterior commissure and ventricle. This localization means that most supraglottic tumours can be excised surgically without resection of the glottis: good functional voice recovery is therefore possible. More extensive surgery does not appear to improve the overall results. However, large, ulcerating lesions may sometimes involve the thyroid cartilage: they are thus 'transglottic' and require treatment by total laryngectomy. Metastasis to lymph nodes rather than recurrence is the common cause of therapeutic failure in these lesions. Cervical lymph node involvement was present in 24 out of 75 cases in one series.[32]

2. Glottic carcinomas. These are the most common laryngeal cancers. The presenting symptom is hoarseness, at first intermittent and later persistent. When the vocal cords become fixed, the glottic space may be greatly reduced and breathing difficulties result. The progression of the disease is usually slow, and metastasis is a late occurrence since the lymphatic drainage of the cords is limited. The most common site within the region is the anterior half of the vocal cords and the anterior commissure. The posterior commissure is rarely involved. The tumour may spread across the midline to involve the opposite cord; it may invade the ventricle, the thyroid cartilage and the soft tissues of the pre-epiglottic area. Direct involvement of the submucosal and muscular tissues and of the conus elasticus is common. However, most tumours remain localized to the larynx for a long time and this accounts for their relatively better prognosis, with high cure rates obtained by either radiation or surgical removal of vocal cord lesions. The proportion of cases with metastasis to lymph nodes is small; it is reported to range from 0–13%.

3. Subglottic carcinomas. The subglottic space consists of: 1) an anterior triangular portion with the apex formed by the common anterior commissure tendon; 2) the undersurface of the vocal cords; and 3) a lateral portion ending at the lower border of the cricoid cartilage. Normally it is lined by respiratory epithelium. Islands of metaplastic squamous epithelium are present in

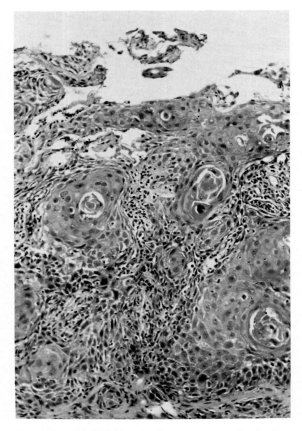

Fig. 11.10 Well-differentiated squamous cell carcinoma showing keratotic 'pearl' formation in the epiglottis of a man of 66. Positive TP1.   Haematoxylin–eosin   × 135

up to 40% of normal, non-smoking individuals.[33] Only about 4% of laryngeal carcinomas arise in the subglottic space (42 out of 1011 in one series).[34] The common presenting symptom is stridor; dyspnoea and hoarseness occur later when the tumour extends to involve the vocal cords. Metastasis to lymph nodes is frequent (in about 50% of cases) although often clinically undetected. The prognosis is poor because of the tendency of the disease to present in an advanced state; the 5-year survival rate is only about 50%. Subglottic carcinomas show a tendency to grow circumferentially, to invade cartilage, and to spread outside the larynx through the cricothyroid membrane[35] (Fig. 11.9).

Histopathology
The majority of carcinomas of the larynx are well

or moderately well differentiated or transitional type squamous neoplasms (Figs 11.10, 11.11, 11.12). As is the practice in dealing with squamous neoplasms in other parts of the body, the laryngeal tumours are graded histologically by taking into account a number of morphological features, of which the following are the most important.

(1) Differentiation is the extent to which the tumour cells resemble normal squamous cells (Fig. 11.10). The presence of prickles (intercellular bridges), keratohyaline granules, and of full keratinization either at the surface of the tumour (as orthokeratosis or parakeratosis) or within the tumour mass as individual cell keratinization and keratin pearl formation (dyskeratosis) are the main features assessed by light microscopy. Electron microscopy may be of further help in identifying desmosomes and tonofilaments as well as

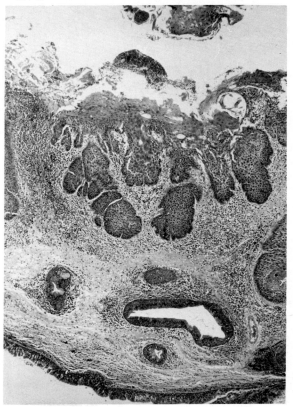

Fig. 11.11 Well-differentiated squamous cell carcinoma invading ventricular fold. Male of 65.

Haematoxylin–eosin   × 35

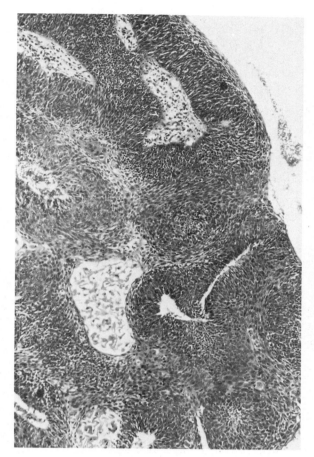

Fig. 11.12 Transitional type squamous cell carcinoma of the vocal cord. Young man of 34.

Haematoxylin–eosin   × 95

keratohyaline and keratin granules, and penetration of the basal lamina (see Fig. 11.7).

(2) Cellular pleomorphism relates to the degree of variation in the size, shape and nucleo-cytoplasmic ratio of the tumour cells, the presence of bizarre, giant or multinucleated cells and the presence of prominent or multiple nucleoli within the nucleus.

(3) Structural or architectural abnormality—for example, loss of normal stratification, anomalous arrangement of the cells into groups, cords or sheets, or their total dissociation from one another.

(4) The mitotic-figure rate is considered an important indication of the rate of growth of the tumour. The presence of abnormal, tripolar,

ring-form or bizarre mitotic figures is usually regarded as a sign of poor prognosis.

(5) The tumour–host interaction: there is considerable variation in the outline of the tumour margins as they meet the adjacent tissues. These tumour edges may be jagged (infiltrative) (Fig. 11.13) or well delineated and rounded ('pushing') (Figs 11.14a,b, 11.15). The extent of penetration of the basal lamina and of the deeper tissues and whether invasion takes place at a small area of the tumour margin or along an extensive front are considered relevant as is the demonstration of vascular, lymphatic and perineural invasion by tumour cells.

(6) The host response, which is perhaps the feature of most doubtful significance. It is manifested by an inflammatory infiltration at the edge of the tumour, usually by plasma cells and lymphocytes.

These parameters are assessed subjectively by pathologists and incorporated into a report which

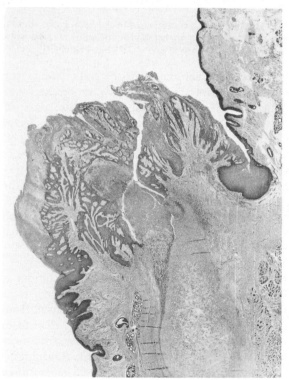

Fig. 11.13 A well-differentiated papillomatous squamous cell carcinoma of the vocal cord displaying jagged edges.

Haematoxylin–eosin   × 13

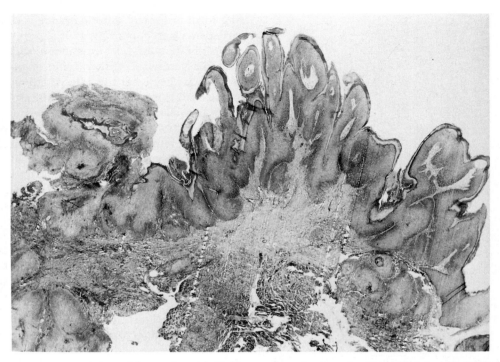

Fig. 11.14a Verrucous carcinoma of the vocal cord (with history of previous negative biopsies). A broadly-implanted, papillomatous, well-differentiated squamous tumour is seen in this biopsy specimen. There is considerable inflammatory reaction in the underlying fibrous tissue.   Haematoxylin–eosin   × 15

is normally summarized by allocating the individual tumours to a well-, moderately- or poorly-differentiated grade. The value of such assessment has stood the test of time. Some careful studies have demonstrated a relationship between the degree of differentiation of the primary tumour and the probability of metastatic involvement of the lymph nodes of the neck and the ultimate rates of cure.[10] There are considerable limitations to the usefulness of this approach because of the subjectivity of the criteria used which inevitably results in variation between observers. The clinician's greatest interest is in obtaining a reliable indication of how the tumour is likely to behave and whether or not metastases have occurred; he requires this information from the diagnostic biopsy specimen rather than from the eventual operation. In this manner, treatment may be selected on a sounder basis. The limitations of the conventional approach, as outlined above, have been successfully overcome at the Karolinska Institute in Stockholm[36] where a point score system of grading the malignant

potential of tumours was devised. Scores of 1 to 4 are given to four features of the tumour cell population (structure, differentiation, nuclear pleomorphism and number of mitoses) and four features of the tumour–host interactions (mode of invasion, stage of invasion, vascular invasion and cellular response to the tumour). Using this system, 230 glottic carcinomas treated by a standard radiotherapy regimen and followed up for at least 5 years were studied; a multivariant analysis with recurrence (local, or metastatic in lymph nodes) as a dependent variable revealed that the most important factors in the prediction of the 5-year recurrence rates were: 1) nuclear pleomorphism; 2) mode of invasion; and 3) total points scored. Regardless of the clinical staging of the tumours, those in which the total score was between 10 and 15 showed a 0% rate of recurrence whereas those with scores of 16–28 had a rate of 20–39%. The figures can be broken down further if the mode of invasion and the nuclear pleomorphism scores are taken into account. The usefulness of this work appears to be very con-

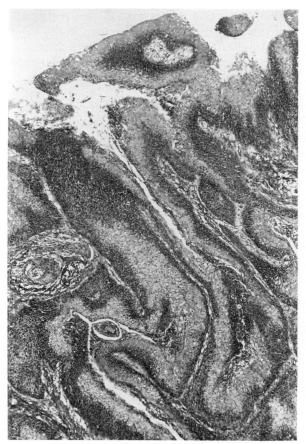

Fig. 11.14b Detail of Figure 11.14a showing the broad 'pushing' papillary structures.

Haematoxylin–eosin × 45

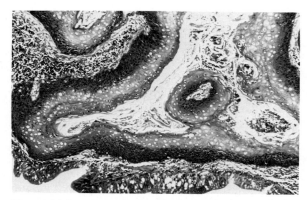

Fig. 11.15 Appears to be 'pushing' towards the ventricular fold covered by stratified columnar epithelium.

Haematoxylin–eosin × 55

siderable, in particular because it is based upon the histological examination of the pretreatment diagnostic biopsy specimen, which tends to produce a lower score than the definitive resected specimen in almost half of the cases.[37] These results, if confirmed by studies of larger series, suggest that the adoption of such a method could considerably improve the value of histological examination of biopsy specimens and its contribution to the management of laryngeal carcinomas.

Prognosis of laryngeal squamous carcinoma

It has already been mentioned that the precise location of the tumour within the larynx, the occurrence of metastasis and the histological type of the tumour are relevant factors influencing the overall prognosis. Many of these factors are included in a clinical staging classification similar to that proposed by the International Union Against Cancer in 1968 and usually referred to as the TNM Classification. A modified example of such a classification applied to glottic carcinomas is given below.[37a]

TNM classification

TIS Pre-invasive carcinoma (carcinoma in situ)

T1 Tumour limited to the glottic region with normal mobility
T1A confined to one cord
T1B involving both cords

T2 Tumour extending to the subglottic or to the supraglottic regions (that is to the ventricles or the vestibular folds) with normal or limited mobility

T3 Tumour limited to the larynx with fixation of one or both vocal cords

T4 Tumour extending beyond larynx (into cartilage, piriform fossa, skin)

N0 No lymph nodes clinically palpable

N1 Palpable, mobile lymph nodes on one side of neck

N2 Palpable, mobile lymph nodes on both sides of neck

N3 Palpable, fixed lymph nodes

M0 No clinical evidence of distant metastasis

M1 Clinical or radiological evidence of distant metastasis.

Such clinical staging is a basic foundation but not suitable for every circumstance. It is clinically oriented and it often lacks precision in the assessment of the extent of the tumour and in the correct interpretation of 'palpable' lymph nodes (many metastatic deposits are not detectable clinically). It is however, a rough guide to the survival rates and as such retains its value in clinical management. It can be usefully and precisely applied to resected specimens.

Following surgery there are two major indications of the failure of treatment—stomal recurrence and distant metastases. While the increasing detection of distant metastases (visceral deposits and lymph node involvement below the level of the clavicles) may be related to the overall improvement in the rate of survival the pathogenesis of stomal recurrence remains unclear. The frequency with which local recurrence occurs is estimated at approximately 5%.[38] Factors that are thought to be of importance in their occurrence include undetected (and therefore unremoved) submucosal extension of tumour to the margin of the resection; there are also such possibilities as the development of a new primary tumour at the stoma and the implantation of malignant cells during the removal of the original tumour. In support of the first of these factors is the observation that patients whose resected specimens have a margin of resection clear of tumour greater than 0.2 cm show a lesser incidence of recurrence and a better 5-year survival rate. Approximately half of the recurrences occur within 6 months of the initial operation. The operative mortality for this type of complication is very high and radiotherapy appears to be ineffective.

It seems likely that the lack of autopsy studies of patients who have had carcinoma of the larynx may account for the low reported incidence of distant metastases from these tumours. The findings of diffuse tumour spread in 16 out of 18 patients with laryngeal carcinoma have been reported.[39] Other series show a smaller percentage but it seems that tumours from the supraglottic area are more likely to spread far and that more than half of the patients with distant metastases have also uncontrolled local disease in the neck. The lungs are the most common site of distant tumour spread, followed by mediastinal lymph nodes, bones and the liver.

Verrucous carcinoma

This now well-established clinicopathological entity was first described by Ackerman[40] who reported, in 1948, 31 cases involving the oral mucosa. Several cases have been reported involving the larynx, the skin and the male and female reproductive organs. The larynx is the most common site within the respiratory tract, where it accounts for approximately 2–3% of all squamous carcinomas. Most cases arise in the glottic region and involve one or both vocal cords. Ferlito & Recher[41] have reported a series of 77 cases from their own clinic at Padua in Italy and reviewed the relevant literature. From these data, it emerges that most patients are men (74 out of their 77; 6 to 1 in other series) aged 29–80 with a peak incidence between 50 and 69 years, and a very high proportion of smokers (90% according to Fechner).[42] Macroscopically the lesion varies in size but is often extensive; it appears as a broadly implanted papillomatous 'fungating' mass, usually interpreted by the clinician as a malignant tumour (Fig. 11.14a). Histologically, the tumour does not show its 'true nature' on a biopsy specimen and hence causes considerable diagnostic difficulty, and even dissension between pathologists and surgeons. The characteristic microscopical features are the presence of well-differentiated keratinizing islands and cords of tumour cells which do not display features of malignancy (for example, nuclear pleomorphism and mitotic activity). The tumour is covered by a thick layer of keratinized cells and shows a papillary infolding with clefts between the folds that reach the deepest layers and are often filled with keratin debris (Fig. 11.14b); typically, the deeper margin is rounded and well-delineated, with an 'advancing' or 'pushing' appearance compressing the underlying stroma, which contains a heavy lymphocytic and plasma cell inflammatory reaction (Fig. 11.15). Commonly, a granulomatous reaction of foreign-body type may be seen at the margins. The biopsy specimens, which often are superficial, usually show none of the characteristic deeper features but only a benign-looking epithelium with much keratosis and papillomatosis. In these circumstances, consultation between pathologist and surgeon is the only way to arrive at the correct diagnosis, and in many cases a second, and adequate, biopsy specimen, including the base of the lesion, may be necessary. The need to recognize this entity is emphasized by its non-aggressive behaviour: it seems that no acceptable example of a verrucous laryngeal carcinoma has given rise to metastases unless after radiotherapy (see below). The tendency of these tumours to extend locally and to destroy adjacent structures is widely recognized. The treatment of choice appears to be surgical removal, which, when complete, results in a very low recurrence rate (4 of the 60 surgically-treated cases in the Italian series referred to above).[41]

Transformation of the verrucous laryngeal carcinoma into a frank squamous carcinoma, with potential for metastatic spread, has been reported in rare instances, sometimes after radiation treatment.

Some verrucous carcinomas are multifocal at presentation.

A recent study of 104 patients with verrucous carcinoma of the oral cavity[43] has drawn particular attention to the finding of 'foci of invasive squamous cell carcinoma which has coexisted within the larger verrucous lesions in 20% of the cases'. The authors emphasize the importance of examining any verrucous carcinoma for the presence of such microscopical foci of invasive carcinoma.

Spindle-cell squamous carcinoma
This interesting tumour is variously named pseudosarcoma, carcinosarcoma and 'collision tumour', as well as spindle-cell squamous carcinoma. The names reflect controversy about its histogenesis. Various theories have been proposed to explain the admixture of malignant epithelial cells and mesenchyme-like spindle-shaped cells. The theories range from interpretation of the spindle cells as a non-neoplastic reaction of the stroma to the presence of the carcinoma (pseudosarcoma), the existence of two synchronous tumours, a sarcoma and a carcinoma from nearby sites ('collision tumour'), the origin of the tumour from a primitive cell capable of differentiation towards squamous epithelium and stromal tissues (carcinosarcoma), and the view that the spindle cells are modified malignant epithelial cells (spindle-cell carcinoma).[44a] Recent studies with the electron microscope and the light microscope support the latter interpretation and disclose features of epithelial differentiation, such as tonofilaments and desmosomes, within the spindle cells which, in addition, show abundant rough endoplasmic reticulum with dilated cisternae and a close association with collagen fibrils;[44, 45] such appearances can be explained if a process of mesenchymal metaplasia of the malignant squamous cells is accepted.[44] Cells with both epithelial and mesenchymal features are seen regularly in the myoepithelial component of pleomorphic salivary gland tumours.

Regardless of the origin of this tumour there are two misconceptions about it that must be corrected. One of these is that the spindle-cell component does not have the potential for metastasis. It has been documented that among four cases in which metastases to the neck and lymph nodes had occurred, two showed both squamous and spindle-cell elements in the secondary deposits and one showed spindle cells alone.[46] Similar findings have been reported by others.[47] The second misconception relates to the often comparatively benign behaviour of these tumours.[48] In a series of 111 cases, the overall mortality was 32%, which is similar to that of typical squamous carcinomas.[48]

These spindle-cell tumours are seen in men more often than in women, with a ratio of 10:1. They present mostly in the sixth and seventh decades (range 42–87 years). Most (72%) originate in the glottis, the remainder in the hypopharynx (14%), the supraglottic region (12%) and the subglottic region. Two-thirds of the tumours are polypoid (Fig. 11.16) and measure from 1 to 3 cm in diameter (some as large as 6 cm have been described). The others are sessile or have a wide attachment area; when cut across they show a greyish, firm, uniform parenchyma. Histologically, the squamous component may be inconspicuous and a diligent search, even with step

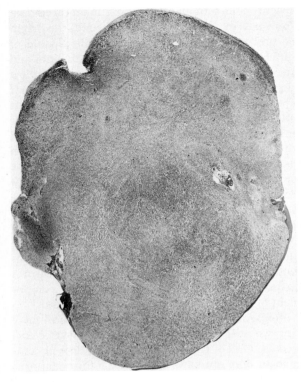

Fig. 11.16 A polypoid spindle-cell carcinoma from the anterior commissure of a 57-year-old man. The covering squamous epithelium is thin and partially ulcerated.

Haematoxylin–eosin   × 8

sections, may be required; it is often seen concentrated at the base or stalk of the tumour and, in some instances, has been reported as carcinoma in situ. 'Streaming' of the squamous cells among the underlying spindle-cell elements can be seen at sites where the basal lamina is disrupted. The spindle-cell component constitutes the greater proportion of the tumour and often reaches the surface or is covered by an attenuated layer of squamous cells (Fig. 11.17); it varies in cellularity from cases in which there is collagenous stroma with sparse malignant spindle cells to others in which the cells are densely packed and may be arranged in whorls or bundles (Fig. 11.18). Multinucleated forms are occasionally present. The frequency with which mitotic figures are seen is variable (Fig. 11.18). Metastasis develops in about 20% of cases, the rate

varying with the location of the primary lesion (15% of glottic tumours, 30% of subglottic tumours and up to 60% of the hypopharyngeal tumours).[47]

The treatment of choice appears to be surgical removal by local excision or, if necessary, by laryngectomy. Irradiation is followed by recurrence in a high proportion of cases.

TUMOURS OF THE SEROMUCOUS GLANDS

Adenomas

Adenomas of the submucosal glands present clinically as a swelling of a few millimetres in diameter, commonly associated with hoarseness. The histological appearances of the lesions often reveal the presence of the so-called oncocytes. This, together with the considerable doubt as to their neoplastic nature, accounts for the multiplicity of names given to them, including oxyphilic adenoma, oncocytoma, oncocytic cyst and oncocytic papillary cystadenoma. Oncocytes are cells with a small, densely staining nucleus and a brightly eosinophilic, coarsely granular cytoplasm; under the electron microscope the cytoplasm is filled with tightly packed abnormal mitochondria with little remaining space for endoplasmic reticulum. Histochemical studies demonstrate high activity of mitochondrial respiratory enzymes. These features are thought to indicate degeneration or 'ageing' of the cells. Oncocytes are commonly found in the ducts of normal salivary glands, in the mucosal glands of the upper respiratory tract and upper parts of the digestive tract; they are also the main component lining the ductal elements of adenolymphomas of salivary glands (Warthin's tumour).

A review of 135 published cases of oncocytic lesions of the larynx[49] showed that they occur most frequently in elderly patients (average age 64) and more commonly in females (62%). The most frequent sites are in the supraglottic region (the ventricles and vestibular folds); some examples have occurred in the subglottic region. The tumours are polypoid masses covered by intact mucosa. They consist of a simple or multi-

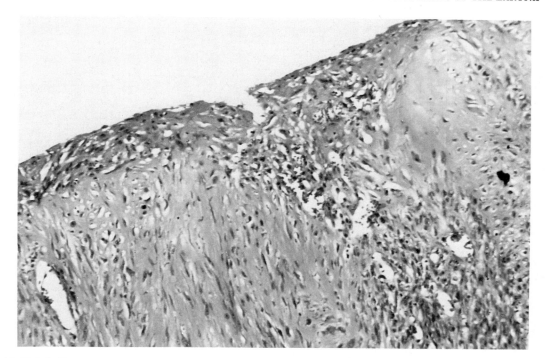

Fig. 11.17 Spindle-cell carcinoma of the larynx to show transition from squamous to spindle-cell type. Haematoxylin–eosin   × 125

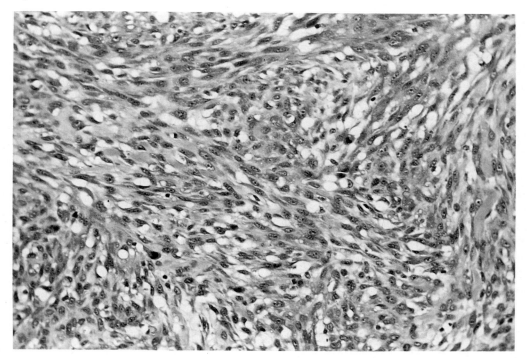

Fig. 11.18 High-power detail of the spindle-cell component forming bundles and whorls. A few mitotic figures are present. Haematoxylin–eosin   × 250

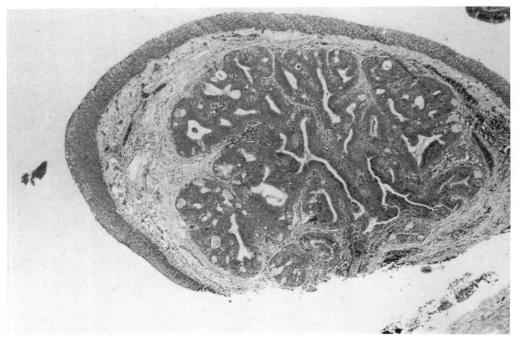

Fig. 11.19 Eosinophilic 'oncocytic' papillary adenoma of the vocal cord. Haematoxylin–eosin   × 40

locular cyst filled with seromucinous fluid; sometimes the cyst lining has a papillary infolding (Fig. 11.19) and is composed of one or two layers of oncocytes and columnar ciliated cells in varying proportions (Figs 11.20, 11.21). It seems widely agreed that the majority of these lesions represent a process of oncocytic metaplasia either in a cystic or hyperplastic gland or in a benign cystadenoma. True oncocytomas are solid lesions and are found only exceptionally in the larynx.

Malignant tumours of the seromucinous glands

Adenocarcinomas of the larynx are rare, representing less than 1% of all malignant laryngeal tumours. Most of the patients are men over the age of 60. Some distinct histological types are recognized: ´

1. Adenocarcinoma

Primary laryngeal adenocarcinomas are often large (1–2 cm in diameter). They present as non-ulcerated supraglottic or transglottic masses that present the usual features of a carcinoma arising from ducts or glands. In spite of treatment their mortality is almost 100% within 2–5 years (Fig. 11.22).[50]

2. Adenoid cystic carcinoma (cylindroma, cribriform adenocarcinoma)

Like their counterparts in the major salivary glands, these tumours of the laryngeal glands are usually characteristic with neatly demarcated islands of epithelial cells around a dense, acellular hyalinized matrix. Two-thirds occur in the subglottic region and most of the remainder in the supraglottic region. Although they have a tendency to recur locally and may metastasize to cervical lymph nodes, long survival after surgery is not uncommon.

3. Mucoepidermoid tumour

This, also, is a tumour that is seen most frequently in the major salivary glands. Occasionally it arises in the epiglottis or, more rarely, elsewhere in the larynx. The typical histological picture of clumps or strands of squamous cells, mucin-containing cells, and intermediate ('trans-

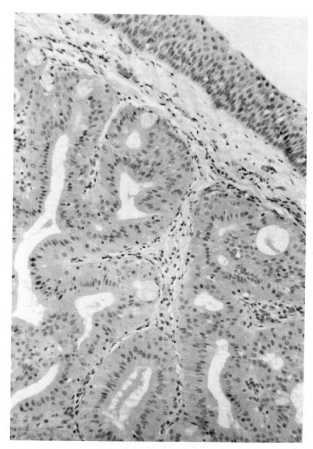

Fig. 11.20 Detail of eosinophilic adenoma formed by twin-layered epithelium.

Haematoxylin–eosin   × 112

itional') cells is seen in a large proportion of the cases. This tumour accounted for 11 cases out of 872 examples of laryngeal cancer (1.2%).[51] It tends to be diagnosed as a squamous carcinoma on biopsy, being reclassified as mucoepidermoid only when the whole tumour is examined.[51] Although some of these tumours are very well-differentiated they should all be regarded as malignant, since metastases have been known to occur even from the best-differentiated examples. The tumours can be classified as of high, moderate or low malignancy, according to histological differentiation.[51]

4. Pleomorphic tumour ('mixed' tumour)
Only an occasional pleomorphic tumour of the type seen in salivary glands has been reported.[52]

It is even rarer for such a tumour to be unequivocally malignant.

When considering the adenocarcinomas that arise in the larynx it is important not to overlook the occurrence of metastatic deposits of renal and—less often—of bronchial, mammary, prostatic and other carcinomas originating elsewhere in the body.[53]

OTHER RARE CARCINOMAS

Giant cell carcinoma
This is a very rare tumour of the larynx.[54] Microscopically, it is composed of pleomorphic multinucleated tumour giant cells with an intensely acidophilic vacuolated cytoplasm in a delicate fibrovascular stroma (Fig. 11.23).

Clear cell carcinoma
The very rare primary clear cell carcinoma of the respiratory tract has a close histological resemblance to the clear cell carcinoma that arises in the kidney. This resemblance may lead to a wrong diagnosis of some consequence to the patient. In the lungs it accounts for 2–3% of all malignant neoplasms. Three cases of primary clear cell carcinoma of the larynx have been reported.[55] The tumour is composed of nests or clusters of large, round, clear cells with a small vesicular central nucleus. The cytoplasm is abundant and vacuolated, appearing so clear that it may be described as 'empty'. Some of the cells are multinucleated and very atypical. Diagnostic certainty rests on electron microscopy, which shows a distinctive pattern of membrane-bound glycogen-filled vesicles in the cells. The behaviour of these tumours is difficult to assess because of their rarity. All three of the patients whose cases are on record presented with extensive metastatic involvement of lymph nodes and died within a comparatively short period.

NEUROENDOCRINE TUMOURS

Paraganglioma (chemodectoma)
The extra-adrenal paraganglia comprise a dispersed group of organs with a common neuro-

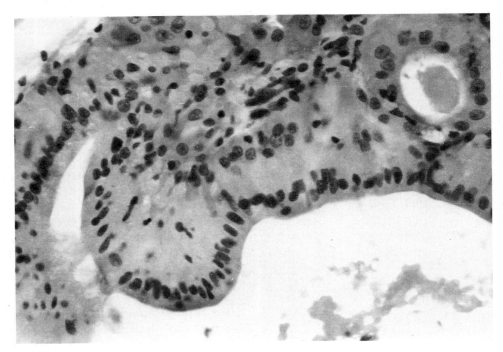

Fig. 11.21 Detail of twin-layered epithelium from an 'oncocytic' adenoma.
Haematoxylin–eosin   × 375

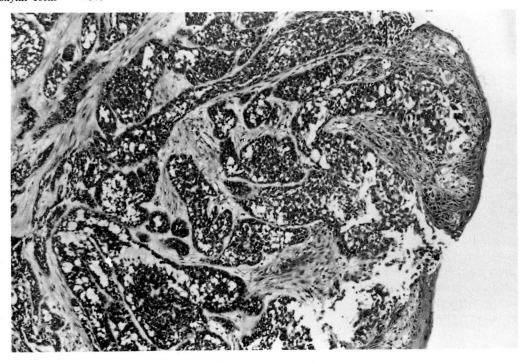

Fig. 11.22 Invasive moderately well-differentiated adenocarcinoma of the larynx.
Haematoxylin–eosin   × 50

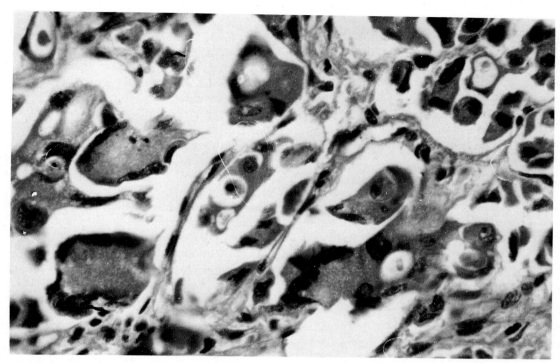

Fig. 11.23 Giant cell carcinoma of the larynx. The tumour is composed of pleomorphic multinucleated giant cells with a vacuolated eosinophilic cytoplasm, in a delicate fibrovascular stroma. Some of the giant cells contain phagocytosed cells or debris.

Haematoxylin–eosin   × 480

Section provided by Professor Alfio Ferlito, University of Padua, Italy.

ectodermal origin. There are two pairs of paraganglia in the larynx, the superior beneath the epithelium on each side of the midline just above the anterior end of the vocal cords and the inferior between the thyroid and cricoid cartilages. It is from these structures that the rare laryngeal paragangliomas arise. The term paraganglioma is preferable to chemodectoma and glomus tumour since it is now established that the cells of the paraganglia contain neurosecretory granules and are derived from the neural crest. They are related to the system of neuroendocrine cells, the APUD system. It is almost certain that paraganglia do not have a chemosensory function: the name chemodectoma is therefore inappropriate for the tumours that arise from them.[56]

In a review of the literature published in English up to the end of 1980 altogether 17 cases of paraganglioma were found.[57] The salient features of these tumours (Figs 11.24, 11.25) are the arrangement of large polyhedral cells in nests and cords separated by fine bands of fibrovascular tissue. The tumour cells have a regular, round central nucleus and granular eosinophilic cytoplasm which almost invariably shows argyrophilia when stained by such methods as the Grimelius technique. Electron microscopy is usually very helpful, demonstrating the presence of dense-core, neurosecretory-type, membrane-bound granules.

Most of the reported tumours were biologically inactive. In one case secretion of adrenaline and noradrenaline and of the calcium-lowering hormone calcitonin has been reported.[58]

The prognosis of laryngeal paraganglioma is uncertain and unrelated to its histological appearance. Malignant behaviour has been reported in one-third of cases; it has been suggested[20]— rightly, we believe—that this may be an overestimate. However, the likelihood of local recurrence and metastasis has to be considered.[59, 60] In the series of 17 cases referred to above, metastasis

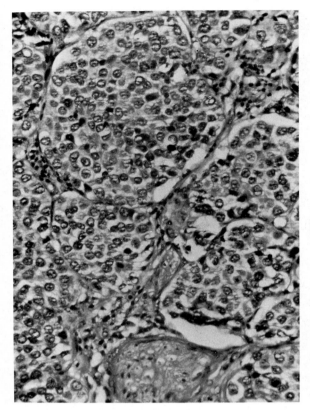

Fig. 11.24 Paraganglioma of the larynx to show the typical alveolar pattern of large round massed cells separated by fibrous septa. Note small nerve haematoxylin–eosin. Male of 70 (Case as Fig. 11.22).

Haematoxylin–eosin   ×175

polygonal cells with a varying amount of eosinophilic, finely granular cytoplasm and a round or oval nucleus. The cells form solid nests and acini surrounded or separated by septa of vascular fibrous tissue. A trabecular pattern is sometimes seen, as in cases of atypical carcinoids of the digestive and respiratory system that lack the characteristic histological pattern usually associated with argentaffinity of the cells (Fig. 11.28). A mixture of these patterns is commonly seen in atypical cases.[64] Amyloid degeneration of the stroma may occur.

Electron microscopy (Fig. 11.29) shows large numbers of membrane-bound neurosecretory granules in the cytoplasm.

It is of interest that some of these cases have been found to contain cytoplasmic material which reacts with antibodies to human polypeptide hormones such as calcitonin, indicating their

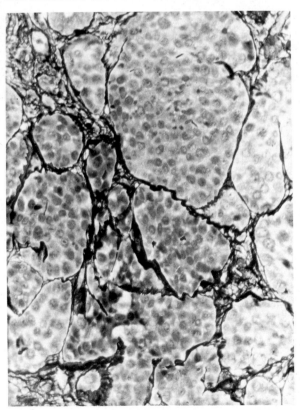

Fig. 11.25 Paraganglioma of the larynx. Reticulin impregnation emphasizing the alveolar pattern. Male of 70 (as Fig. 11.24).

Haematoxylin–eosin   ×175

to lymph nodes had occurred in 4, and 3 caused the death of the patients. In 8 of the cases there had been no recurrence of the tumour after its initial resection.[57]

Carcinoid tumours

The carcinoid tumours are closely related to paragangliomas, although they differ in histology. They are sometimes referred to as neuroendocrine carcinomas. They were first described in the larynx by Goldman et al in 1967[61] and a review published in 1983 included 8 cases altogether,[62] including a malignant example in the subglottic region.[63] Macroscopically, the neoplasm has no distinctive features and may be mistaken for a carcinoma. Microscopically (Figs 11.26, 11.27, 11.28), it is composed of small

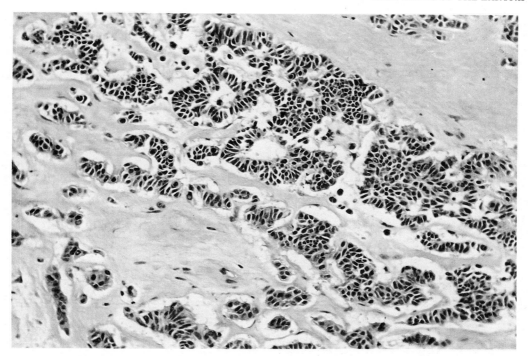

Fig. 11.26a Carcinoid tumour of the larynx; the small regular cells are arranged in a trabecular pattern, forming ribbons. Haematoxylin–eosin   × 250

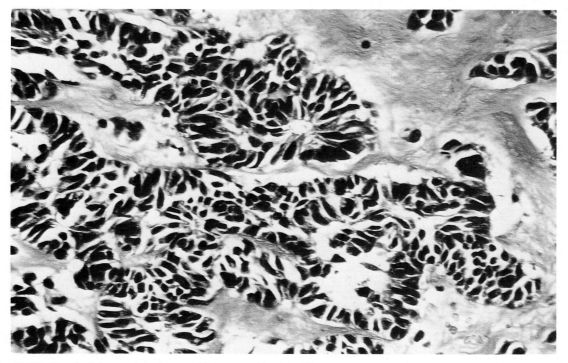

Fig. 11.26b Detail of the previous figure at higher magnification. The pseudoglandular arrangement of the cells at the centre of the picture is noticeable.   Haematoxylin–eosin   × 500

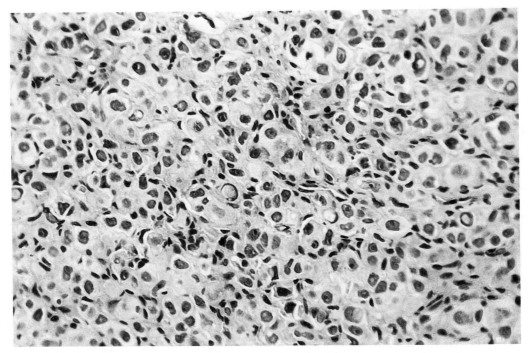

Fig. 11.27 A different carcinoid tumour of the larynx of a much more undifferentiated type.
Haematoxylin–eosin   × 500

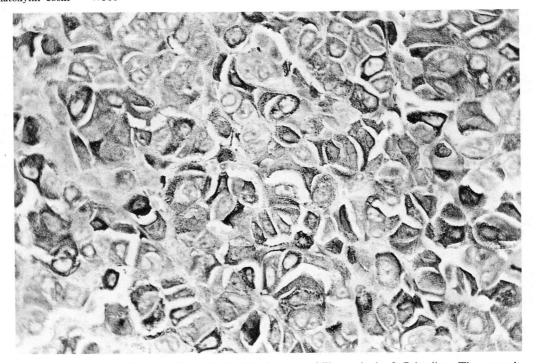

Fig. 11.28 Same case as in Figure 11.27 stained with the argyophilic method of Grimelius. The strongly positive intracytoplasmic granules are clearly visible.
Grimelius   × 500

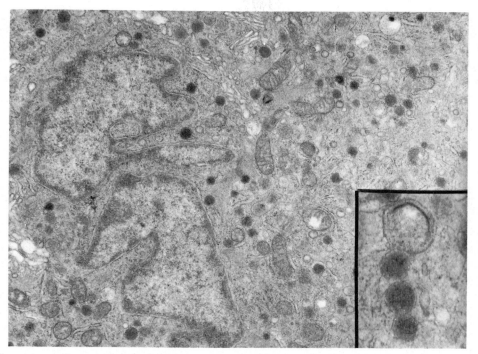

Fig. 11.29 Low-power electron micrograph of the same tumour illustrated in Figures 11.27, 11.28. Note the membrane-bound neurosecretory-type cytoplasmic granules seen at higher power in the inset.   × 4 200 (inset × 21 000)

origin from cells of the neuroendocrine–APUD system.[65] Such cells are widespread throughout the respiratory system.

Small cell anaplastic carcinoma ('oat-cell' carcinoma)[66]

There is increasing evidence, as is the case with carcinoid tumours, that APUD cells may be the source of the small cell anaplastic carcinomas, the so-called 'oat-cell' carcinomas of the bronchus, some of which are known to synthesize polypeptide hormones and can be shown by electron microscopy to contain neurosecretory-type granules. Tumours of identical appearances have been reported in the larynx.[67] Microscopically, the typical 'oat cell' tumour is composed of small, oval cells with dark staining nucleus and scanty cytoplasm; the cells may be arranged in ribbons and there may be pseudorosette formation. Of the 16 cases reported up to 1981,[60] 55% were supraglottic, 33% were subglottic, and only 12% involved the vocal cords; metastases were evident in 72% of the patients at the time of presentation and the median survival was only 10 months.

SECONDARY TUMOURS

Secondary tumours of the larynx are rare, probably due to the relatively terminal position of the larynx in the normal lymphatic and vascular circulation[68] but may occur either by lymphatic dissemination or through the blood stream.

An analysis of 72 cases of metastatic tumours in the ear, nose and throat included 9 instances involving the larynx.[53]

Renal adenocarcinoma and cutaneous melanoma account for most examples of metastasis to the larynx; others include carcinoma of breast, lung, gastrointestinal tract and genito-urinary tract.[69–71]

MULTIPLE PRIMARY MALIGNANT TUMOURS

Tumours of identical histological type

Multiple squamous carcinomas of the larynx occur frequently; they may develop simultaneously or consecutively.[72, 73] They may occur spontaneously, or following irradiation;[26, 74, 75] they have also been observed in patients who had had surgical treatment. In a series of 44 cases of multiple primary cancers in the head and neck the site of the first cancer was the larynx in 11; in 6 patients the larynx was the site of the second primary cancer.[76] The occurrence of separate primary tumours in the larynx and in the lungs has been reported, including one series of 21 cases.[77]

Tumours of different histological types

Multiple primary malignant tumours of the larynx of different cell origin are rare. When two different tumours develop synchronously they may form a 'collision tumour'. In all the cases that we know of one of the neoplasms was a squamous carcinoma; the other was either epithelial (also adenocarcinoma or small cell anaplastic carcinoma) or of mesenchymal type (fibrosarcoma, rhabdomyosarcoma, malignant fibrous histiocytoma, haemangiopericytoma or malignant lymphoma). The association of anaplastic small cell carcinoma ('oat-cell' carcinoma) with squamous carcinoma in the larynx is of particular interest.[78]

MESENCHYMATOUS TISSUE TUMOURS

Most malignant neoplasms of the larynx are epithelial; the incidence of malignant mesenchymal tumours is low (1–2% of all malignant neoplasms[79]). The majority of the latter are fibrosarcomas, and these must be distinguished from the spindle-cell anaplastic carcinomas ('pseudosarcomas') referred to above. Chondrosarcomas are next in frequency; rhabdomyosarcoma, liposarcoma and angiosarcoma are among tumours that have been recorded occasionally.

Lymphomas have been recognized in the larynx. In most cases the larynx seems to have been involved secondarily.

Fibrosarcoma

Fibrosarcoma of the larynx is infrequent. In a study of 40 patients with fibrosarcoma arising in the head and neck there was only one laryngeal example.[80] It is seen particularly in elderly men. The usual site is the anterior third of the vocal cord and the anterior commissure. Less often it arises in the ventricular fold and subglottic region. Macroscopically, the neoplasm is hard, greyish and nodular or pedunculated. The usual microscopical picture consists of slender spindle cells with fine tapering nuclei forming intertwining bands; occasionally a 'herring-bone' pattern or perivascular palisading may be seen.

Cartilaginous tumours

Up to 200 cases of cartilaginous tumours of the larynx have been reported in the literature in English. There is a male to female ratio of 4:1; most patients are aged between 40 and 60 but some have been much younger, including a boy and a girl aged 15. The cricoid cartilage is involved in 70% of the cases and the thyroid cartilage in 20%; tumours of the arytenoids, the epiglottis and, more rarely, the vocal cords account for the rest.[81] As with tumours of cartilage arising elsewhere in the body, the distinction between benign chondroma and chondrosarcoma is not always feasible and may be related to the location and size of the growth, the age of the patient and the histological characteristics (Figs 11.30, 11.31). It is widely accepted that the following features are indicative of the potentially malignant nature of an individual tumour: pronounced irregularity of the size of the cells and their nuclei; increased cellularity and clustering; marked hyperchromasia of the nuclei; and the presence of large or giant cells, with or without multinucleated forms. At the other end of the spectrum, the microscopical appearances of a benign chondroma differ little from those of normal cartilage, with very uniform small cells regularly distributed throughout the tumour.

As already indicated the histological diagnosis must be made with caution since the biopsy procedure—often a difficult operation—may yield unrepresentative, superficial fragments of the lesion. It is not uncommon that the diagnosis of malignancy is made only in retrospect, after recurrence of a tumour thought to be benign on first observation. Of 33 cartilaginous tumours of the larynx seen at the Mayo Clinic from 1919 to 1979, 31 were chondrosarcomas and 2 were chondromas (both in men, aged 36 and 72). A diagnosis of chondroma had been made originally in

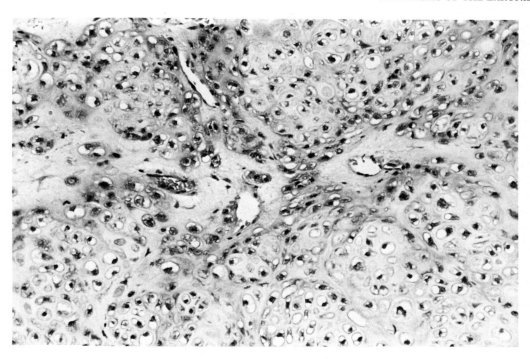

Fig. 11.30 Chondrosarcoma of the arytenoid cartilage. There is marked hypercellularity with pleomorphism and loss of orientation of the cells. Binucleated chondrocytes are easily seen.

Haematoxylin–eosin   × 250

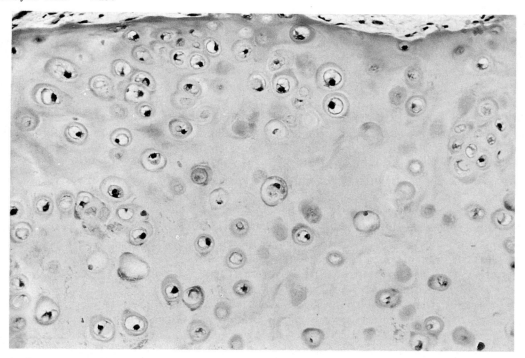

Fig. 11.31 Same case as in Figure 11.30, but this area shows almost normal histological appearances.

Haematoxylin–eosin   × 250

2 of the other cases but had later to be changed to chondrosarcoma.[82] This distinction may not be as critical as in other circumstances since even the malignant chondrosarcoma of the larynx is usually non-aggressive and only exceptionally gives rise to metastasis. When metastasis occurs the secondary deposits are usually in the neck or in the lungs.

The treatment of choice appears to be local surgical removal of the tumour and its capsule to minimize the chances of recurrence. However, surgery must be adapted to the best interests of the individual patient rather than related primarily to the histological appearances; it should be as conservative as possible. Involvement of more than half of the cricoid cartilage and the presence of multiple chondromas are indications that laryngectomy may be advisable to avoid laryngeal stenosis.[83] Recurrence, which develops in about 25% of cases and is often of late onset, can usually be treated locally.

Clinicopathological correlation is essential in the diagnosis of cartilaginous tumours of the larynx or elsewhere in the body. Treatment should be based on the most unfavourable features of the tumour, be they clinical, radiographical or histological. The tumours almost always recur and gradual extension into the surrounding tissues is commonly a feature of chondrosarcomas of the upper respiratory tract.

Tumours of adipose tissue

Although common elsewhere in the body, benign and malignant lipomas are rare in the larynx.[83, 84] Histologically simple lipomas resemble mature adipose tissue. Most liposarcomas have two main components—fat cells of varying maturity and spindle cells in a mucoid background.

Osteosarcoma (osteogenic sarcoma)

Osteosarcomas are among the rarest malignant mesenchymal neoplasms of the larynx.[85, 86]

Macroscopically, the osteosarcoma usually presents as a polypoid tumour. Microscopically, it is composed of frankly malignant, usually spindle-shaped mesenchymal cells, associated with the formation of osteoid and immature neoplastic bone. Osteoblastic elements may predominate but other components, such as chondroblastic and fibroblastic tissue, may be present. The amount of osteoid or bone formation by the tumour cells is variable. There may be areas of fibrochondrosarcomatous or angiosarcomatous pattern.

TUMOURS OF MUSCLE DERIVATION

Leiomyomas and leiomyosarcomas are extremely rare in the larynx.[87] They have been found in the glottic and supraglottic regions. They occur mainly in middle-aged men.

Tumours of smooth muscle

Leiomyomatous tumours form interlacing bundles of spindle cells with fibrillary cytoplasm and elongated, blunt, baton-shaped nuclei. The diagnosis of malignancy is based on cellularity, cellular and nuclear irregularities and the frequency of mitoses, though none of these features is totally reliable.

Leiomyosarcoma has a tendency both to invade locally and to metastasize. Secondary deposits are most frequent in the lungs.

Rhabdomyoma

Tumour-like lesions referred to as rhabdomyomas are least rare in the heart and their nature is debatable. Rhabdomyomas have also been found in the larynx, usually presenting as polypoid lesions on the vocal cords.[88] In some cases[89] the condition appears to be multifocal. The appearances on light microscopy and electron microscopy (Fig. 11.32) are characteristic, with typical cross-striation of the cytoplasm of the spindle-shaped muscle fibres and large ovoid or rounded cells with eosinophilic granular cytoplasm (Fig. 11.33). The electron microscope demonstrates the bands and intercalated discs of striated muscle. This remarkable condition of the larynx is benign. Its nature and pathogenesis are obscure.

Rhabdomyosarcoma

Rhabdomyosarcoma of the larynx is rare. Only three of a series of 83 rhabdomyosarcomas in the head and neck were in the larynx.[90] In most cases the patients have been children in the first de-

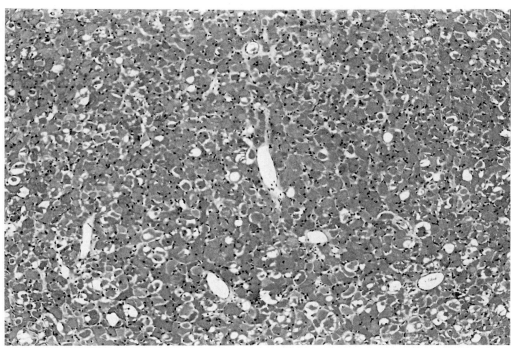

Fig. 11.32 Rhabdomyoma of the vocal cord. The low power view shows the characteristic, round, regular tumour cells with small, peripheral nuclei.   Haematoxylin–eosin   × 80

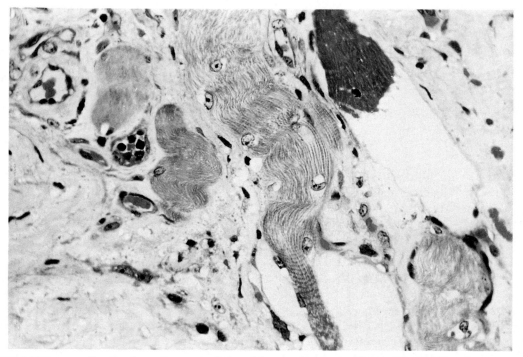

Fig. 11.33 A higher magnification shows the cross-striation of the cytoplasmic myofibres (as Fig. 11.32).
Haematoxylin–eosin   × 500

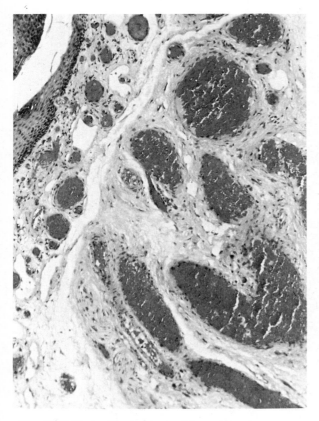

Fig. 11.34 Benign haemangioma of the vocal cord.
Haematoxylin-eosin　　× 85

cade. The tumours may be associated with squamous carcinoma and present as a collision tumour (see p. 227).[91]

Malignant fibrous histiocytoma

The tumour described as 'malignant fibrous histiocytoma'[92] (see page 122) may appear in the larynx as a soft-tissue mass, usually of fibrous consistency.[93]

VASCULAR TUMOURS

Benign haemangioma

Haemangioma of the larynx is rare. Most of the lesions that have been so diagnosed were probably angiomatoid polyps. However, true haemangiomas occur in children and may cause severe bleeding during attempted intubation of the larynx. They are hamartomas rather than true neoplasms (Fig. 11.34).

Haemangiopericytoma[94]

The region of the head and neck accounts for 15–25% of all haemangiopericytomas.[95] Stout[96] presented 197 cases of haemangiopericytoma, only one of which was located in the larynx. The literature contains references to 5 other cases.[97] Some ultrastructural studies have been reported.[98]

Angiosarcoma (malignant haemangioendothelioma)

Until 1974 only 16 cases of angiosarcoma of the larynx have been described.[98, 99, 100] The incidence was greatest amongst males of 30–60 years of age. The tumour presents as a pedunculated mass. It is composed of poorly-cohesive cells forming vascular channels lined by atypical large pleomorphic endothelial cells. Mitotic figures may be numerous and atypical. Areas of necrosis may be seen. The tumour is extremely aggressive and is liable to metastasize to distant parts.

LYMPHOMA

Lymphomas account for less than 1% of all laryngeal neoplasms. A review of the world literature published in 1970 revealed only 19 cases of laryngeal lymphoma.[101] Since then further cases have been reported.[102–104] There is no significant difference in incidence between the sexes. The condition occurs most frequently from the fifth to the seventh decades, although some younger patients have been affected. It involves the supraglottic region, in particular the epiglottis and the aryepiglottic folds; the vocal cords may be involved.

Macroscopically, the tumour appears as a swelling, usually covered by intact but oedematous mucosa. Microscopically, most laryngeal lymphomas are of the lymphocytic types. Hodgkin's disease very rarely involves the larynx.[105] An adequate biopsy specimen is essential for diagnosis of the presence and of the type of lymphoma.

Mycosis fungoides

Involvement of the larynx in the terminal stage of dissemination of mycosis fungoides is well recognized.[106] Exceptionally, involvement of the larynx may be the presenting manifestation of the disease.[107]

Leukaemia

Any part of the larynx may be the site of a leukaemic infiltrate. The cytological features depend on the type of leukaemia.

Plasmacytoma

The name plasmacytoma is given to a localized tumour of plasma cells in the absence of myelomatosis. It is not a common tumour in the larynx but it is by no means rare. At least 82 cases are on record in the world literature.[108] Patients from 40 to 60 are most frequently affected and most are men. The epiglottis is the most common site. Other locations are the vocal cords and the laryngeal ventricles.

Macroscopically, the tumour may present as a polypoid or pedunculated mass, with a smooth surface and intact mucosa. Occasionally there are multiple tumours. Microscopically, the tumour is composed of clusters of plasma cells forming an alveolar pattern; the cells are supported by a delicate stroma containing numerous dilated capillaries. Binucleated and multinucleated plasma cells may be present. Russell bodies may be found (see p. 33). It must not be overlooked that myelomatosis may present clinically with laryngeal involvement. In such cases the myeloma is usually of either the IgG type or the IgA type; it is only exceptionally of the IgD type.[109]

The prognosis of plasmacytoma is uncertain. Myelomatosis may develop after many years.[108]

PERIPHERAL NERVE TUMOURS

Granular cell tumour (granular cell myoblastoma)

This tumour was described by Abrikossoff,[110] who observed it in the tongue and elsewhere.

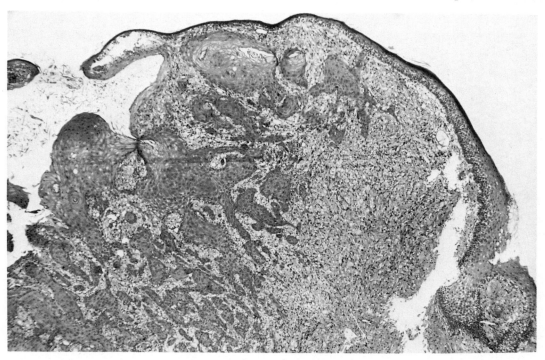

Fig. 11.35 Granular cell tumour of the vocal cord showing extensive (reactive) pseudoepitheliomatous hyperplasia initially mistaken for squamous cell carcinoma in a middle-aged woman.

Haematoxylin–eosin   × 35

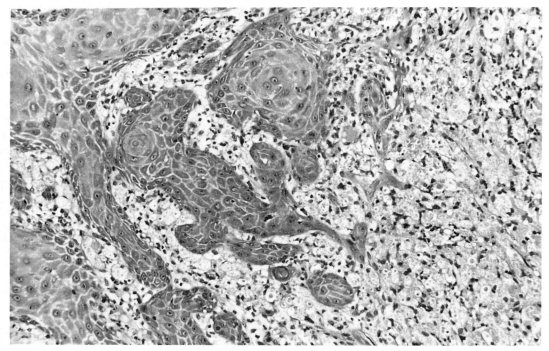

Fig. 11.36 Detail of Figure 11.35 revealing granular cells surrounding the squamous epithelial processes.
Haematoxylin–eosin   × 180

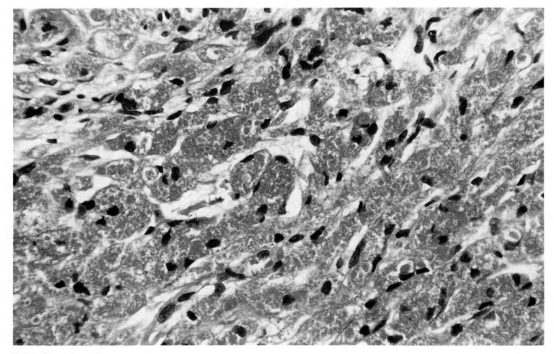

Fig. 11.37 Granular cells.
Haematoxylin–eosin   × 450

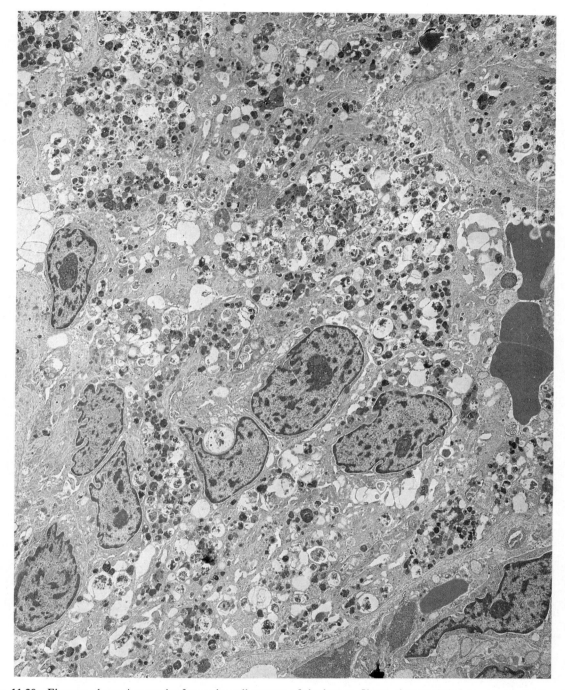

Fig. 11.38a Electron photomicrograph of granular cell tumour of the larynx. Shows characteristic large rounded cells with granular cytoplasm.

× 7000

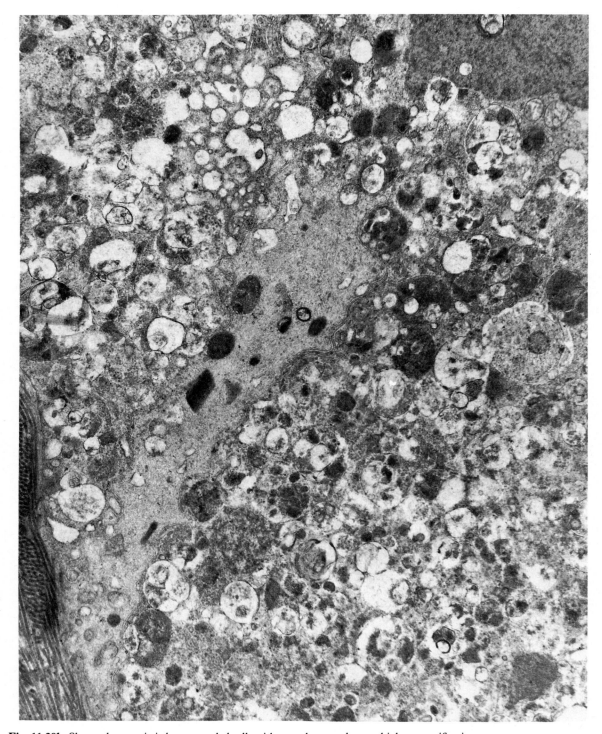

Fig. 11.38b Shows characteristic large rounded cells with granular cytoplasm at higher magnification.
× 17 500

Many cases have now been reported in which the lesion developed in a site devoid of voluntary muscle.

About 10% of all granular-cell tumours occur in the larynx, which is the commonest site of its presence in the respiratory tract. Up to 1970 at least 69 cases of laryngeal involvement had been reported.[111] Occasionally the tumours are multiple. In most instances the tumour has been located on the middle or posterior third of the vocal cords or on the posterior commissure or arytenoids. The lesion has commonly been mistaken for a laryngeal polyp or granuloma, its true nature being found on histological examination.

Histopathology (Figs 11.35, 11.36, 11.37, 11.38)
The histological appearances are characteristic. The lesion is circumscribed but not encapsulated, and at the margins the characteristic granular cells are seen between muscle fibres and around nerves, and closely associated with the overlying epithelium. The cells are large and vary from polyhedral to spindle-shaped. Their abundant, granular cytoplasm (Fig. 11.37) is palely eosinophilic and gives strongly positive PAS and Sudan Black reactions. The nucleus is small and usually central. Pseudocarcinomatous hyperplasia (Figs 11.35, 11.36) of the overlying squamous epithelium is not uncommonly present and may be misinterpreted as squamous carcinoma, particularly in a superficial biopsy specimen: it has been suggested that carcinoma should never be diagnosed in the presence of a granular cell tumour.[111]

Under the electron microscope the most striking feature is the presence of large numbers of complex granular phagosomes (also known as myelin figures) (Fig. 11.38a,b). The presence of the so-called angulate body described by Bangle[112] has been confirmed.

Although there are some well-documented cases of malignant varieties of the granular-cell tumour arising elsewhere in the body none has been reported as arising in the larynx.[20] The neoplastic nature of these lesions has been questioned. They have been regarded as degenerative or regenerative lesions of muscle fibres.[113] Evidence has been collected that indicates the possibility that the granular material

in the cytoplasm of the tumour cell consists of myelin: this suggests that the tumour has a neurogenic origin.[114] It is interesting that nests of granular cells identical with those in the granular cell tumour have been found in a typical Schwannoma.[115] The demonstration by immunoperoxidase staining methods that the neuroectodermal protein S-100 is present in the cells has provided further evidence for the possible Schwann cell origin of the granular cell tumours.[116]

Schwannomas (neurilemmomas) and neurofibromas
Histologically, these tumours in the larynx are identical to their counterparts elsewhere. They are described on pages 338 to 345.

Other neural tumours and tumour-like conditions

Neurofibrosarcomas
Neurofibrosarcomas in the larynx appear not to have been documented.

Laryngeal involvement in von Recklinghausen's disease is unusual.[20]

Occasionally, the larynx is one of the sites of multiple mucosal neuromas (similar to traumatic neuromas) in association with phaeochromocytomas and medullary thyroid carcinoma in patients in a familial syndrome.[117]

REFERENCES

1. Ullman EV. Acta Otolaryngol (Stockh) 1923; 5: 31.
2. Incze JS, Lui PS, Strong MS, Vaughan CW, Clemente MP. Cancer 1977; 39: 1634.
3. Lack EE, Vawter GF, Smith HG, Healy GB, Lancaster WB, Jenson AB. Lancet 1980; ii: 592.
4. Anon. Lancet 1981; i: 367.
5. Olofsson J. Bjelkenkrantz K, Grontoft O, Nordstrom G. J Otolaryngol 1978; 7: 353.
6. Bewtra C, Krishnan R, Lee SS. Arch Otolaryngol 1982; 108: 114.
7. Yoder MG, Batsakis JG. Otolaryngol Head Neck Surg 1980; 88: 745.
8. Fechner RE, Mills SE. Am J Surg Pathol 1982; 6: 357.
9. Crissman JD. Head Neck Surg 1979; 11: 386.
10. McGavran MH, Bauer WC, Ogura JH. Cancer 1961; 14: 55.
11. Crissman JD. Arch Otolaryngol 1982; 108: 445.
12. Broders AC. JAMA 1932; 99: 1670.
13. Buckley CH, Butler EB, Fox H. J Clin Pathol 1982; 35: 1.

14. Miller AH. In: Alberti PW, Bryce DP eds. Centennial Conference on Laryngeal Cancer. New York: Appleton–Century–Crofts, 1976; 161
15. Hellquist H, Lundgren J, Olofsson J. Clin Otolaryngol 1982; 7: 11.
16. Ferlito A, Polidoro F, Rossi M. J Laryngol Otol 1981; 95: 141.
17. Hellquist H, Olofsson J, Grontoft O. Acta Otolaryngol 1981; 92: 543.
18. Auerbach O, Hammond EC, Garfinkel L. Cancer 1970; 25: 92.
19. Park WW. The Histology of Borderline Cancer, with Notes on Prognosis. Berlin: Springer-Verlag 1980; 383.
20. Batsakis JG. Tumours of the Head and Neck. 2nd ed. Baltimore: Williams and Wilkins 1979; 200.
21. Muller KM, Krohn BR. J Cancer Res Clin Oncol 1980; 96: 211.
22. McMichael AJ. Lancet 1978; ii: 1244.
23. Lund V, Sawyer R, Papavasiliou A. Clin Oncol 1982; 8: 201.
24. Goolden AWG. Br J Radiol 1957; 30: 626.
25. Rabbet WF. Ann Otol Rhinol Laryngol 1965; 74: 1149.
26. Baker DC, Weissman B. Ann Otol Rhinol Laryngol 1971; 80: 634.
27. Newman RK, Byers RM. Otolaryngol Head Neck Surg 1982; 90: 431.
28. Gindhart TD, Johnston WH, Chism SE, Dedo HH. Cancer 1980; 46: 1683.
29. Webber P. J Laryngol 1984; 98: 901–904.
30. Lederman M. J Laryngol 1970; 84: 867–896.
31. Michaels L, Hassmann E. Clin Otolaryngol 1982; 7: 165.
32. Som ML. J Laryngol Otol 1970; 84: 655.
33. Stell PM, Gudrun R, Watt J. Clin Otolaryngol 1981; 6: 389.
34. Steel PM. In: Alberti PW, Bryce DP eds. Centennial Conference on Laryngeal Cancer. New York: Appleton–Century–Crofts 1976; 682.
35. Olofsson J. In: Alberti PW, Bryce DP eds. Centennial Conference on Laryngeal Cancer. New York: Appleton–Century–Crofts 1976; 626.
36. Jakobsson PK. In Alberti PW, Bryce DP eds. Centennial Conference on Laryngeal Cancer. New York: Appleton–Century–Crofts 1976; 847.
37. Fisher HR. In: Alberti PW, Bryce DP eds. Centennial Conference on Laryngeal Cancer. New York: Appleton–Century–Crofts 1976; 843.
37a. Maran AGD, Stell PM eds. Clinical Otolaryngology. Oxford: Blackwell Scientific 1979; 384.
38. Batsakis JG, Hybels R, Rice DH. In: Alberti PW, Bryce DP eds. Centennial Conference on Laryngeal Cancer. New York: Appleton–Century–Crofts 1976; 868.
39. Harrer WV, Lewis PL. Arch Otolaryngol 1970; 91: 382.
40. Ackerman LV. Surgery 1948; 23: 670.
41. Ferlito A, Recher G. Cancer 1980; 46: 1617.
42. Fechner RE. Arch Otolaryngol 1981; 107: 454.
43. Medina JE, Dichtel MC, Luna MA. Arch Otolaryngol 1984; 110: 437–440.
44. Battifora H. Cancer 1976; 37: 2275.
44a. Brodsky G, Otolaryngologic Clinics of North America. Vol. 17. 1984: 185.

45. Harris M. Histopathology 1982; 6: 197.
46. Hyams VJ. In: Alberti PW, Bryce DP eds. Centennial Conference on Laryngeal Cancer. New York: Appleton–Century–Crofts 1976; 489.
47. Lambert PR, Ward PH, Berci G. Arch Otolaryngol 1980; 106: 700.
48. Gowing NFH. Colour atlas of tumour histopathology. London: Wolfe Medical 1980; 24.
49. Lundgren J, Olofsson J, Hellquist H. Acta Otolaryngol (Stockh) 1982; 94: 335.
50. Fechner RE. In: Alberti PW, Bryce DP eds. Centennial Conference on Laryngeal Cancer. New York: Appleton–Century–Crofts 1976; 466.
51. Ferlito A, Recher G, Bottin R. ORL 1981; 43: 280.
52. Batsakis JG. Ann Otol Rhinol Laryngol 1982; 91: 342.
53. Friedmann I, Osborn DA. J Laryngol Otol 1965; 79: 576.
54. Ferlito A. J Laryngol Otol 1976; 90: 1053.
55. Pesavento G, Ferlito A, Recher G. J Clin Pathol 1980; 33: 1160.
56. Glenner GG, Grimley PM. In: Atlas of tumour pathology, Series 2, Fascicle 9, Washington, DC: Armed Forces Institute of Pathology 1974.
57. Wetmore RF, Tronzo RD, Lane RJ, Lowry LD. Cancer 1981; 48: 2717.
58. Justrabo E, Michiels R, Calmettes C, et al. Acta Otolaryngol (Stockh) 1980; 89: 135.
59. Gallivan MV, Chun B, Rowden G, Lack EE. Am J Surg Pathol 1979; 3: 85.
60. Levene A. Clin Otolaryngol 1981; 6: 209.
61. Goldman NC, Hood I, Singleton GT. Arch Otolaryngol 1967; 90: 90.
62. Duvall E, Johnston A, McLay K, Piris J. J Laryngol Otol 1983 (in press).
63. Ferlito A. Acta Otolaryngol (Stockh) 1977; Suppl 342; 31.
64. Friedmann I, Galey FR, House WF, Carberry JN, Ward PP. J Laryngol Otol 1983; 97: 465.
65. Paladugu RR, Nathwani BN, Goodstein J, Dardi LE, Memoli VE, Gould VE. Cancer 1982; 49: 343.
66. Gnepp DR, Ferlito A, Hyams VJ. Cancer 1983; 51: 1731.
67. Hay JH Busuttil A. J Laryngol Otol 1981: 95; 1081.
68. Quinn FB, McCabe BF. Ann Otol Rhinol Laryngol 1957; 66: 139.
69. Whicher JH, Carder GA, Devine KD. Arch Otolaryngol 1972; 96: 182.
70. Glanz H, Kleinsasser O. HNO 1978; 26: 163.
71. Freeland AP, van Nostrand AWP, Jahn AF. J Otolaryngol 1979; 8: 448.
72. Epstein SS, Shaw HJ. Cancer 1958; 11: 3236.
73. Olofsson J, van Nostrand AWP. Acta Otolaryngol (Stockh) 1973; Suppl 308: 1.
74. Lawson W, Som M. Ann Otol Rhinol Laryngol 1975; 84: 771.
75. Brown M. J Laryngol Otol 1978; 92: 991.
76. Cohn AM, Peppard SB. Am J Otolaryngol 1980; 1: 411.
77. Ferlito A, di Bonito L. J Otol Rhinol Laryngol 1976; 38: 230.
78. Ferlito A, Polidoro F. J Otol Rhinol Laryngol 1980; 42: 146.
79. Batsakis JG, Fox JE. Surg Gynec Obstet 1970; 131: 989.

80. Swain RE, Sessions DG, Ogura JH. Ann Otol Rhinol Laryngol 1974; 83: 439.
81. Hyams VJ, Rabuzzi DD. Laryngos cope 1970; 80: 755.
82. Neel HB, Unni KK. Otolaryngol Head Neck Surg 1982; 90: 201.
83. Friedmann I. In: Alberti PW, Bryce DP eds. Centennial Conference on Laryngeal Cancer. New York: Appleton–Century–Crofts 1976; 479.
84. Fu YS, Perzin KH. Cancer 1977; 39: 195.
85. Dahm LJ, Shaeffer SD, Carder HM, Vellios F. Cancer 1978; 42: 2343.
86. Gorenstein A, Neel B, Weiland LH, Devine KD. Arch Otolaryngol 1980; 106: 8.
87. Wolfowitz BL, Schnaman A. S Afr Med J 1972; 47: 1189.
88. Ferlito A, Frugoni P. J Laryngol Otol 1975; 89: 1131.
89. Neville BW, McConnell FMS. Arch Otolaryngol 1981; 107: 175.
90. Feldman BA. Laryngoscope 1982; 92: 424.
91. Srinivasan U, Talvalker GV. J Laryngol Otol 1979; 93: 1031.
92. Kauffman SL, Stout AP. Cancer 1961; 14: 469.
93. Ferlito A. Cancer 1978; 42: 611.
94. Zimmerman KW. Ztschr Anat 1923; 68: 29.
95. Batsakis JG, Rice DH. Head Neck Surg 1981; 3: 231.
96. Stout AP. Lab Invest 1956; 5: 217.
97. Pesavento G, Ferlito A. J Laryngol Otol 1982; 96: 1065.
98. Battifora H. Cancer 1973; 31: 1418.
99. Pratt LW, Goodof II. Arch Otolaryngol 1968; 87: 484.
100. Triplet I, Vankemme B, Madelain M. Lille Med 1974; 19: 743.
101. De Santo LW, Weiland LH. Laryngoscope 1970; 80: 966.
102. Anderson HA, Maisel RH, Cantrell RW. Laryngoscope 1976; 86: 1251.
103. Ferlito A, Carbone A, Volpe R. Otol Rhinol Laryngol 1981; 43: 61.
104. Gregor RT. J Laryngol Otol 1981; 95: 81.
105. Meyer-Breitting E. Laryngol Rhinol Otol 1975; 54: 897.
106. Rappaport H, Thomas LB. Cancer 1974; 34: 1198.
107. Hood AF, Mark GJ, Hunt JV. Cancer 1979; 43: 1527.
108. Maniglia AJ, Xue JW. Laryngoscope 1983; 93: 741.
109. Ferlito A, Carbone A, Volpe R, Recher G. J Laryngol Otol 1981; 96: 759.
110. Abrikosoff A. Virchows Arch (Pathol Anat) 1926; 260.
111. Booth JB, Osborn DA. Acta Otolaryngol (Stockh) 1970; 70: 279.
112. Bangle R. Cancer 1952; 5: 950.
113. Willis RA. The pathology of tumours. London: Butterworth 1953; 745.
114. Azzopardi JG. J Pathol Bacteriol 1956; 71: 85.
115. Sobel HJ, Marquet E, Schwarz R. J Pathol 1973; 109: 101.
116. Armin A, Connelly EM, Rowden G. Am J Clin Path 1983; 79: 37.
117. Gorlin RJ, Sedano HO, Vickers RA, Cervenka J. Cancer 1968; 22: 293.

PART FIVE

I. Friedmann

The ear

12

Introduction and anatomy
Congenital abnormalities

INTRODUCTION

The ear has not attracted sufficient attention from pathologists, who, with few exceptions, have fought shy of the apparently barren regions of the temporal bone. Only quite recently have aural surgeons begun to appreciate the practical importance of regular pathological examination of all specimens taken at operations on the ear. Hitherto, the so-called 'aural polyps' have been the commonest specimens sent for histological examination, and even those often continue to be dismissed as of little account, for it is not always appreciated how easily they hide much that proper study shows to be important. Only when all aural specimens are subject to routine histological examination is it possible to detect all the cases of occult carcinoma or glomus jugulare tumour, or of tuberculosis and other infections of the middle ear, that otherwise might be unrecognized and untreated.

If the pathologist possesses a basic knowledge of the various pathological conditions that occur in the ear, he can play an important part in the prevention of potentially disastrous delays in treatment. The ear still presents many problems, often peculiar to them, that await solution by the application of the general principles of pathology. In the past, theoretical considerations of the pathology of otitis, for example, have been based largely on clinical observations and impressions. In recent years, however, considerable advances have been made in our knowledge of the pathology of the ear, and many of these are incorporated in the following chapters, presenting a practical account of the pathology of diseases of this organ.

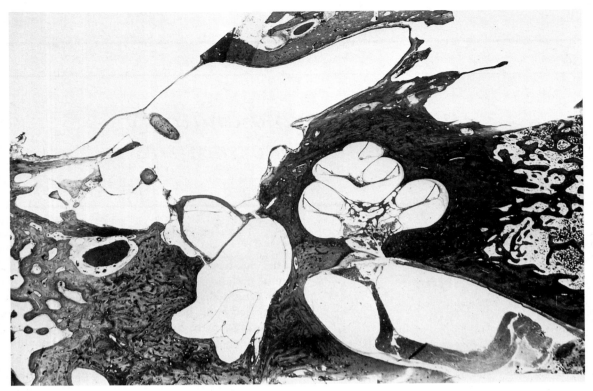

Fig. 12.1a Photomicrograph of a midmodiolar or horizontal section of the temporal bone showing the principal regions of the ear.   Haematoxylin–eosin   × 6.5

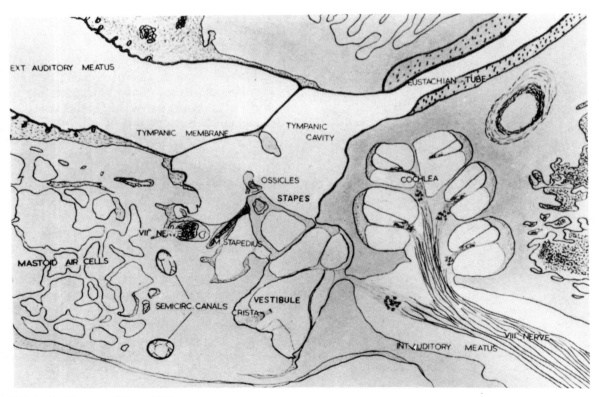

Fig. 12.1b Diagram of Figure 12.1a.

The incidence of both acute and chronic otitis media has not abated and has remained a world-wide health problem.[1] The same is true of neoplasms of the ear and even more of various congenital syndromes associated with hearing loss. There has been understandable questioning of the changes which seem to have occurred in the pathology of the ear but the study of various familiar clinicopathological problems by means of new techniques has failed to provide the answers.

GROSS ANATOMY OF THE EAR

The delicate structures of the ear (Fig. 12.1a,b) are housed in a comparatively inaccessible part of the skull.

Anatomically the ear is usually divided into:

1. the *external ear* consisting of the auricle or pinna and the external auditory meatus; it is separated by the tympanic membrane from
2. the *middle ear* or tympanic cavity, which communicates anteriorly with the nasopharynx through the auditory tube (pharyngotympanic or Eustachian tube) and posteriorly with the mastoid antrum and through it with the intricate and important air-cell system of the mastoid process; and
3. the *internal ear* which harbours the sensory apparatus of hearing and equilibrium. Certain aspects of the microscopical anatomy of the ear will be mentioned when considering the pathology of the relevant parts.

CONGENITAL ABNORMALITIES[2]

Abnormalities of the auricle
The shape and size of the auricle vary widely. Frequent variations include the pointed auricle ('satyr ear'), which is often accompanied by a well-developed Darwinian tubercle a minor variation of the auricular shape forming a small elevation on the lateral edge of the helix; the macacus auricle ('monkey ear'); the pointed helix; the drooping or roll ear ('dog ear'); cleft lobule; absent lobule; and various degrees of abnormal protrusion of the auricle or its anatomical parts.

One or both auricles may be absent. In contrast, there may be supernumerary auricles (polyotia). An association of anomalies of the auricle with nephroblastoma (Wilms' tumour) has been described.

Malformations of the external ear are usually associated with multiple malformations of the skull. Malformations of the ear were engraved on the tablets of ancient Babylonian scribes.[3] Among the rarer malformations of the external ear is duplication of the external auditory meatus.[4, 5]

Abnormalities of the external acoustic meatus
The most important malformation of the external meatus is atresia. This occurs in two forms. In one the ectodermal core does not undergo canalization in the normal manner: this is associated with deformation of the tympanic cavity. In the other there is partial or complete stenosis of the meatus as a manifestation of abnormal encroachment of bone, which may obliterate the meatus completely.

Abnormalities of the middle ear
There is a great range of differences in the size, shape and layout of the tympanic cavity—'Each ear is as different as is each human face.'[6]

Anomalies of the middle ear, in the presence of a normal tympanic membrane, are very frequent. Each or any of its anatomical parts may be in some degree malformed or lacking, with effects that range from the undetectable to complete functional failure.

Dehiscence of the tympanic ring is an anomaly of particular importance because it exposes the jugular bulb to a special risk of injury during surgical operations on the middle ear.

REFERENCES

1. Meyerhoff WL, Kim CS, Paperella MM. Ann Otol Rhinol Laryngol 1978; 87: 749.
2. Sando I, Suehiro S, Wood RP. In: Bluestone CD, Stool SE, eds. Pediatric Otolaryngology. Chicago: W.B. Saunders, 1983.
3. Warkany J. Arch Pathol 1963; 75: 579.
4. Beck C. HNO 1970; 18: 307.
5. Stennert E, Arold R. HNO 1973; 21: 293.
6. Hough JVD. Arch Otolaryngol 1963; 78: 335.

13

Inflammatory diseases of the ear

OTITIS EXTERNA

Anatomical and physiological factors relating to otitis externa

The external acoustic meatus consists of cartilaginous and osseous portions lined by skin. The cartilaginous portion possesses sebaceous glands and the so-called ceruminous glands. The latter are saccular glands consisting of cuboidal secretory cells and provided with myoepithelial cells. They are considered to be modified sweat glands, akin to the apocrine glands found elsewhere in the skin. They lie deep in the subcutaneous tissue; some of them open on to the surface of the skin, and some into the ducts of sebaceous glands. They usually contain brownish, lipoprotein granules; similar granules are often seen in apocrine glands elsewhere. The granules do not contribute to the secretion, which is a clear, colourless, watery fluid that is devoid of lipids. The mixture of this secretion with the lipid-rich sebum, together with dust and desquamated epithelium, forms the cerumen. Its brown colour is probably due to oxidation of some of its constituents, including aminoacids and lipids. Two types of cerumen have been recognized in different populations. Wet and sticky cerumen is common in Caucasians and Blacks; dry flaky cerumen is more common among Oriental races, the Eskimo and some Indian tribes of North America.[1, 2]

The physiological role of cerumen is not clearly understood, though its antibacterial and antifungal properties may be important (see below). An investigation of the relation between cerumen production and the occurrence of otitis externa showed that the inflammatory process in this disease is not confined to the surface of the skin of the external acoustic meatus, but also affects the underlying glands. The consequent fall in the production of cerumen deprives the skin of a natural protection and creates conditions that predispose to infection. A vicious circle develops that may lead to chronic otitis externa and, eventually, to complete cessation of the formation of cerumen.

The results of investigations into the bacteriostatic and fungistatic properties of cerumen have been discordant. Earlier workers were unable to demonstrate that it has any antimicrobial action. Recently, however, cerumen has been shown to be capable in most instances of inhibiting the growth of *Streptococcus pyogenes*, although it has no such effect on *Staphylococcus aureus* or *Pseudomonas aeruginosa*. It is noteworthy that the two last named organisms are the commonest of the infective causes of otitis externa (see also below).

Various fungi, including species of *Aspergillus* and *Penicillium* and of the zygomycetes, have been found to be unaffected by cerumen. In contrast the growth of most species of *Trichophyton* is inhibited by most specimens of cerumen.

Gonococcal external otitis has been reported in a young man suffering from gonococcal urethritis. *Neisseria gonorhoeae* was cultured from both situations. The occurrence of the aural infection in such a case may be due to autoinfection.[3]

Progressive or non-healing external otitis (malignant external otitis)

Clinical features
This rare form of external otitis, first described by Meltzer & Kelemen[4] in 1959, was defined by Chandler[5] as a severe form of external otitis occurring in elderly diabetic patients and caused by *Ps. aeruginosa*. The disease affects mainly the elderly, 55 years of age or older.[6] Factors that predispose to the development of the disease, in addition to diabetes mellitus, are old age, minor trauma to the external auditory meatus, and blood diseases.[7] The disease causes serious complications such as extension of the infection to cartilage, bone, nerve and soft tissue resulting in osteomyelitis of the skull, multiple nerve palsies and death.[8] The most common complication in the reported cases was facial nerve palsy.[6, 9, 10]

Light microscopy shows necrosis of the bone of the floor of the meatus covered by acute or chronic inflammatory granulation tissue. Once osteomyelitis of the temporal bone has developed, the disease may spread into the base of the skull.[11] Necrotizing external otitis[12] has been reported in a non-diabetic patient. In some cases the clinical appearances have been mistaken for those of cancer of the external acoustic meatus and auricle.

Relapsing perichondritis
Relapsing perichondritis is a rare, often dramatic, inflammatory disease of cartilage of unknown cause affecting the auricular cartilage, the nasal septum and the glottic and subglottic cartilages of the larynx. It occurs mainly in persons over 40 years of age and its course is characterized by spontaneous remissions and recurrence.[12a] The auditory tube may be affected and swelling of its cartilaginous portion may cause conductive hearing loss. The effects of the long-standing relapsing course of the condition led a 73-year-old woman to suicide.[13]

Microscopy shows loss of metachromasial necrotic cartilage in which chondroblasts are still recognizable and some non-specific inflammatory granulation tissue infiltrated by lymphocytes and plasma cells. The involved cartilage degenerates and is eventually replaced by fibrous tissue.

Otomycosis
When otitis externa is associated with the growth of fungi in the meatus, the condition is known as otomycosis. There are several varieties of the disease and they are all chronic, recurrent, non-contagious infections, characterized by pruritus, a sensation of pressure or fullness in the ear and sometimes impairment of hearing. Otomycosis is worldwide in distribution, and in various recorded series has accounted for 5–20% of all cases of infective otitis externa. The external acoustic meatus comes to contain a mass formed of epithelial debris, exudate, cerumen and the fungus: the colour of the mass, which is usually grey or black, is mainly determined by the type of fungus concerned. The surface of the meatus and of the tympanic membrane is reddened and

scaly and may be eroded or ulcerated. The tympanic membrane itself may be oedematous.

Aspergillus niger is the most frequent cause of otomycosis; *A. fumigatus*, *A. flavus* and *A. nidulans* have also been isolated. Some of the dermatophytes, such as *Trichophyton violaceum*, *T. schoenleinii* and *T. mentagrophytes*, may infect the skin of the auricle and on occasion may spread into the meatus: however, as noted on page 256 cerumen has a fungistatic effect on these organisms and this probably explains the rarity with which they infect the meatus. In a few cases otomycosis may be due to infection by species of *Candida* or of various zygomycetes or of *Penicillium*.

INFLAMMATORY OR INFECTIOUS DISEASES: OTITIS MEDIA AND ITS COMPLICATIONS

Anatomy of the tympanic cavity

The *roof* or *tegmen* of the tympanic cavity, the cranial or meningeal wall, is in immediate contact with the dura. In the infant, the petrosquamosal suture forms a portal of entry of infection in purulent otitis media. The malleus and incus are attached by their ligaments to the tegmen tympani.

The *floor* or jugular wall is in close contact with the jugular bulb.

The *anterior wall* (tubal wall) contains the tympanic orifice of the Eustachian tube and is close to the internal carotid artery.

The *posterior wall* (mastoidal wall) contains the antral aditus. Mucosal folds surrounding the malleus, incus and chorda tympani nerve form delicate supporting ligaments for the ossicles and outline the pouches first described by Prussak[14] and von Tröltsch.[15] Prussak's pouch is a triangular space limited by the pars flaccida of the tympanic membrane, the short process of the malleus and the lateral malleolar fold.[16] The pouches of von Tröltsch lie adjacent to the malleus. The importance of these delicate mucosal folds between the ossicles has been emphasized; they leave very narrow channels of communication between the mesotympanum and the attico-antral segments.[17] Adhesions, mucosal hypertrophy and

polyposis easily obstruct them, thus contributing to the development of infections of the epitympanic recess (attic) of the tympanic cavity, a common site of epidermoid cholesteatoma.[18, 19]

The mastoid process

The air-cell system of the mastoid process has been an important subject in the past and has been attracting renewed attention because of its surgical importance. The extent of pneumatization varies considerably from a partial or limited air-cell system to the pneumatization of the entire temporal bone.[20, 21, 22]

If pneumatization is arrested, the bone remains diploic in type (Cheatle's infantile diploic type of mastoid): this diploic bone may be transformed into compact bone as a result of the laying down of lamellar bone in the marrow spaces. The result, clinically and radiologically, will be an 'acellular mastoid'. Microscopically, this normal compact bone differs from the pathological sclerotic bone that is the result of reconstruction in the course of repeated and alternating cycles of absorption and deposition. The cyclical processes lead to a readily recognizable change in the microscopical pattern. Infection occurring in any of the normal types of mastoid bone—pneumatized, infantile diploic or compact—may convert it partly or completely into bone that is sclerotic in the pathological sense. The occurrence of some degree of pneumatization, usually limited in extent and patchy in distribution, probably explains why sclerotic mastoid processes do not always appear acellular at operation.

Acute otitis media and mastoiditis

Otitis media, a dreaded disease of childhood before the antibiotic era, has retained its great social and economic importance as a frequent cause of hearing loss. Moreover, certain sequelae of otitis media known to earlier authors have been gaining in importance—for example the 'glue ear' syndrome, epidermoid cholesteatoma, cholesterol granuloma and tympanosclerosis. Intracerebral complications still occur and must not be ignored.[23, 24]

Histopathology

The tympanic cavity and the air cells of a pneu-

Table 13.1 Histopathology of otitis media: a summary of the microscopical changes occurring in the tissues of the infected middle-ear cleft. The clinical diagnosis of otitis media may disguise some specific granulomas such as tuberculosis. Also, Wegener's granuloma, eosinophilic granuloma and neoplasms may present with aural pain and discharge.

Acute or subacute purulent mastoiditis	Chronic purulent mastoiditis
Mucosa	
Necrosis and suppuration Granulation tissue (Fig. 13.2)	Columnar secretory epithelium contributing to secretory or catarrhal otitis—'glue ear' (Figs 13.5 and 13.7)
Columnar epithelium with goblet cells: early reversal of the mucosa to respiratory secretory type	Fibrous granulation tissue (infiltrated by inflammatory cells) Dense hyalinized fibrous tissue with calcification (tympanosclerosis) Adhesions (Figs 13.8–13.11)
	Cholesterol granuloma (Figs 13.14–13.16)
	Epidermoid cholesteatoma (Figs 13.12 and 13.13)
	Suppuration: recurrent infection (acute or chronic infection)
	Specific granulomas Wegener's granuloma Carcinoma
Bone	
Osteoclastic activity and bone resorption (Fig. 13.3)	Reconstruction of bone and obliteration of air spaces
Necrosis	Multiplication and condensation of lines of apposition
Osteoblastic activity New bone formation (Fig. 13.4)	Mosaic pattern of cement lines (Fig. 13.6)

matized mastoid process are lined by a very thin mucosa consisting of a layer of fibrous tissue covered by flattened cells of respiratory epithelial origin (Fig. 13.1). The earliest microscopical signs of infection occur in the mucosa (Table 13.1). The initial congestion and oedema are quickly followed by the formation of a purulent exudate, often with haemorrhage, and pus soon fills the tympanic cavity and the mastoid cells (Fig. 13.2).

The inflammatory process may extend beyond the middle ear, giving rise to thrombosis and suppuration in the lateral sinus, with resulting pyaemia, or to the development of an extradural abscess, suppurative meningitis, or an abscess in the cerebellum or in the temporal lobe of the cerebrum. Occasionally penetration of the mastoid process results in the formation of *Bezold's abscess*[25] beneath the periosteum or in the digastric fossa. In rare cases the suppurative process spreads forward beside the auditory tube and a retropharyngeal abscess (*internal Bezold abscess*) results.

Bone is involved early in the course of infections in the middle ear. The affected areas become necrotic, osteoclasts accumulate, and granulation tissue develops (Fig. 13.3). Fragments of necrotic bone form small sequestra in the suppurating granulation tissue. Organization of the granulation tissue begins early in the tympanic cavity and mastoid cells and slender trabeculae of newly formed osteoid tissue make their appearance in the marginal areas. These gradually form a dense spongework of trabecular bone, replacing the granulation tissue in the attic and in the mastoid antrum and the mastoid cells (Fig. 13.4). Neighbouring air cells may present different stages of the inflammatory process ranging from persistent suppuration to fibroblastic organization and ossification. In some cases there is a great deal of haemorrhage and bone destruction. The formation of new bone, which usually takes place on a luxuriant scale, frequently leads to obliteration of all the air spaces in the mastoid.

Otitis media is strictly defined as an inflammation of the middle ear that may or may not be of infectious origin and that may or may not be associated with effusion in the tympanic cavity. The term may be modified further as 'acute', 'subacute' or 'chronic'. Effusion when present, may be characterized by the terms 'serous', 'purulent' or 'mucoid'. There are differences in the terminology used by various workers.[26]

Bacteriology

The principal microorganisms causing acute purulent otitis media have remained *Streptococcus pneumoniae*, *Str. pyogenes* and *Haemophilus influenzae*. The role of *Staphylococcus aureus* is more difficult to assess, although its role in the

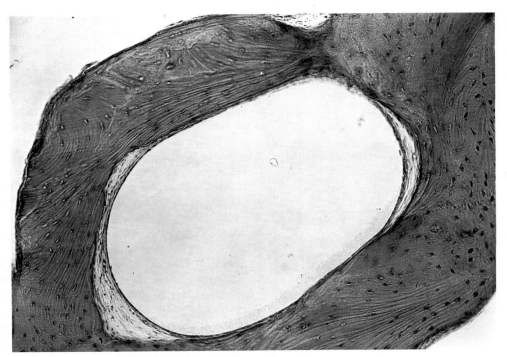

Fig. 13.1 Normal mastoid air cell lined by a thin layer of fibrous tissue covered by flat epithelial cells.
Haematoxylin–eosin   × 150

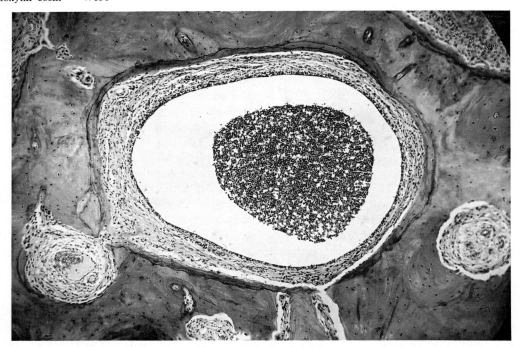

Fig. 13.2 Acute suppurative mastoiditis. A pus-filled mastoid air cell. The contents and lining have shrunk apart during the histological processing of the specimen. The connective tissue of the mucosa is conspicuous, hyperaemic, and infiltrated by neutrophils.
Haematoxylin–eosin   × 60

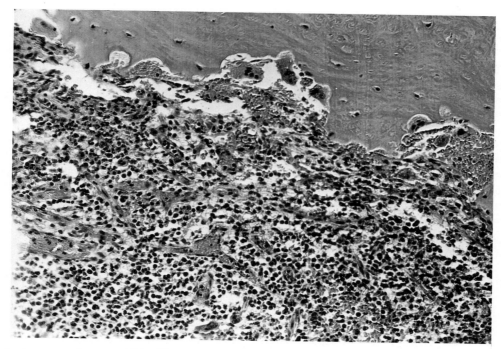

Fig. 13.3 Acute suppurative mastoiditis. There are osteoclasts in Howship lacunae at the surface of the bone. There is purulent exudate in the granulation tissue.

Haematoxylin–eosin   × 225

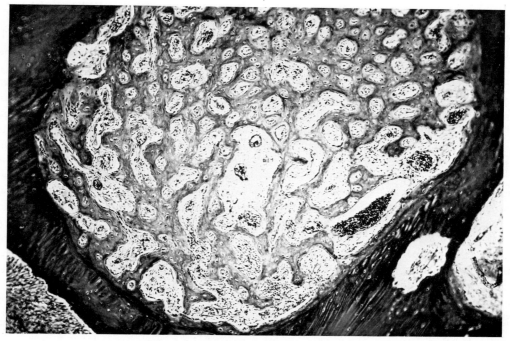

Fig. 13.4 Subacute mastoiditis. The air cell has been obliterated by newly formed trabecular bone which contrasts markedly with the surrounding normal lamellar bone.

Masson's trichrome stain   × 50

various stages of otitis media cannot be doubted.

Recent world-wide reports have confirmed that the relative incidence of the principal causative microorganisms has not changed.[27–31] A Norwegian study in 1980[27] of 505 patients with acute otitis media has shown the following results: *Str. pneumoniae* grown from 33% of patients; *H. influenzae* from 17%; *Str. pyogenes* from 7%. A Japanese study[31] of 586 cases resulted in the isolation (after paracentesis) of 425 strains of pathogenic microorganisms. These were: *Str. pneumoniae* (49.9%); *H. influenzae* (23.5%); *Str. pyogenes* (14%); *Staph. aureus* (5.9%).

H. influenzae causes about 20% of otitis media in children.[32, 33] Its incidence declines with increasing age, but *H. influenzae* is important in all age groups. There has been an increasing proportion of *H. influenzae* strains (15–30%) that have been β-lactamase-producing and therefore ampicillin-resistant.[34, 35] *Branhamella* (formerly *Neisseria*) *catarrhalis* accounts for fewer than 10% of the cases. In about 25% of the effusions no bacteria or only apparently non-pathogenic organisms may be cultured. Care must be taken to avoid contamination from the skin of the auditory meatus.

Anaerobic bacteria may play a minor role in the causation of acute otitis media.[28, 36–38] The significance of the respiratory syncytial virus and of some other viruses has not been fully established although they have been identified by enzyme immuno-assay techniques or grown in middle-ear fluids.[39] Recurrence of the disease may be enhanced by respiratory syncytial virus, adenovirus and influenza A or B viruses.[40] *Chlamydia trachomatis* can infect the middle ear.[41]

Immunological studies
Immunological studies have been contributing to the investigation of the pathogenesis of infective middle-ear diseases. The presence of immunologically-competent cells has been interpreted as indicative of enhanced activity of the normal defence mechanisms of the mucosa of the middle ear leading to the local production of antibodies. This property of the middle ear matures with age. The level of immunoglobulin production is low at 6 months, then increases rapidly to the age of 2 years and thereafter slowly to the age of 6 years, thus correlating with the decreasing incidence of otitis as children grow older. The rapid increase with age of the amount of IgA and IgG in middle-ear effusions suggests that the immunoglobulins may be of local origin.

It is interesting to note that when the antibody response in serum and middle-ear fluid was studied in 40 children under 2 years of age, with otitis media due to *Haemophilus influenzae*, IgG and IgA antibodies occurred with equal frequency, but IgA antibody was found more often in middle-ear fluids and was absent in the serum. Thus infants with otitis media seem to respond systemically and locally with specific antibody to *H. influenzae*.[42] In another study IgA antibodies to measles, mumps, rubella, and polio viruses were determined in serum and middle-ear fluid of 103 patients with otitis media: the occurrence of IgA viral antibody in middle-ear fluid and its absence in simultaneously drawn serum was used as an indicator of local antibody production and showed 41 instances in which IgA antibody was found exclusively in middle-ear fluid, indicating local antibody production.[43]

Intracranial complications of otitis media
The incidence of purulent meningitis and of abscesses of the central nervous system has fallen. The mortality rate of otogenic meningitis has been reduced, as a result of antibiotic therapy and improved surgery, from 80 to 22% and that of otogenic cerebral abscess from 34 to 4%.[44] Nevertheless the seriousness of these complications of otitis media—intracranial or extracranial—cannot be overstated. The intracranial complications include cerebral and cerebellar abscess, purulent meningitis, lateral sinus thrombosis, otitic hydrocephalus and the posterior fossa syndrome (pseudotumour syndrome).* Although less frequent than in the pre-antibiotic era, these complications still occur.[46, 47] The extracranial complications—facial palsy and labyrinthitis causing hearing loss and impairment of balance—have remained more common.

---

*The term 'posterior fossa syndrome' was coined by Rogers[45] in 1933 for a syndrome that was the result of rapidly increased intracranial pressure below the tentorium cerebelli. It may be caused by a cerebellar abscess, intracranial tumour or cerebellar haemorrhage.

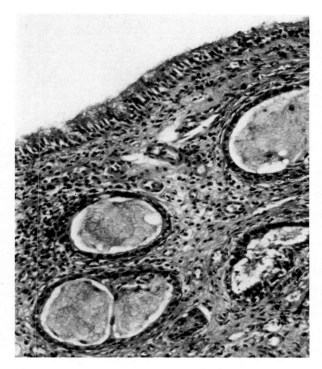

Fig. 13.5 Biopsy of mucosa of middle ear in a case of chronic catarrhal otitis media ('glue ear'). The tall columnar secretory epithelium is characteristic of the condition. Gland-like structures, filled with thick mucus are seen in the granulation tissue.

Haematoxylin-eosin   × 105

Haemophilus influenzae and certain anaerobic micro-organisms, particularly *Bacteroides fragilis*, play a significant role in the causation of intra-cerebral complications, such as brain abscesses, and in malignant or non-healing external otitis. They may perhaps have a role also in chronic otitis media, in which the Gram-negative flora, particularly *Proteus vulgaris* and *Pseudomonas aeruginosa*, predominate.

The chances of isolating an anaerobic micro-organism causing an abscess depend on prompt inoculation of the culture media and prompt incubation. The patient's survival may depend on the early successful isolation of such a pathogen.[47]

Purulent meningitis, an equally serious complication of otitis media, may result in ossifying labyrinthitis, causing deafness.[48, 49] Recurrent meningitis may be the presenting symptom of a congenital defect of the footplate of the stapes.[50, 51] Purulent otitis media may provide the portal of entry for *Clostridium tetani*.[52]

Other complications and sequelae of acute otitis media

A recent comprehensive review of acute otitis media in children has drawn renewed attention to some of the complications and sequelae that may occur in the tympanic cavity and in the temporal bone of such patients; for example adhesive otitis, ossicular damage and epidermoid cholesteatoma affecting the quality of life of these children.[53]

Chronic petrositis, an inflammation of the petrous portion of the temporal bone, is a rare complication, presenting with persistent aural discharge, headache and diplopia (Gradenigo's syndrome).[54]

Chronic otitis media and mastoiditis

Mucosal changes (Table 13.1)
The formation of oedematous, hyperaemic granulation tissue containing mononuclear inflammatory cells is a prominent feature of chronic otitis media and frequently this gives rise to polypoid masses (aural polyps) that may hinder drainage of the exudate and encourage persistence of infection.[48] The stroma of the mucosa becomes greatly thickened and fibrotic, and there is some degree of accompanying lymphocytic and plasma cell infiltration. The flat endothelial-like surface epithelium reverses to columnar and ciliate epithelium containing globlet cells. Gland-like structures may be formed (Fig. 13.5).

These changes have been interpreted as an irreversible differentiation of the epithelial lining[48] playing an important role in the maintenance of the discharge and in the pathogenesis of a 'glue ear'; moreover they provide a medium that favours the growth of bacteria and re-infection. Bone chips removed at operations on the mastoid process are often found to be covered by tall columnar epithelial cells or to include strings or groups of gland-like structures filled with thick mucous secretion.

Middle-ear effusion can persist after an attack of acute otitis media in children and it may be

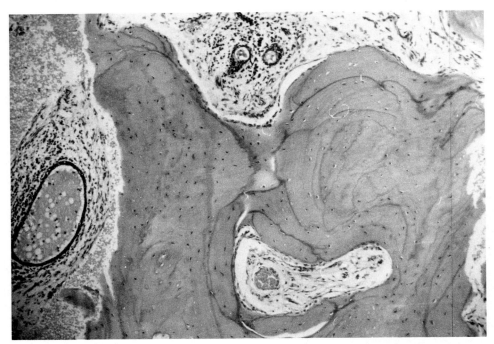

Fig. 13.6a Fragments of bone from the mastoid process of a 5-year-old boy operated for chronic otitis media (recent case). There is the characteristic pattern of irregular lines of apposition in the reconstructed bone. Note the row of osteoblasts and some inflammatory granulation tissue containing gland-like structures. A residual air space is lined by cuboidal cells and contains much muco-purulent secretion. It is surrounded by inflammatory granulation tissue.

Haematoxylin–eosin   × 240   *Provided by Mr K.P. Ferris, All Saints' Hospital, Chatham, UK.*

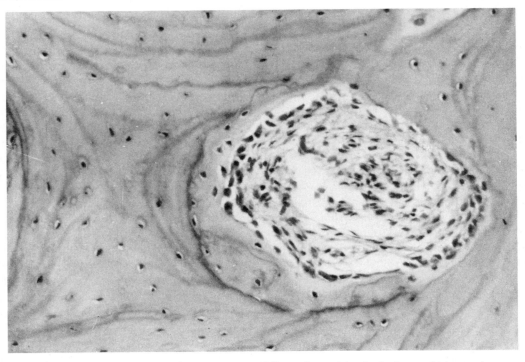

Fig. 13.6b As Figure 13.6a, showing the irregular pattern of lines of apposition in the bone which contains a vessel with some fibrous tissue surrounded by osteoblasts covering a narrow seam of osteoid tissue.

Haematoxylin–eosin   × 800

associated with impaired hearing.[55] This is caused by the described changes of the middle-ear mucosa.

Bone changes

The structure of the bone of the middle ear and mastoid process undergoes considerable change in the presence of infection. In the acute stage of otitis media or mastoiditis, destructive processes predominate at first, but it is not long before the reparative efforts of the bone supervene.

It has been postulated that the mechanism of the localized destructive process was chemical in origin and that bone resorption was induced by collagenase, lysosomal enzymes, prostaglandins and other cell mediators.[56] Osteoclasts play the major role in bone absorption but the cells from which they are derived and the mechanism by which their activity is controlled remain uncertain. It has been shown that calcitonin specifically altered the behaviour of osteoclasts, rendering them inactive in contrast to osteoblasts, peritoneal macrophages and inflammatory giant cells.[57]

Bone chips removed at operation for chronic otitis media show microscopical evidence of repeated alternation of absorption and deposition of bone, leading to reconstruction of the bone pattern. A variety of pictures may result, one of the most frequent being described as a glacier-like pattern of haematoxyphile lines of new bone apposition, with or without a mosaic of irregular cement lines reminiscent of Paget's disease (Fig. 13.6a,b).

In chronic otitis media the formation of new bone and bone reconstruction must be regarded as fundamental processes that lead to alteration of the whole internal structure of the affected mastoid bone. Moreover, the altered microscopical pattern enables a reasonably accurate distinction to be made between sclerotic bone (pathological), with its irregular pattern, and compact bone (normal) with its regular Haversian systems of lamellar bone. It is surprising that this very important aspect of the pathology of otitis media has been overlooked until recently. It is noteworthy that these histopathological findings have been confirmed on specimens operated on recently (Fig. 13.6a,b).

The site of initial mineralization of lamellar bone is at the junction of mineralized bone with osteoid. This area is usually referred to as the calcification front. It may be demonstrated by different apparently specific staining methods and also by administering a tetracycline label and studying undecalcified sections by fluorescence microscopy.[58]

Catarrhal otitis media ('glue ear syndrome')

'Glue ear' is a form of middle-ear catarrh—the name 'catarrhal otitis media' is used here in the sense that it is characterized by the presence in the tympanic cavity of a sterile mucoid fluid containing only comparatively few inflammatory cells and desquamated columnar cells. Other synonyms include *otosalpingitis*, *tubotympanitis*, *secretory otitis media*, *serous otitis media*, *chronic exudative otitis media* and *otitis media with effusion*.

It may be of interest to recall that the mucous membranes were first described by Schneider (1614–1680),[59] who disproved the theory that mucus originated in the pituitary and developed the catarrhal theory based on the flowing qualities of mucus to be accumulated in cavities (*kata* = down; *rheîn* = to flow). Since mucoid secretion is an important element in the production of the glue ear syndrome, the term 'catarrhal' has a historical pedigree and was used by Politzer in 1869[60] in his term 'otitis media catarrhalis'.

Aetiology

There are various reasons for the accumulation of fluid in the middle ear. For instance, serous or mucoid fluid sometimes collects in the tympanic cavity when the auditory (Eustachian) tube is occluded by enlarged nasopharyngeal lymphoid tissue or by a nasopharyngeal neoplasm. Chronic tubal malfunction may lead to further complications.[61] It has been suggested that inadequate antibiotic prophylaxis in the course of simple respiratory infections may predispose to the development and persistence of catarrhal otitis media and its occasional complication by chronic adhesive otitis. As pointed out, the epithelium of the middle-ear cleft undergoes characteristic changes during chronic otitis media, overt or

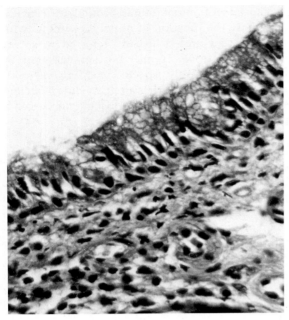

Fig. 13.7 Catarrhal otitis, so-called 'glue ear'. Biopsy of tympanic cavity of child with clinical signs of 'glue ear'. The surface epithelium is tall and stratified, consisting of secretory columnar epithelium with goblet cells.

Periodic-acid/Schiff reaction   × 230

latent, resulting in the 'reversal' or 'transformation' into a secretory-type epithelium.[48]

The increased goblet-cell population of the middle-ear mucosa in chronic otitis media contributes greatly to the amount of mucoid secretion and forms the basic substrate of the glue-ear syndrome or catarrhal otitis media (Fig. 13.7). It has been shown experimentally that the epithelial lining of the middle ear of the guinea pig, chinchilla and nude mouse may undergo considerable transformation following infection with various organisms, the surface of the inflamed mucosa becoming covered by tall ciliated columnar cells interspersed with goblet cells. It is interesting to note that the transformation of the lining of the pulmonary alveoli from their habitually flat type to cuboidal- or columnar-type cells is a common accompaniment also of disordered repair of the lungs.

The human middle-ear mucosa may regenerate following surgical removal, e.g. at tympanoplasty, and be lined by cuboidal to pseudo-stratified secretory epithelium containing secretory granules; their cells are endowed with cilia and microvilli.[63]

The transformed mucosa of the middle ear can behave like that of the nose and nasal sinuses; consequently some of the aetiological factors that lead to nasal discharge, including allergy, may enhance the production of mucous secretion of high viscosity in the tympanic cavity. While the term 'glue ear' may be used to refer to a fairly clear-cut clinical picture, it cannot be regarded as relating to a pathological entity definable more precisely than as a type or phase of chronic otitis media.[48] Secretory or catarrhal otitis media may form part of the immotile ciliary syndrome.[63]

Chronic adhesive otitis media

The formation of adhesions between the tympanic membrane and the bony walls of the middle ear or ossicles is common. It has been suggested that inefficient antibiotic treatment of local infection may be a significant factor encouraging the organization of purulent exudate, with the development, in some cases, of fibrous adhesions. On the other hand, histological sections of the temporal bones obtained at necropsy have not infrequently displayed fibrous bands crossing the middle-ear cavity, suggestive of some previous lurking infection.

Otitis nigra

Otitis nigra is a rare condition, characterized by haemorrhagic and serous otitis media. Ultrastructural studies have demonstrated enhanced permeability of the congested vessels.[63a] This permits increased migration of the red blood corpuscles. Following the breakdown of the cells, haemoglobin is transformed into haemosiderin and ferritin, which in turn are absorbed by various cells, thus giving rise to the dark appearance of the mucosa that gives the condition its name. The clinical features are caused by these changes.

Tympanosclerosis

Tympanosclerosis is a frequent sequela of otitis media. First recognized a century ago by von Tröltsch (1881),[64] it remained in almost total obscurity until it was rediscovered by Zöllner & Beck.[65] With the introduction of microsurgery it has been gaining in interest and importance.

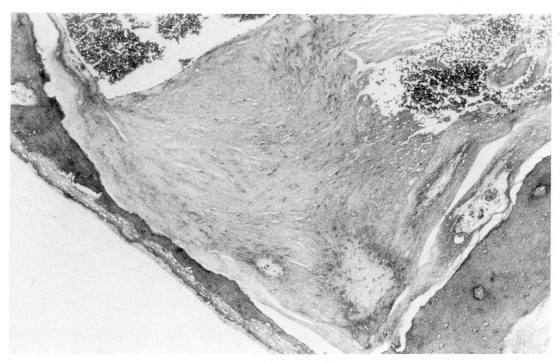

Fig. 13.8 Tympanosclerosis. Lamellar fibrous tissue fills the intercrural space of the stapes. This may reduce its mobility. Haematoxylin–eosin   × 100

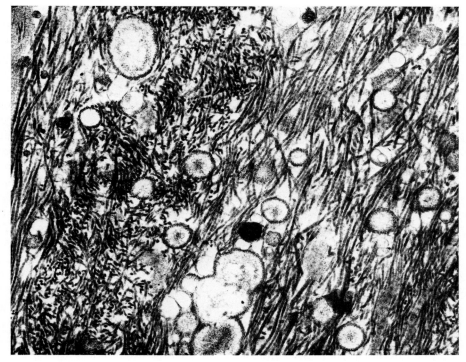

Fig. 13.9 Tympanosclerosis. Electron micrograph of tympanosclerotic tissue showing the collagenous matrix and many scattered matrix vesicles.   × 19 950

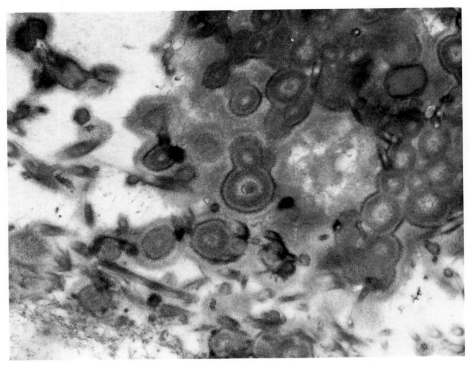

Fig. 13.10a Tympanosclerosis. Aggregated, probably fused calcospherules outlined by the lamina limitans. There is calcification in the large plaques formed.   Electron micrograph   × 12 745

Clinically, the extent of the lesion varies from small plaques on the tympanic membrane or in the oval window niche to a diffuse process enveloping the entire tympanic cavity in whitish fibrous tissue, which may cover the ossicles, thus impeding their movement (Fig. 13.8).

Light microscopy of a specimen reveals a rather monotonous picture contrasting with the more dramatic clinical features. It is composed of dense layers and bundles of collagenous fibrous tissue arising from the granulation tissue covering and replacing the mucosa of the middle-ear cavity. The lesion undergoes hyalinization and profuse calcification; ossification may ensue.

Electron microscopy shows a storiform network of criss-crossing bundles of collagen fibres of normal periodicity. There are vast numbers of plain vesicles in the collagenous tissue which form the primary site of calcification (Fig. 13.9). Calcification starts in the centre of these membrane-bound vesicles, called 'matrix vesicles' by Anderson and Bonucci.[66-68] The process spreads to the rest of the vesicle resulting in the

formation of calcospherules of various size and shape[69] (Figs. 13.10a,b). Some may be ring-shaped or serpiginous, others doughnut-like structures which may coalesce to form large plaques.[70-72]

The pathogenesis of tympanosclerosis has remained obscure but some general agreement has emerged. Tympanosclerosis is considered to be a healing process or a reparative process closely linked with chronic otitis media and it resembles the fibrotic healing process in other organs. Clearly, degenerative processes in otitis media may trigger off the release of a factor (or factors) in the matrix vesicles acting as fibrogenetic stimulants and primary sites of calcification.

The matrix vesicles contain calcium and phosphate ions and alkaline phosphatase. The membrane of the matrix vesicles may become altered, followed by loss of water and supersaturation inside the matrix vesicles. Supersaturation leads to incipient calcification and crystal formation and will proceed spontaneously, resulting in the production of calco-

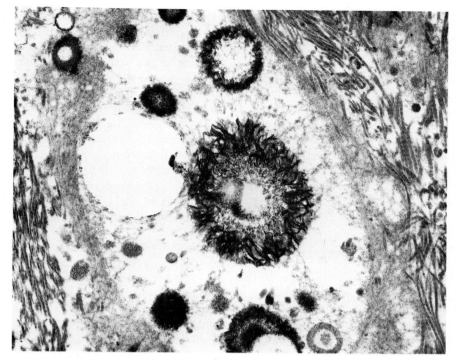

Fig. 13.10b Tympanosclerosis. Solitary calcospherules formed by hydroxy-apatite crystals in collagen.
Electron micrograph   × 19 950

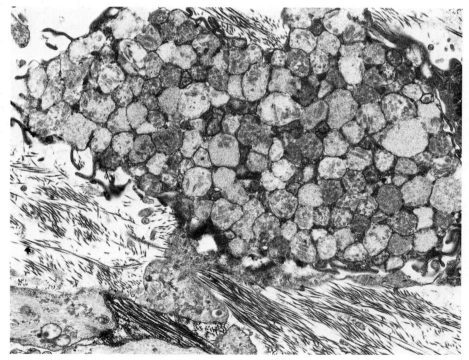

Fig. 13.11 Tympanosclerosis. Fibroblast with cytoplasmic or matrix vesicles being released into the tympanosclerotic stroma.
Electron micrograph   × 18 900

spherules (Fig. 13.10a,b). Vesicular degeneration of cells, e.g. fibroblasts, leads to the formation of the matrix vesicles released into the fibrous tissue in which calcium carbonate or apatite is deposited (Fig. 13.11). Similar processes of mineralization occur in nodular fasciitis and other fibroproliferative lesions showing calcification or metaplastic bone formation.[73] In osteoarthritis, apatite crystal deposition on collagen bundles of the articular cartilage resembles the features of tympanosclerosis,[74] and it is interesting to note that in both processes, as well as in various fibrotic diseases, immunological mechanisms may be active.[75, 76]

EPIDERMOID CHOLESTEATOMA

The so-called 'cholesteatoma of the ear' has been the subject of much argument and discussion since Cruveilhier[77] in 1829 described the 'pearly tumours' which Johannes Muller[78] was to name in 1838 'cholesteatoma'. It is an important and irreversible complication of chronic otitis media, and surgical treatment is usually necessary. It is not a neoplasm and may be regarded as an epidermoid cyst.

The 'cholesteatoma' appears most commonly in the area of the epitympanic recess (attic) and mastoid antrum and in the mastoid process. The epitympanic recess or attic is an upward extension of the tympanic cavity behind the roof of the external acoustic meatus. It accommodates the head of the malleus and the body of the incus. Attico-antral infection may ensue and because of the poor drainage from the attic, impeded by the ossicles and folds, a serious disease of the middle ear may develop. Cholesteatoma often forms here. In exceptional cases it may form in the petrous part of the temporal bone, or it may present in the antero-inferior part of the tympanic cavity.

Microscopically it is a cystic structure lined by keratinizing stratified squamous epithelium resting on a fibrous stroma of variable thickness; the stroma may contain certain elements of the original mucosa lining (Fig. 13.12). The keratinized layers of the epithelium are innermost and are shed into the cavity of the cyst, forming its contents (Fig. 13.13), often with an admixture of neutrophile leucocytes. The lesion enlarges very slowly, encircled by the surrounding inflammatory granulation tissue containing some agents of absorption of the surrounding bone.[48]

The question of the extension of epidermoid cholesteatoma has remained unanswered. There is evidence that it is assisted by the proteolytic and bone resorbing activity of the inflammatory granulation tissue forming part of the matrix. Epithelial-mesenchymatous interaction is an important factor in this process[80] and enhanced collagenase and proteolytic activity may further the expansion of the lesion at the cost of the surrounding bone and other tissues of the middle-ear cleft.[81-83]

Erosion of the surrounding bony structures may open up a channel through which infection by aerobic and/or anaerobic organisms can spread. The possible presence of anaerobic organisms in infected cholesteatomas is important in relation to the choice of appropriate antibiotic treatment.[82, 83] In some cases it may include foci of cholesterol granuloma and large numbers of desquamated cells in the inflammatory tissue. The keratinized cells can provoke a foreign-body type reaction; usually this is less developed than in the areas of cholesterol granuloma.

Pathogenesis of epidermoid cholesteatoma

The origin of the squamous epithelium forming the epidermoid cholesteatoma and its role have occasioned fierce arguments, and such arguments have been based often on emotional rather than on basic biological principles or on experimental evidence.[84-89] Various theories have been advanced to explain its presence in the middle-ear cleft—the congenital theory, the immigration theory, the metaplasia theory and the implantation theory.

The congenital theory

The rare intracranial epidermoid cysts or cholesteatomas are considered to arise from epithelial rests displaced during defective closure of the neural tube between the third and fifth week of embryonic development. It is relevant that some intracranial cholesteatomas remain asymptomatic during life and may be discovered only at post

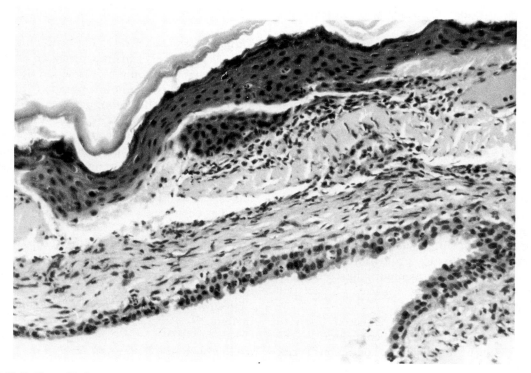

Fig. 13.12 Epidermoid cholesteatoma showing the keratotic squamous epithelium of the cyst. It is separated by a layer of hyalinized collagenous tissue and some inflammatory granulation tissue from the secretory epithelium of the tympanic cavity. This feature argues against the metaplastic origin of the squamous epithelium.

Haematoxylin–eosin   × 480

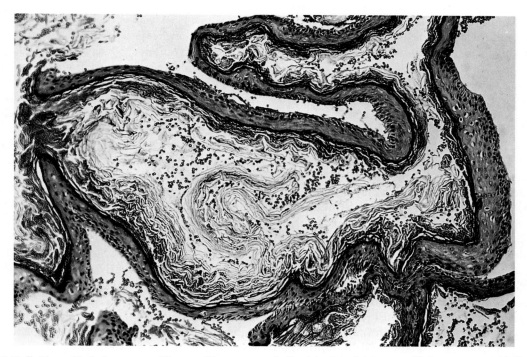

Fig. 13.13 Epidermoid cholesteatoma. The cyst-like structure is lined by keratinizing stratified squamous epithelium and filled with keratotic material.

Haematoxylin–eosin   × 165

mortem.[90] In a listing of the most frequent sites of intracranial cholesteatomas, the middle-ear cleft was not mentioned.[91] I have failed to find any embryonic cell nests in the course of examining a large number of temporal bones sectioned. Epidermoid cholesteatomas in the petrous-pyramidal portion of the temporal bone are usually of secondary (to otitis media) and not of congenital origin.[92]

The immigration theory

This theory covers three processes: 1) the immigration of the squamous epithelium through the perforated tympanic membrane; 2) the attic-retraction theory; and 3) proliferation of the basal epithelial cells of the squamous epithelium of the tympanic membrane (the apparently intact tympanic membrane).

The immigration theory is based upon the well-known pathological phenomenon of ingrowth of epithelium from the contiguous surface to form the lining of sinus or fistula tracks. According to this view, the lesion results from the ingrowth of keratinizing epidermis from the external acoustic meatus into the tympanic cavity through a perforation or defect in the tympanic membrane and/or by direct migration or proliferation of the basal epithelium or the tympanic membrane. The theory was challenged when cases were described in which the drumhead appeared to be intact; however in view of the difficulty of assessing the integrity of the tympanic membrane by clinical examination, such reports scarcely constituted indisputable evidence against this explanation.

The composition of the tympanic membrane has to be considered in this context. It consists of three layers: outer, epidermal, middle lamina propria and inner mucous layer. The middle lamina propria of the para tensa is formed mainly of outer radial and inner circular fibres arranged in an orderly way. The fibre arrangement in the middle lamina propria of the diseased human tympanic membranes is disturbed, affecting the healing process and the structure of the perforated tympanic membrane.[93] Furthermore, complete closure of the perforation may be impeded by the spreading squamous-cell epithelium around the margins of the perforation.

The attic-retraction theory. The attic-retraction of Bezold (1890)[94] explains the formation of the epidermoid cholesteatoma by retraction of the pars flaccida of the tympanic membrane (Shrapnell's membrane) into the epitympanic cavity where it may become attached to its wall.[95] Occlusion of the Eustachian tube and consequent atelactasia of the middle-ear spaces play an important contributory role causing Shrapnell's membrane to retract. A retraction pocket forms a cyst-like structure lined by keratinizing squamous epithelium (and has been described clinically as a 'Mikimoto pearl').[96] Microscopic studies have confirmed that the epithelium is derived from the squamous epithelial lining of the tympanic membrane.[97, 98] Perforation of the retraction pocket is considered to be a factor in the production of an epidermoid cholesteatoma by the spreading squamous epithelium.[95]

Proliferation of the basal-cell layer of the tympanic membrane. It has been shown that basal-cell proliferation occurred during low-grade infections of the middle ear causing no perforation of the tympanic membrane, although penetrating its fibrous layer.[99] Experimental evidence by various authors has been disregarded by those relying on the clinical impression of the apparently intact tympanic membrane.[100] I have described in man and the guinea-pig proliferating squamous epithelial cones extending from the tympanic membrane into the underlying inflammatory granulation tissue frequently forming small epidermoid cysts (micro-cholesteatomas).[48, 84]

Palva et al[101] have noted, in the right temporal bone of a 69-year-old woman suffering from chronic otitis media, that the squamous epithelium of the thickened but intact tympanic membrane formed papillary projections deep into the stroma. Such papillary projections form 'the structural basis from which cholesteatoma may develop behind an (apparently) intact tympanic membrane'[101] as previously recognized by Friedmann (1959)[84] and by Ruedi (1978).[102]

The metaplasia theory

Squamous metaplasia has been suggested as a possible source of epidermoid cholesteatoma[103] but is uncommon. The usual absence of hyperkeratinization when there is squamous metaplasia of the bronchial epithelium suggests that squamous metaplasia of respiratory type epithelium in the middle ear would not necessarily be followed by keratinization and the formation of an epidermoid cholesteatoma, although it may occur. Equally, the simultaneous presence in the matrix of the two different layers of epithelial cells, columnar deep to squamous (Figs 13.12, 13.13) and separated by inflammatory granulation tissue, argues in a given case against the metaplastic origin of the squamous epithelium.[84, 103]

The exponents of the metaplasia theory rely on the dubious clinical evidence of an intact tympanic membrane. The importance of even small 'temporary' defects in the lamina propria of the tympanic membrane has to be appreciated.[100, 104] This is easily overlooked on clinical examination alone, leading to the erroneous assessment that the tympanic membrane is intact with all the theoretical implications of that assumption.[105] Basal-cell hyperplasia and proliferation of the squamous epithelium of the tympanic membrane are common[106, 107] and may occur in an apparently intact tympanic membrane (see above).[100]

The implantation theory

Traumatic cholesteatoma. The development of post-traumatic cholesteatoma was described in non-infected middle ears following perforation of the tympanic membrane by gun-blast trauma associated with a displacement of squamous epithelial fragments into the middle-ear cleft.[108, 109] Such epithelial fragments may remain viable for many years behind the healed tympanic membrane and produce a cholesteatoma many years later.[110] Three cases of cholesteatoma as a late complication of extralabyrinthine fracture of the temporal bone were described.[111] These fractures offer a portal of entry for the invasion of the middle-ear cleft by squamous epithelium. It is suggested that such acquired cholesteatoma can display a very aggressive behaviour and the surgical management may be difficult. For example, in a series of 12 cases tympanoplasty preceded the development of epidermoid cholesteatoma by 5 months to 3 years.[112, 113]

The development of epidermoid spinal tumours after previous lumbar puncture is of some relevance to the implantation theory of epidermoid cholesteatoma.[114–116] Spinal epidermoid tumours can develop even years after a lumbar puncture from implanted fragments of the epidermis.

Neonatal otitis. Neonatal otitis may be mentioned in this context. The pharyngo-tympanic tube is patent at birth and amniotic squames may be found in the cavity of the ear of infants. Aschoff in 1897[117] described neonatal otitis caused by amniotic squamous debris in the middle ear. Squamous cells reaching the middle ear *in utero* can persist for several days after birth, provoking a foreign-body type reaction. Occasionally secondary infection results and aural polyps are formed.[118]

Latent epidermoid cholesteatoma. There occur clinically unrecognized cases of aural cholesteatoma where only the specimen obtained at operation or at necropsy might furnish the definite histopathological evidence of a latent or occult epidermoid cholesteatoma.[113, 119, 120]

Experimental cholesteatoma

Experimental studies have thrown light on the origin of squamous epithelium in the middle ear.[86, 102, 121, 122] The experimental injection of bacterial cultures into the tympanic bulla of guinea pigs, in particular *Pseudomonas aeruginosa*, was followed by the prompt development of otitis media, reversal of the middle-ear mucosa of the tympanic bulla to a secretory type of epithelium and, in about 10% of the animals, by the immigration of squamous epithelium and the development of epidermoid cysts.[52]

The experimental application of various mildly irritant substances into the ear of rabbits may be followed by the formation of epidermoid cholesteatoma.[121, 122] Similarly the lesion has been reproduced by transplanting human cholesteatoma membranes into the middle-ear cavity of the immunodeficient 'nude mouse'.[123] Spontaneous aural cholesteatoma is a frequent occurrence in the adult Mongolian gerbil, *Meriones unguiculatus* arising from the tympanic membrane and the

Table 13.2 'Epidermoid cholesteatoma'—terminological chaos.

'Pearly tumour'	Cruveilhier[77]
Cholesteatoma	Muller[78]
Margaroid or margaritoma*	Craigie [79]
Cholesteatosis	Young[128]
Black cholesteatosis	Birrell[129]
Epidermosis or pre-epidermosis	Tumarkin[130]
Epidermoid cholesteatoma	Friedmann[84]
Epidermoid cyst	Ferlito[131]
Keratocyst	Schuknecht [132]
Keratoma	Goodhill[133]

* from the Greek for 'pearl'

external auditory meatus.[124] Since the cholesteatoma of the gerbil erodes bone and invades the labyrinth and the cranial cavity, it provides an animal model for investigating the destructive properties of cholesteatoma in man.[125]

Terminological chaos

The term 'cholesteatoma' appears to have been accepted by most authors, although it has invited a good deal of speculation both on the role of cholesterol in the production of the lesion and on the possibility that the latter is neoplastic. It cannot be emphasized too strongly that the 'epidermoid cholesteatoma' is an epithelial structure, the product of hyperkeratosis of stratified squamous epithelium. It is not a granuloma or neoplasm and cholesterol plays no part in its genesis—in fact, the term 'cholesteatoma' is a misnomer. Table 13.2 is an indication of the terminological chaos arising from the attempts of various authors to invent a more accurate term. The term 'cholesteatosis' eliminated the neoplastic interpretation but perpetuated the equally incorrect implication of cholesterol. More recent terms include 'epidermosis', 'squamous cholesteatosis' and 'squamous epitheliosis'. These, even when they have the advantage of eliminating the reference to cholesterol, are inadmissible because they may be thought to imply that the condition is a disease of the epithelium itself.

It could be argued that it might be best to dispense altogether with the term 'cholesteatoma', and call the condition by a name that describes what in fact it is, *epidermoid cyst* (or *kera-*

tinic cyst) of the middle ear. Although these are correct descriptions of the pathological findings, I have adopted the combined term *epidermoid cholesteatoma* based on the clinicopathological aspects of the lesion.[84]

Summarizing, epidermoid cholesteatoma results mainly from the spread of pre-existing keratinizing squamous epithelium into the middle ear;[126] metaplasia plays a minor aetiological role; and the congenital type is at most a curiosity of rare occurrence.[127]

CHOLESTEROL GRANULOMA

The cholesterol granuloma is not a clinical or pathological entity but merely a particular form of granulation tissue developing as part of the varied tissue reaction in cases of otitis media.[84] It is associated with chronic mastoiditis but may also develop quite rapidly in cases of acute haemorrhagic mastoiditis in children. The histopathology of cholesterol granuloma differs fundamentally from that of the 'epidermoid cholesteatoma'. It is a granulomatous lesion in which crystals of cholesterol esters (represented by distinct cleft-like spaces in paraffin wax sections) are surrounded by foreign-body giant cells in the fibrotic granulation tissue (Fig. 13.14). There is frequently convincing evidence of recent or recurrent haemorrhage (Figs 13.15, 13.16) and more often some blood pigment or inflammatory exudate is present, suggesting that the granuloma may be a reaction to the presence of breakdown products of blood, and of inflammatory and other cells in the tissues. Crystals of cholesterol esters are very resistant and provoke the formation of foreign-body giant cells and the development of fibrosis. Free cholesterol is intensely sclerogenic.[134]

It must be stressed that the term 'cholesterol granuloma' is a histological one and that the condition can only be recognized with accuracy by microscopical examination, although at operation the finding of haemorrhagic matter in the mastoid cells and shimmering crystals floating in the blood or effusion may suggest its presence.[135]

Experimental evidence points to blood as the main but not the sole source of cholesterol.[86, 136, 137] The formation of cholesterol

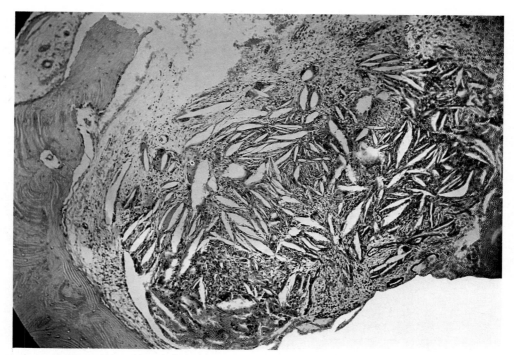

Fig. 13.14 Cholesterol granuloma in a mastoid air cell (chronic otitis media). The pointed clefts contained crystals of cholesterol esters that have been dissolved during histological processing of the specimen. Multinucleate giant cells of 'foreign-body' type have formed round some of the crystals. There are many lymphocytes in the fibrotic granulation tissue.

Haematoxylin–eosin   × 60

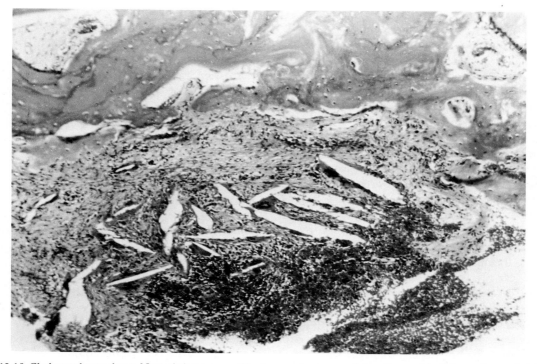

Fig. 13.15 Cholesterol granuloma. Necrotic bone covered by haemorrhagic granulation tissue with cholesterol crystals (chronic otitis media) some of which are clearly formed in the blood.

Haematoxylin–eosin   × 100

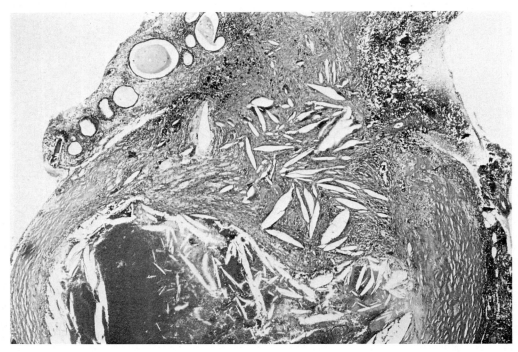

Fig. 13.16 Tympanosclerosis and cholesterol granuloma—chronic otitis media. Complex lesion removed from the middle ear forming a large cyst-like structure containing blood. Cholesterol clefts are seen in the haemorrhagic content of the cyst and embedded in the surrounding lamellar (tympanosclerotic) fibrous tissue, which also contains gland-like structures.

Haematoxylin–eosin   × 70

crystals from the breakdown products of the blood has been confirmed by many authors.[138–140] The formation of cholesterol granuloma has been induced by chronic obstruction of the auditory tube.[141] Cholesterol granuloma[84, 135] may also develop in serous or catarrhal otitis media, idiopathic haemotympanum, and in a xanthoma.

The ultrastructure of giant cells in cholesterol granuloma has been studied with particular reference to their role in the absorption of cholesterol needles.[134, 142] The giant cells are rich in lysosomes and resemble actively phagocytic histiocytes. They seem to be well equipped for an active role in the absorption of cholesterol crystals formed in the affected tissues of the middle ear. In semi-thin sections, the smaller needles of cholesterol can be recognized inside the giant cells, a feature overlooked in earlier descriptions (Fig. 13.17).[134, 142] The giant cells frequently contain one, two or more rhomboid or short dart-shaped or needle-shaped inclusions of cholesterol appearing as empty spaces ranging

from about 0.5–2 μm in length. Electron microscopy shows the needles in the inflammatory granulation tissue of the cholesterol granuloma surrounded not only by plasma cells, lymphocytes and histiocytes but also by many red blood corpuscles—further evidence of the role of haemorrhage in the pathogenesis of cholesterol granuloma (Fig. 13.18).

Ochronosis

Ochronotic alkaptonuria (ochronosis) may cause thickening and dark discoloration of the tympanic membrane combined with high-frequency hearing loss.[142a]

OTHER INFECTIONS

Tuberculosis of the middle ear

Tuberculous infection has been recognized as an occasional cause of chronic middle-ear disease.[48] Early diagnosis and treatment are very impor-

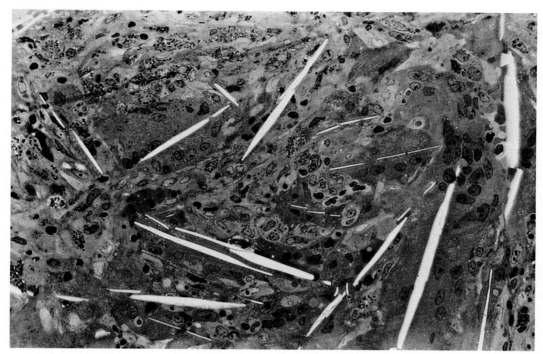

Fig. 13.17 Cholesterol granuloma. Giant cells with fine needle-shaped cholesterol crystals in their cytoplasm. Araldite-embedded tissue.   Gentian violet   × 400

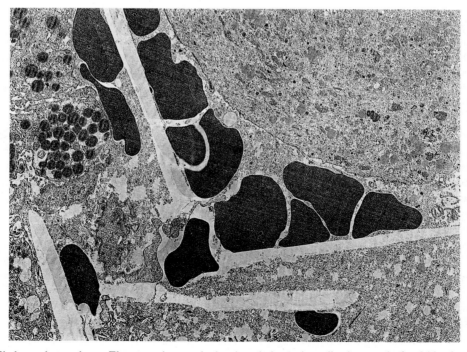

Fig. 13.18 Cholesterol granuloma. Electron micrograph showing cholesterol needles in a pool of red blood cells. Part of a giant cell is also seen; contains large numbers of mitochondria.   × 9945

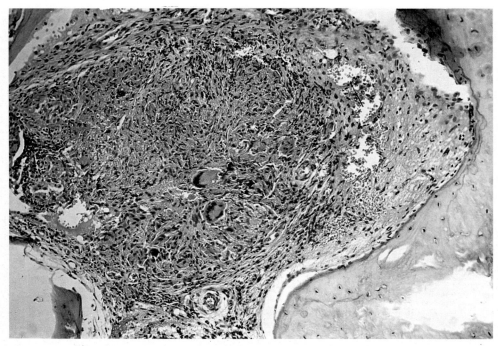

Fig. 13.19 Tuberculous mastoiditis. Typical tuberculous granulation tissue fills the air cell. There is early caseation. Haematoxylin–eosin × 100

tant, and the comparative rarity of the condition should not preclude its consideration in the differential diagnosis of otitic infections.[143, 144] The onset of otitis media in a patient known to be suffering from pulmonary tuberculosis should always lead the clinician to suspect the possibility of spread of the infection to the ear. Early correct diagnosis of the disease is less likely in patients whose initial symptoms are aural. In many such cases there are no clinical features that specifically indicate the true nature of the infection: instead, the symptoms are those of any nonspecific, acute or chronic, otitis media. The mastoid is often cellular and pneumatized.

The microscopical picture is essentially that of a tuberculous lesion in any location, characterized by tubercles composed of epithelioid cells, Langhans-type giant cells, plasmacytes and lymphocytes (Fig. 13.19). Caseating necrosis is not a marked feature but secondary infection may obscure the primary lesion. Acid-fast bacilli may or may not be demonstrable.

The diagnosis depends not only on the classical histological picture but, more important, on the isolation of the causal organism by culture and guinea pig inoculation. Attention has been drawn[145] to the fact that whereas previously the characteristic tubercle has been regarded as pathognomonic of tuberculosis, this was no longer true since the pattern of interpretation has undergone a profound change. There has been an increasing awareness of other 'tuberculoid' lesions, especially in the upper respiratory tract, with the result that pathologists have become reluctant to diagnose tuberculosis solely on histopathological grounds. A variety of conditions may give rise to a 'tuberculoid granuloma', the commonest being sarcoidosis but fungal or nocardial infection may occasionally be involved. It must be emphasized that the finding of tuberculoid lesions calls for extensive investigation, including clinical, radiological and bacteriological examinations.

Syphilis

Gummatous osteitis of the otic capsule is the basic lesion of both congenital and acquired syphilis of the inner ear. In cases of congenital

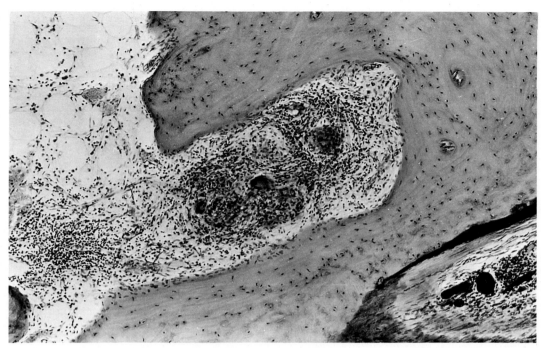

Fig. 13.20 Congenital syphilis. Small giant cell granuloma in the temporal bone of a patient suffering from deafness all his life due to congenital syphilis. The differential diagnosis from other giant cellular specific granulomas is difficult. The patient, a 60-year-old man when he died, was treated for congenital syphilis at the age of 16.

Haematoxylin–eosin   × 100

syphilis it may not become manifest until many years after birth (Fig. 13.20). Progressive sensorineural hearing loss and symptoms and signs resembling Ménière's disease may ensue. Endolymphatic hydrops is common.[146, 147] Ossifying labyrinthitis may develop (Fig. 13.21).

Mycoses

Aspergillosis of the external ear is a common disease causing *otomycosis* particularly in warmer climates, but the temporal bone can also be affected in opportunistic and other systemic fungal infections. A histopathological study of the temporal bone changes in three patients with fatal systemic fungal infections was reported.[148] All three patients were compromised hosts who failed to respond to chemotherapy. One patient with cryptococcosis presented with a unilateral hearing loss as the sole manifestation of cerebral cryptococcosis. In the other two, a case of aspergillosis and one of mucormycosis, the most common histopathological change consisted of a fungal infiltration of the nerves in the internal auditory meatus, with moderate infiltration of the sense organs of the membranous labyrinth.

Primary infection of the middle ear by *Histoplasma capsulatum* and followed by disseminated histoplasmosis has been reported from Thailand.[148a]

MISCELLANEOUS LESIONS

Sarcoidosis

Sarcoidosis is a systemic granulomatous disease of unknown aetiology which may affect the ear. Systemic lesions occur in the skin, lymph nodes, lungs, bones, eyes and nose. Deafness or labyrinthine disturbance may be due to sarcoidosis even in the absence of evident involvement of the central nervous system. The facial nerve is frequently affected.[149] Sarcoid lesions of the auricle are occasionally seen, usually as a manifestation of more widespread cutaneous sarcoidosis.

Microscopy shows epithelioid tubercles surrounded by lymphocytes. Caseation is absent

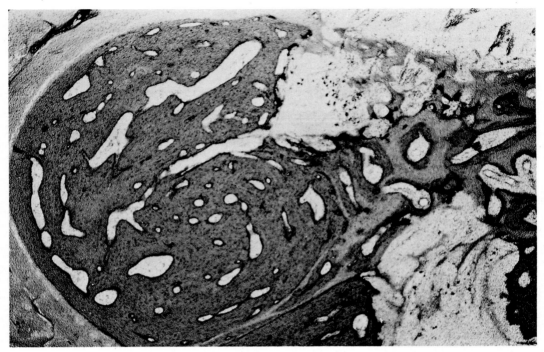

Fig. 13.21 Ossifying labyrinthitis. The totally-ossified basal coil of the cochlea is expanded and forms a large, moon-shaped mass.
Haematoxylin–eosin   × 100

and giant cells may be numerous or scanty and may contain asteroid inclusion and Schaumann bodies. Reticulin stain shows fibres within the sarcoid nodules in contrast to true tuberculous nodules. The Kveim test may assist in the diagnosis.

Wegener's granulomatosis

The middle ear is a rare site of the initial lesions in Wegener's granulomatosis, a condition likely to be overlooked unless the microscopist keeps its possibility in mind. Such cases are being recognized more often than hitherto. The middle ear becomes filled with the type of giant-cell granulomatous tissue that is characteristic of the disease[150–152] (Figs 13.22, 13.23).

Among 112 patients with Wegener's granulomatosis treated at the Mayo Clinic from 1970 to 1980, 21 were found to have aural involvement.[151] Conductive hearing loss was caused by various lesions including granulation tissue in the middle-ear cleft. In the cases of several patients with sensorineural hearing loss, there was at least some improvement in the deafness as an accompaniment of the treatment given for the underlying disease.

'Xanthoma' (xanthogranuloma)

Accumulations of lipid-laden macrophages with the appearances characteristic of 'xanthoma' are a rare finding in the temporal bone:[48] they occur least infrequently in the mastoid process, where they may simulate chronic mastoiditis.

Malakoplakia of the middle ear

Malakoplakia is a peculiar granulomatous lesion characteristically occurring in the urinary bladder. It has been recognized in other organs. Malakoplakia of the mastoid cavity of a 10-year-old Iranian boy has been reported.[153] The patient had repeated episodes of aural infection and an attack of meningitis. Mastoidectomy was performed, the ear continued to discharge and the patient developed a large postauricular swelling and peripheral facial palsy. The granulation

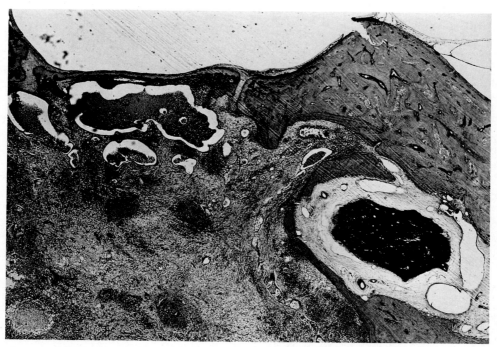

Fig. 13.22 Wegener's granulomatosis presenting as sudden deafness. The middle ear is filled with partly necrotic granulation tissue in which giant cells are present.

Haematoxylin-eosin   × 160

tissue removed from the ear was found to contain numerous intracellular inclusions in the macrophages, the *Michaelis–Gutmann bodies* first described in 1902.[154]

The histochemical features and the origin of the Michaelis–Gutmann bodies have attracted great interest. It has been concluded that they are formed by a process of phagolysosomal coalescence and mineralization of the phagocytosed cellular matter.[155–157] Lysosomes play the role of a digestive system of the cell and discharge various enzymes which digest foreign matter phagocytosed by the cell. Foreign particles phagocytosed by the cell are enclosed in membrane bound vesicles, the phagosomes which fuse with a lysosome to form the phagolysosome. The aetiology of the condition has remained obscure. Electron microscopy has shown some microorganisms in phagolysosomes in about 50% of the studied cases.[157]

It is perhaps noteworthy that von Hansemann, in 1903,[158] noted short bacilli attached to some of the cells, probably macrophages, which now bear his name. Malakoplakia of the urinary tract and possibly of the ear may be regarded as a peculiar response to infection by coliform bacteria.[157]

Amyloid deposits in the temporal bone
Amyloid deposits occur fairly frequently in the larynx and comparatively rarely in the nasal cavity. Such deposits in the temporal bone were first reported in 1983.[159] The patient was a 75-year-old man whose entire mastoid on one side was found to contain extensive deposits of a hyalinized tissue. This was identified as amyloid at necropsy when the right temporal bone and the occipital area of the same side were found to be infiltrated by an amyloid mass (amyloidoma) that also enclosed the internal carotid artery. Microscopy showed homogeneous infiltration of granulation tissue by amyloid. There were many scattered giant cells present, as frequently noted in amyloid deposits elsewhere. In sections stained with Congo red the homogeneous material showed dichroism under polarized light, typical of amyloid.

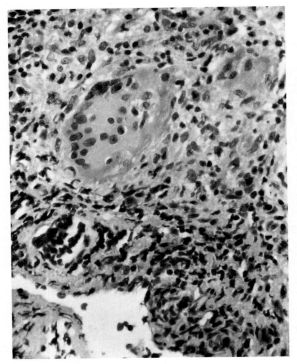

Fig. 13.23 Wegener's granulomatosis. Biopsy specimen from the middle ear showing giant cells near an inflamed vessel infiltrated by lymphocytes and plasma cells.

Haematoxylin–eosin   × 260

REFERENCES

1. Bass EJ, Jackson JF. Am J Phys Anthropol 1977; 47: 209.
2. Matsunagac E. Ann Hum Genet 1962; 25: 273.
3. Pareek SS. N Eng J Med 1979; 300: 1490.
4. Meltzer PE, Kelemen G. Laryngoscope 1959; 69: 1300.
5. Chandler JA. Laryngoscope 1968; 78: 1257.
6. Zaky DA, Bentley DW, Lowy K, et al. Am J Med 1976; 61: 298.
7. John AC, Hopkin NB. J Laryngol Otol 1979; 92: 259.
8. John AC, Cheesman AD. Hosp Update 1979; 5: 589.
9. Chandler JA. Ann Otol Rhinol Laryngol 1972; 81: 648.
10. McDonald TJ, Neel HB. Post Med 1975; 57: 95.
11. Sando I, Harada T, Saito B, et al. Ann Otol Laryngol 1981; 90: 109.
12. John AC, Hopkin NB. J Laryngol Otol 1979; 92: 259.
12a. McCaffrey TV, McDonald TJ, McCaffrey Lee. Ann Otolaryngol 1978; 86: 473.
13. N Eng J Med 1982; 307: 1631 (Clinical Pathological Conference).
14. *See* Ballantyne JC, Groves J. Scott Brown's Diseases of the ear, nose and throat. 4th ed. Vol. 1. London: Butterworth, 1978: 15–16.
15. Von Tröltsch AF. Surgical diseases of the ear. London: New Sydenham Soc, 1881.
16. Wullstein SR. Acta Otolaryngol (Stockh) 1976; 81: 197.
17. Proctor B. J Laryngol Otol 1964; 78: 631.
18. Wullstein SR. Laryngol Rhinol Otol (Stuttg) 1975; 54: 32.
19. Tumarkin A. J Laryngol Otol 1958; 72: 610.
20. Allan AF. Ann Otol Rhinol Laryngol 1969; 78: 49.
21. Diamant M. Acta Otolaryngol (Stockh) 1954; (Suppl. 118): 54.
22. Tumarkin A. J Laryngol Otol 1961; 75: 487.
23. Ingham HR, Selkon JB, Robxy CM. Br J Med 1977; ii: 991.
24. Ingham HR, Selkon JB, Roxby CM. J Antimicrob Chemother 1978; 4 (Suppl. C): 63.
25. Bezold F. Ohr etc. Heilk 1878; 13: 26.
26. Feigin R. N Eng J Med 1982; 306: 1417.
27. Haugsten P, Lorentzen P. J Laryngol 1980; 94: 169.
28. Brook R, Schwartz R. Acta Otolaryngol (Stockh) 1981; 91: 111.
29. Friedmann AD, Fleishe GR, Henretic F, et al. Ann Emerg Med 1982; 11: 181.
30. Luotonen J, Herva E, Karma P, et al. Scand J Infect Dis 1981; 13: 177.
31. Sugita R, Kawamura S, Fujimaki Y, et al. Pract Otol (Kyoto) 1982; 75: 921.
32. Lim D, DeMaria TF. Laryngoscope 1982; 92: 278.
33. Karma P, Luotonen J, Pukander J, et al. Acta Otolaryngol (Stockh) 1983; 95: 105.
34. Schwartz R, Rodriguez W, Khan W, Ross S. J Am Med Assoc 1978; 239: 320.
35. Schwartz RH, Rodriguez WJ, Khan WN. Ann Otol Rhinol Laryngol 1982; 91: 328.
36. Brook I, Schwartz R. Acta Otolaryngol (Stockh) 1981; 91: 111.
37. Luotonen J, Jokipii AMM, Sipila P, et al. Acta Otolaryngol (Stockh) 1982; 94 (suppl. 1): 386.
38. Thore M, Burman LG, Holm SE. J Infect Dis 1982; 145: 822.
39. Klein BS, Dollete FR, Yolken RH. J Pediatr 1982; 101: 16.
40. Henderson FW, Collier AM, Sanyal MA, et al. N Eng J Med 1982; 306: 1377.
41. Chugg V, Coelen R, et al. Br Med J 1984; 288: 114.
42. Sloyer JL, Cate CC, Howie VM, et al. J Infect Dis 1975; 132: 685.
43. Sloyer JL, Howie VM, Ploussard JH, et al. J Immunol 1977; 118: 248.
44. Data Bank of the Am J Otolaryngol 1983; 4: 268.
45. Rogers L. Brit Med J 1933; ii: 100.
46. Pfaltz CR. Orl 1982; 44: 301.
47. De Louvais J, Gortvai P, Hurley R. Br Med J 1977; ii: 981.
48. Friedmann I. Pathology of the ear. Oxford: Blackwell, 1974; pp. 128, 362.
49. Hoffman RA, Brookler KH, Bergeron RT. Ann Otol Rhinol Laryngol 1979; 88: 253.
50. Hipskind MM, Lindsay JR, Jones TD, et al. Laryngoscope 1976; 86: 682.
51. Schindler RA. Trans Pac Coast Otol Soc 1976; 57: 275.
52. Boussagol C, Marchand J. Ann Otolaryngol Chir Cervicofac 1977; 94: 331.
53. Bluestone C. N Eng J Med 1982; 306: 1399.

54. Gillanders DA. J Otolaryngol 1983; 12: 169.
55. Shurin PA, Pelton SI, Finkelstein J. N Eng J Med 1977; 296: 412.
56. Gantz BJ, Maynard J, Bumstead RM, Huang CC, Abramson M. Ann Otol Rhinol Laryngol 1979; 88: 693.
57. Chambers TJ, Magnus CJ. J Pathol 1982; 136: 27.
58. McLure J. J Clin Pathol 1982; 35: 1278.
59. Schneider V. De catarrhis (5 parts). Wittebergae: 1660.
60. Politzer A. Diseases of the ear. London: Baillière, Tindall & Cox, 1902.
61. Tos M. Acta Otolaryngol (Stockh) 1981; 92: 51.
62. Gamoletti R, Zini C, Sanna M, Bellomi A. ORL 1982; 44: 310.
63. Ernstson S, Afzelius BA, Mossberg B. Acta Otolaryngol (Stockh) 1984; 97: 83.
63a. Arnold W, Von Ilberg C. Arch Klin Exp Ohren Nas Kehlkopfheilk 1974; 208: 15.
64. Von Tröltsch A. Lehrbuch der Ohrenheilkunde. 1st ed. Leipzig: Vogel, 1869 (8th ed. 1881).
65. Zollner F, Beck C. Ztschr Laryngol 1955; 34: 137.
66. Anderson HC. J Cell Biol 1969; 41: 59.
67. Anderson HC. Fed Proc 1976; 35: 105.
68. Bonucci E. Clin Orthop 1971; 78: 108.
69. Friedmann I, Galey FR, Odnert S. Am J Otol 1981; 3: 144.
70. Chang IW. Acta Otolaryngol (Stockh) 1969; 68: 62.
71. Sorenson H, True O. Acta Otolaryngol (Stockh) 1971; 73: 18.
72. Friedmann I, Hodges GM, Graham M. Ann Otol Rhinol Laryngol 1979; 89 (Suppl. 68): 241.
73. Daroca PJ, Pulitzer DR, Lockero J. Arch Pathol Lab Med 1982; 106: 682.
74. Doyle DV. J Pathol 1982; 136: 199.
75. Schiff M, Poliquin JF, Catanzaro A, Ryan AF. Ann Otol Rhinol Laryngol 1980; 89 (Suppl. 70).
76. Fleischmajer R, Perlish JS, Duncan M. Arch Dermatol 1983; 119: 957.
77. Cruveilhier J. Anatomie pathologique du corps humain. Paris: Baillière 1829; 341.
78. Muller J. Ueber den feinren Bau und die Formen der krankhaften Geschwülste. Berlin: G. Reimer, 1838; 50.
79. Craigie D. Cited by: Virchow R: Elements of general and pathological anatomy adapted to the present state of knowledge in that science. 2nd ed. Edinburgh: Black, 1828; 343.
80. Jackson DG, Lim DJ. Acta Otolaryngol (Stockh) 1978; 86: 71.
81. Abramson M. Ann Otol Rhinol Laryngol 1969; 78: 112.
82. Gantz B, Maynard J, Bumsted R, Huang CC, Abramson M. Ann Otol Rhinol Laryngol 1979; 88: 693.
83. Harker LA, Kontz FP. Arch Otolaryngol 1977; 97: 183.
84. Friedmann I. Ann Otol Rhinol Laryngol 1959; 68: 57.
85. Friedmann I. In: McCabe BF, Sade J, Abramson M, eds. Cholesteatoma. First International Conference. Birmingham, Ala: Aesculapius Publishing Co, 1977; 10.
86. Friedmann I. Pathol Annu 1978; 13: 373.
87. Sade J. In: McCabe BF, Sade J, Abramson M, eds. Cholesteatoma. First International Conference. Birmingham, Ala: Aesculapius Publishing Co, 1978; 212.
88. Sade J. J R Soc Med 1978; 71: 716.
89. Sade J. J Laryngol Otol 1982; 96: 685.
90. Love JG, Kernohan JW. J Am Med Assoc 1936; 107: 1876.
91. Banna M. Clin Radiol 1977; 28: 161.
92. Martin CH. Ann Otolaryngol 1984; 101: 77.
93. Hiraide F, Sawada M, Inouye T, Miyakogawa N, Tsubaki Y. Arch Otorhinolaryngol 1980; 226: 93.
94. Bezold F. Zbl Obrenheilk 1890; 20: 5.
95. Day KM. Arch Otolaryngol 1941; 34: 1144.
96. Ballantyne JC. In: Ballantyne JC, Groves J. Diseases of the ear, nose and throat. 4th ed. 1978. Vol. 3. London: Butterworth.
97. Zechner G. In: Sade J, ed. Cholesteatoma and mastoid surgery. Amsterdam: Kugler, 1982.
98. Wells M, Michaels L. Clin Otolaryngol 1983; 81: 39.
99. Ojala L, Saxen A. Acta Otolaryngol (Stockh) 1952; (Suppl. 100): 33.
100. Smith R, Moran WB. Laryngoscope 1977; 87: 237.
101. Palva T, Johnsson LG. Acta Otolaryngol (Stockh) 1984; 98: 208.
102. Ruedi L. Acta Otolaryngol (Stockh) 1978; (Suppl. 361) 1: 45.
103. Sade J, Avraham S, Brown M. Acta Otolaryngol (Stockh) 1981; 92: 501.
104. Friedmann I. Bull Int Pathol 1975; 16: 9.
105. Boedts D. Acta Otorhinolaryngol Belg 1978; 32: 295.
106. Juers AL. Arch Otolaryngol 1965; 81: 1.
107. Buckingham RA. Ann Otol Rhinol Laryngol 1968; 77: 1054.
108. Kelemen G. Acta Otolaryngol (Stockh) 1934; 20: 211.
109. Seaman RW, Newell RC. Arch Otolaryngol 1971; 94: 440.
110. Brookes GB. Clin Otolaryngol 1983; 8: 31.
111. Freeman J. Ann Otol Rhinol Laryngol 1983; 92: 558.
112. Schwerdtfeger FP. HNO 1981; 29: 47.
113. Wullstein HL. HNO 1977; 25: 389.
114. Choremis C, Economos D, Papadatos C, Gargouhas A. Lancet 1956; ii: 437.
115. Manno NJ, Uihlein A, Kernohan JW. J Neurosurg 1962; 19: 754.
116. Shaywitz BA. J Pediatr 1972; 4: 638.
117. Aschoff L. Z Ohrenheilk 1897; 31: 295.
118. DeSa DJ. Arch Dis Child 1973; 48: 872.
119. Goodhill V. Ann Otol Rhinol Laryngol 1960; 69: 1199.
120. Pfaltz CR, Redli M. ORL 1978; 40: 23.
121. Ruedi L. Acta Otolaryngol (Stockh) 1959; 50: 233.
122. Steinbach E. Laryngol Rhinol Otol (Stuttg) 1978; 57: 724.
123. Bretlau P, Sorensen CH, Jorgensen MB, Dabelsteen E. Ann Otol Rhinol Laryngol 1982; 91: 131.
124. Chole RA, Henry KR, McGinn MD. Am J Otol 1981; 2: 204.
125. McGinn MD, Chole RA, Henry KR. Acta Otolaryngol (Stockh) 1982; 93: 61.
126. Habermann J. Schwartze's Handbuch der Ohrenheilkunde. Leipzig: F.C.W. Vogel, 1892; Vol. 1: 255.
127. Friedmann I. In: Silverberg SG, ed. Principles and practice of surgical pathology. New York: Wiley & Sons, 1983; 1521.
128. Young G. J Laryngol 1950; 64: 271.
129. Birrell JF. J Laryngol 1956; 70: 260.
130. Tumarkin A. J Laryngol 1961; 75: 487.
131. Ferlito A. Ann Otolaryngol 1973; 90: 697.

132. Schuknecht HF. The pathology of the ear. Boston: Harvard University Press, 1974.
133. Goodhill V. Arch Otolaryngol 1973; 97: 183.
134. Bayliss OB. Br J Exp Pathol 1976; 57: 610.
135. Sheehy JL, Linthicum FH, Greenfield EC. Laryngoscope 1969; 79: 1189.
136. Beaumont GD. J Laryngol Otol 1966; 80: 236.
137. Goycoolea MV, Paparella MM, Juhn SK, et al. Laryngoscope 1980; 90: 2037.
138. Sakamoto T. J Rhinol Otol Laryngol Soc Jap 1967; 70: 1926.
139. Lim DJ, Birck M. Ann Otol Rhinol Laryngol 1971; 80: 838.
140. Arnold W, Von llberg C. Archiv klin exp Ohr Nas Kehlkopfheilk 1974; 208: 15.
141. Hiraide F, Inouye T, Miyalogawa N. J Laryngol Otol 1982; 96: 491.
142. Friedmann I, Graham MD. J Laryngol Otol 1979; 93: 433.
142a. Pau HW. Laryngol Rhinol Otol 1984; 63: 541.
143. Emmett JR, Fischer ND, Biggers WP. Laryngoscope 1977; 87: 1157.
144. Glover SC, Tranter RMD, Innes JA. J Laryngol Otol 1981; 95: 1261.
145. McCaffrey TV, McDonald TY, Facer GW, DeRemee RA. Otolaryngol Head Neck Surg 1980; 88: 586.
146. Goodhill V. Ann Otol Rhinol Laryngol 1939; 48: 676.
147. Karmody CS, Schuknecht HF. Arch Otolaryngol 1966; 83: 18.
148. McGill TJL. Arch Otolaryngol 1978; 104: 140.
148a. Kancharak C, Ruckphaopunt K. Ear Nose Throat J 1984; 63: 602.
149. Friedmann I, Osborn DA. In: The pathology of granulomas and neoplasms of the nose and paranasal sinuses. Oxford: Blackwell, 1982; 36.
150. Friedmann I, Bauer F. J Laryngol Otol 1973; 87: 449.
151. McCaffrey TV, McDonald TJ, Pacer GW, DeRemee RA. Otolaryngol Head Neck Surg 1980; 88: 586.
152. Hybášek I. Cesk Otolaryngol 1981; 30: 49.
153. Azadeh B, Ardehali S. Histopathology 1983; 7: 129.
154. Michaelis L, Gutmann C. Z Klin Med 1902; 47: 208.
155. Underwood JCE, Durrant TE, Coup AJ. J Pathol 1982; 138: 41.
156. Stevens S, McClure J. J Pathol 1982; 137: 119.
157. McClure J. J Pathol 1983; 140: 275.
158. Von Hansemann D. Arch Path Anat 1903; 173: 302.
159. Giordano A, Donna Horne G, Gudbrandsson F, Meyerhoff W. Otolaryngol Head Neck Surg 1983; 91: 104.

Bone diseases affecting the ear

OTOSCLEROSIS

It is more than 100 years since Joseph Toynbee[1] first applied the term 'otosclerosis' to the condition characterized by the early onset of progressive and intractable deafness associated with pathological changes in the temporal bone. Ankylosis of the stapes has been known for considerably longer: it was noted by Valsalva in 1704.[2]

Distribution of the lesions
The site of predilection is the region of the otic capsule, between the cochlea and the vestibule and just anterior to the footplate of the stapes (Fig. 14.1). From this site the disease may extend to affect the basal turn of the cochlea and reach the round window (Figs 14.2a,b). Part or the whole of the footplate and part of one or both of the crura of the stapes may be involved (Figs 14.3–14.5).[2a]

Foci of otosclerosis are present much less often in other parts of the labyrinthine capsule or in the wall of the internal acoustic meatus. The disease is bilateral in about 70–80% of cases and then usually presents a striking symmetry in the distribution and extension of the lesions.

The disease may be present for years without causing deafness. Should deafness develop, it is usually due to otosclerotic ankylosis of the footplate of the stapes; however, hearing loss may also be due to the encroachment of large foci on the cochlea. Otosclerotic changes have also been found in bone removed from the ampulla of the horizontal canal. Ossification in the scala tympani in the basal turn of the cochlea, causing degeneration of the labyrinth, has been regarded as a sequel to otosclerosis.

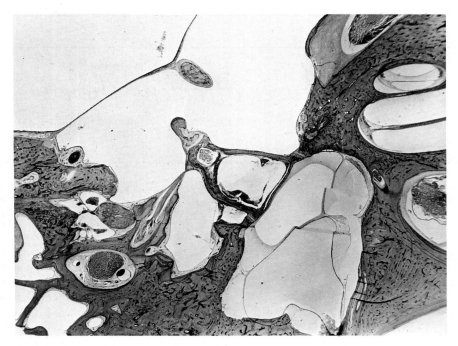

Fig. 14.1 Normal temporal bone. Stapes, stapedial muscle and facial nerve and fissura ante fenestram are seen. These are the usual sites of the primary otosclerotic lesion.

Haematoxylin–eosin   × 10

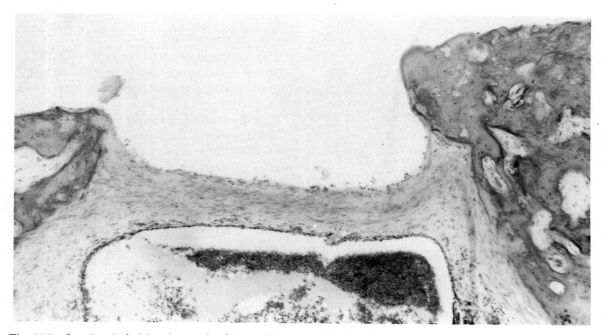

Fig. 14.2a Otosclerotic foci in otic capsule of the cochlea, protruding into the scala tympani near the round window. Note round window membrane.

Haematoxylin–eosin   × 100

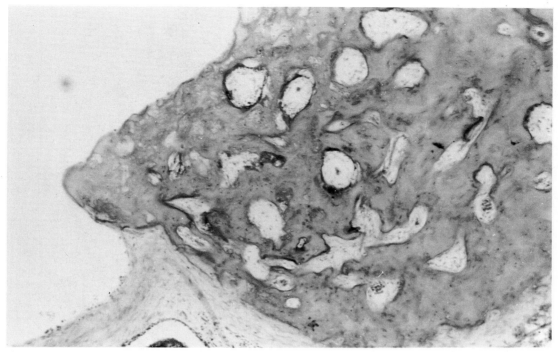

Fig. 14.2b Detail of large otosclerotic focus in Figure 14.2a.

Haematoxylin–eosin   × 140

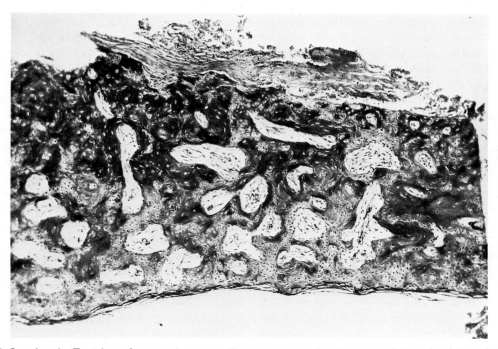

Fig. 14.3 Otosclerosis. Footplate of stapes: the sponge-like woven bone that has replaced the normal bone is seen to be vascular. There is considerable osteoclastic activity.

Haematoxylin–eosin   × 70

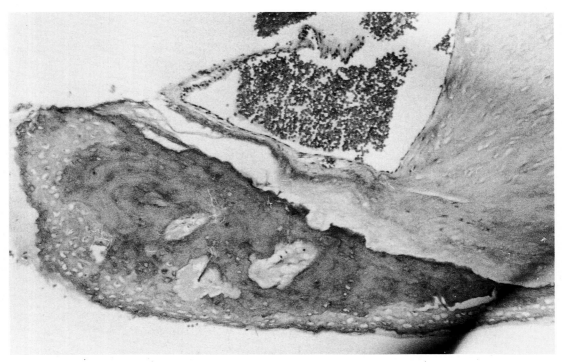

Fig. 14.4 Otosclerosis. Footplate of stapes showing partly active vascular otosclerotic change. The remainder of the footplate has been converted into compact bone (inactive phase). Partly covered by tympanosclerotic tissue.
Haematoxylin–eosin   × 160

The disease is commoner in women than in men. It may develop at any age, but it is rarely recognized before adult life. It is said to affect 3–10 per 1000 White adults.[3] Caucasian races are most frequently affected by otosclerosis: it is therefore, a frequent cause of deafness in Europe, the Middle East, Israel and India. It is equally common in the Caucasian peoples of the Americas, South Africa, Australia and New Zealand. Otosclerosis is rare in the African races but may occur in the Black population of North America, presumably due to intermarriage. It is rarely found in Mongoloids and is uncommon in the Japanese.[4]

Histopathology
Otosclerosis is a peculiar dystrophy of the bony labyrinth. The distinctive pathological feature in the active stage of the disease is not so much sclerosis as a 'spongification' of the bone (otospongiosis in the French literature). The compact lamellar bone, which normally may include fibrous and cartilaginous islands (the 'globuli in-

terossei', see Fig. 14.8), is replaced by woven bone, which can be identified with the aid of polarized light. The woven bone is vascular, its spongy appearance being due to the number of marrow spaces that it encloses (Fig. 14.6).

The osteocytes are more numerous than in normal bone and appear to be misshapen. There is an increase in the number and activity of the cells in the marrow spaces, and in particular there are resorptive changes caused by osteoclasts. At the same time, and sometimes in the same space, osteoblasts are seen, with new bone apposition. The amount of the basophilic cement is increased and the intercellular fibrillar substance undergoes alteration. The basophilia of the cement causes it to be stained intensely blue by certain haematoxylins and is due to the altered chemical composition of the ground substance first described by Mayer. This characteristic is reflected in the term 'blue mantles' that has been applied to such bone, formed particularly round blood vessels.[5, 6] It has been suggested that otosclerotic foci result from fusion of these mantles of 'blue bone', but against

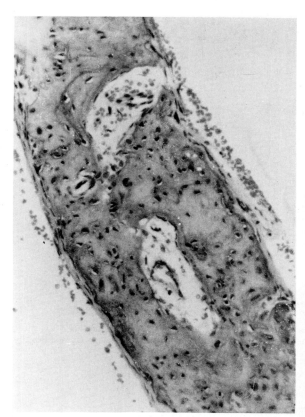

Fig. 14.5 Otosclerosis. Thickened anterior crus of stapes showing otosclerotic change in active phase. Note light cellularity of the vascular otosclerotic tissue. The crura are often affected by the otosclerotic process.

Haematoxylin–eosin   × 208

the line of demarcation of the otosclerotic focus in which the fibrils run in an irregular or woven pattern. This resembles the first bone appearing in the course of embryonic development, and all early membrane bone is called woven bone because it contains an interlaced tangle of calcifiable fibres (Fig. 14.9). This woven bone appears whenever bone formation is re-activated in the adult.

The fundamental pathological process of otosclerosis can be summarized as lacunar resorption of bone by osteoclasts, initiated by an unknown pathological stimulus affecting the cartilaginous rests at certain sites of predilection of the otic capsule. This, however, does not explain how and why an entirely new type of bone is laid

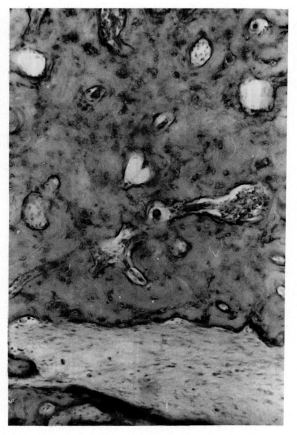

Fig. 14.6 Otosclerosis. Detail of active otosclerotic lesion near the fissula ante fenestram which was filled with fibrous tissue. There are areas of rich vascularization and also dark, irregularly calcified patches.

Haematoxylin–eosin   × 240

this theory is the fact that similar 'blue mantles' are not uncommonly found in chronic mastoiditis and in other diseases affecting the bony parts: 'blue mantles' seem, in fact, to be a non-specific feature.[7]

There is, as a rule, a sharp boundary between the diseased bone and the normal bone (Fig. 14.7). The active stage may be followed by intermissions in which the histological appearances show little or no recognizable evidence of the lesion. Apparently inactive otosclerosis may be re-activated if an infection or other disease develops in the middle ear. The otosclerotic foci enlarge by a process of lacunar erosion alongside the small capillary blood vessels (Fig. 14.8).

In polarized light the straight fibrils of the healthy collagen can be seen ending abruptly at

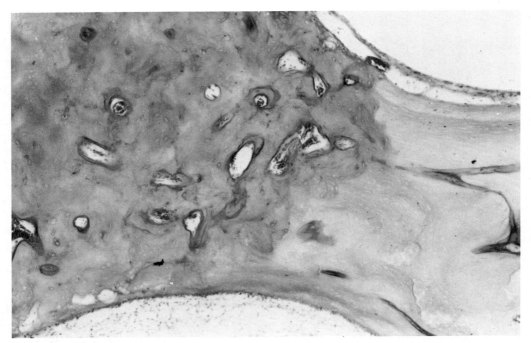

Fig. 14.7 Otosclerosis. The well-defined, moderately-active vascular focus has spread between the vestibule (below) and the cochlea (above) in the otic capsule. The demarcation between the darkly stained abnormal bone and the palely stained healthy bone is distinct.

Haematoxylin–eosin   × 100

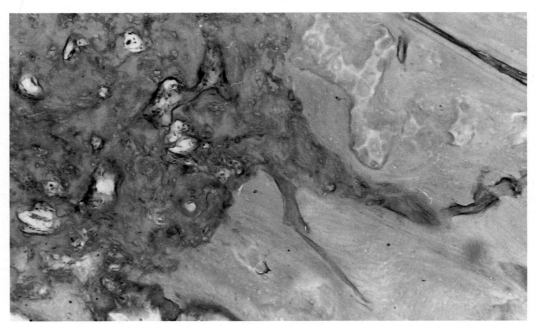

Fig. 14.8 Otosclerosis, showing the spread of the otosclerotic lesion alongside blood vessels into the normal lamellar bone of the otic capsule. There are cartilaginous remnants present (such structures are called 'globuli interossei') which have been considered to form the basis of the otosclerotic process.

Haematoxylin–eosin   × 100

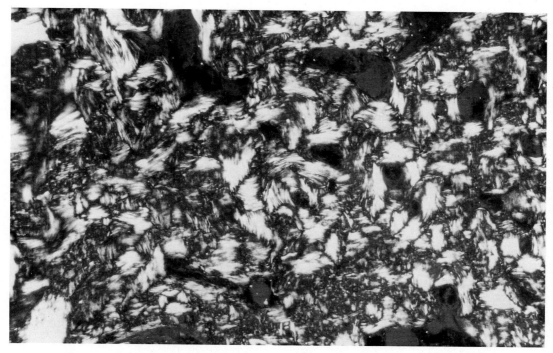

Fig. 14.9 Otosclerosis. Woven pattern of otosclerotic bone seen in polarized light. × 100

down, with a different fibrillar and cellular pattern and the characteristic basophilic appearance of its intercellular substance.

Aetiology

The cause of otosclerosis has remained a mystery. Infection and toxic substances can be dismissed immediately on grounds of lack of evidence. Ingenious concepts, including the assumption of the upright posture during evolution, have been advanced to explain stresses and strains in the temporal bone.[8] However, this assumption is negated by the occurrence of primary otosclerosis in the stapes. Disturbance of the vascular supply to the temporal bone has been postulated. Although this theory is still supported by some, it has not been generally accepted. The undoubted histological resemblance between otosclerosis and Paget's disease of bone has led to the suggestion that the former is a localized example of the latter. The lack of significant clinical association between the two conditions lends no support to this view.

A suggestion that otosclerosis is a metabolic disorder can be disposed of more readily in some of its aspects than in others. In spite of previous claims by some authors regarding abnormal plasma calcium and phosphorus levels, there is no evidence to suggest that otosclerosis is in any way related to abnormal parathyroid function. The possibility of disordered or deficient enzyme function is less easily ruled out and would be the ultimate mechanism of a genetic abnormality. The general feeling at the moment is that the mechanism of inheritance may involve a Mendelian dominant with relatively low penetrance. It has been noted that there is a good correlation between HLA antigen (human leucocyte histocompatibility antigen) frequencies and the incidence of otosclerosis.[9] These findings seem to support the role of genetic factors in the pathogenesis of otosclerosis.

Whatever its aetiology, it seems likely that hereditary factors exert their influence on local peculiarities. There are certain local anatomical features of the osseous labyrinth, for example,

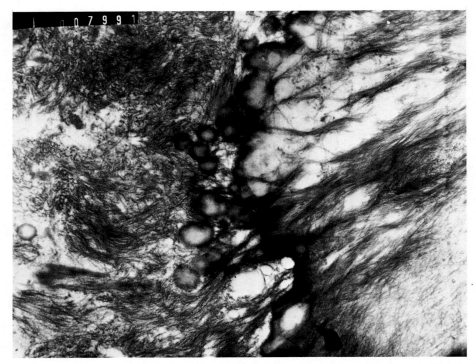

Fig. 14.10 Otosclerosis. Electron micrograph of otosclerotic footplate showing matrix vesicles along the line of calcification.
× 10 250

the fissula ante fenestram and the cartilaginous islands of the enchondral bone of the otic capsule near the oval window (the 'globuli interossei') which may offer a locus minoris resistantiae to the cytochemical agents and/or mechanical influences of stress and strain affecting such areas (Figs 14.6–14.8). The concept that otosclerosis resulted from an autoimmune reaction of the otic capsule to the cartilaginous tissue of the 'globuli interossei'[10] seemed to have been confirmed by recent experimental studies. Otosclerotic changes were produced by the implantation of human cartilaginous material from the 'globuli interossei' into the otic capsule of rats.[11] Moreover, the disease has been inherited by the litters of the otosclerotic rats. These intriguing observations will have to be confirmed.

Electron microscopy has provided further insight into the histopathological features of this common disease.[12] It has been suggested that the active phase of otosclerosis causing destruction of the bone could best be explained on the basis of an enzymatic process initiated by hydrolytic enzymes released from histiocytes or genetically inferior osteocytes and their lysosomes.[13, 14] It is well recognized that lysosomes are closely associated and indeed responsible for cell injury and necrosis.

This activity may be enhanced by various inflammatory and neoplastic processes.[14] It may be assumed that the lysosomal membranes of such cells might be less resistant to systemic influences such as hormones, especially oestrogens, and more liable to rupture. This enzymatic concept has been gaining acceptance.

The appearance of lysosomes and of matrix vesicles from the cells in the collagenous matrix (fibroblasts; inflammatory cells and epithelial cells) (Fig. 14.10) is a characteristic feature of otosclerotic and tympanosclerotic tissue.[14a, 14b, 15] The matrix vesicles are the primary site of calcification and contain ionic calcium and phosphate and alkaline phosphatase. The membrane of matrix vesicles may become altered and the consequent loss of water leads to the supersaturation of the vesicle with calcium. This

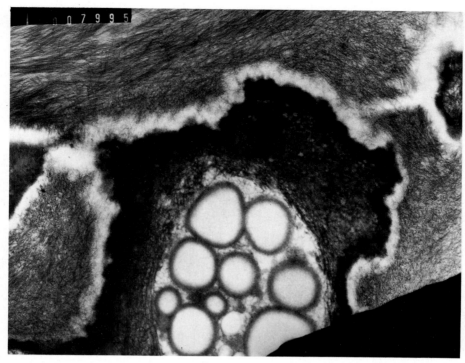

Fig. 14.11a Otosclerosis. Electron micrograph shows calcified focus in collagen with a group of matrix vesicles surrounded by a layer of dense, calcified tissue.   × 21 000

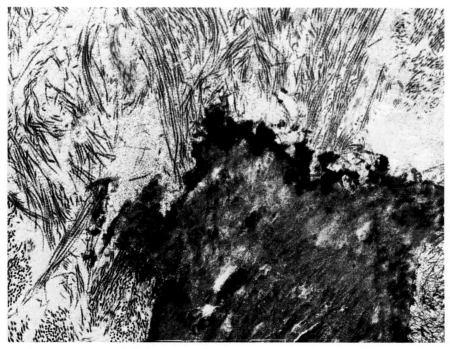

Fig. 14.11b Otosclerosis. Electron micrograph showing otosclerotic plaque expanding into collagen.
× 12 375

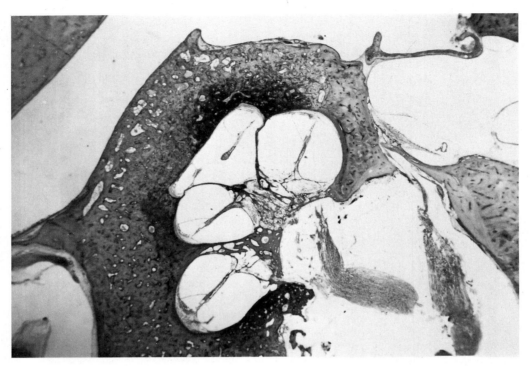

Fig. 14.12 Midmodiolar section showing diffuse otosclerotic change of the otic capsule surrounding the cochlea. The footplate of the stapes (right upper corner) lies freely in the oval window and there is no evidence of ankylosis.

Haematoxylin–eosin   × 12   *Provided by Dr F.H. Linthicum, House Ear Institute, Los Angeles, USA.*

leads to incipient calcification and the formation of hydroxyapatite crystals, proceeding spontaneously to the production of calcospherules in the collagenous tissue. As mineralization progresses, the number of inclusions will increase, frequently accompanied by mineralization beyond the matrix vesicles (Fig. 14.11a). Eventually confluent mineralized masses or plaques are formed (Fig. 14.11b).

The otosclerotic lesion might be set off by a vascular process causing ischaemic necrosis of the bone.[16] It is, however, obvious that an adequate blood supply carrying the initiating or activating agents of a metabolic or hormonal nature is an essential condition and it is worth pointing out that the active otosclerotic focus is very vascular and contains much blood.

Due to its enhanced vascularity, the bone involved in otosclerosis has a greater affinity for sodium fluoride. Administration of sodium fluoride has been advocated for the treatment of otosclerosis.[17] Sodium fluoride administration may reduce the osteoblastic activity in the otosclerotic focus and prevent progression of the disease.

The relation between the histological stage of otosclerosis and the age of the patient at the time of stapedectomy shows a slight upward trend with passage from the more to the less active lesion but the overlap is obviously very great. This underlines the fact, illustrated by many cases, that otosclerosis is a disease of varying behaviour with alternating phases of activity and quiescence.

Otosclerosis of the cochlea

Non-clinical otosclerosis is the condition in which otosclerotic foci are formed in the otic capsule apart from the oval window region and therefore remain 'silent'. Highly vascular foci of this kind have been described in the lateral semi-circular canal.[18, 19] The next commonest sites are the region of the round window and then the various aspects of the cochlear capsule. It is still a matter of debate how far such lesions may give rise to clinical signs in the absence of sta-pedial fixation (Fig. 14.12). Large otosclerotic foci may reach the cochlea and damage the spiral ligament (Fig. 14.2) and cause endolymphatic hy-drops.[20]

SYSTEMIC BONE DISEASES

The temporal bone may be the site of various systemic bone diseases and these may therefore present with hearing loss. These conditions in-clude Paget's disease, osteogenesis imperfecta tarda, osteopetrosis, fibrous dysplasia, histiocy-tosis X, eosinophilic granuloma (presenting as an 'aural polyp') and giant cell reparative granu-loma.

Paget's disease
Paget's disease of the temporal bone may involve the entire temporal bone, although the cochlea usually escapes total obliteration by the dis-ease.[21, 22–24] Sarcomatous change develops in the skull, including the facial bones, in about 10% of cases.[25, 26] Progressive sensorineural hearing loss has been observed in a 79-year-old man with a 26-year history of Paget's disease: as in other cases the cochlea appeared to be histologically normal.[21, 24] Pagetic bone had obliterated the in-ternal auditory meatus, compressing the cochlear division of the auditory nerve and caused severe neural degeneration which may have accounted for the hearing loss.

Osteogenesis imperfecta
Osteogenesis imperfecta may involve the tem-poral bone and stapes.[27]

Osteopetrosis
Osteopetrosis is known to involve the temporal bone in some instances.[28]

Fibrous dysplasia[29]
The temporal bone may be the site of monostotic, or less frequently, of polyostotic fibrous dysplasia causing increasing narrowing of the external au-ditory meatus and consequent conductive deaf-ness. Occasionally, keratosis obturans or epider-moid cholesteatoma of the meatus may develop. Sarcomatous change is a rare complication.

Fibrous dysplasia in the middle ear can re-semble a vascular tumour and any surgical inter-vention might prove hazardous.[29]

MISCELLANEOUS LESIONS

Lipidosis (histiocytosis X)
Lipid storage diseases that affect the skeleton, particularly Hand–Schüller–Christian disease, may present with chronic aural discharge. In such cases a lesion in the temporal bone forming an 'eosinophilic granuloma' is responsible for the aural manifestations.[30, 31] The diagnosis may be made from the histological finding in an aural polyp of large numbers of eosinophils and large palely stained histiocytes, including foam cells and multinucleate cells.

Giant-cell reparative granuloma[32, 33]
Giant-cell reparative granuloma is an infrequent condition in the temporal bone. The changes may involve several cranial nerves.[33]

Rheumatoid arthritis of the ossicles
Rheumatoid arthritis may be accompanied by conductive deafness caused by involvement of the joints of the ossicular chain.[34]

Sensorineural deafness was found in 16 patients in a series of 76 with rheumatoid arth-ritis.[35] Its cause was thought to be neuropathy of the auditory nerve resulting from arteritis of the vasa nervorum.

REFERENCES

1. Toynbee J. The diseases of the ear. London: Churchill, 1860.
2. Valsalva AM. Opera. Hoc est tractatus de aure humana. 4th ed. Venice: F. Pieter, 1740: 1–123.
2a. Iver PV, Gristwood RE. Pathology 1984; 16:30.
3. Guild SR. Ann Otol Rhinol Laryngol 1944; 53: 246.
4. Beales PH. Otosclerosis. Bristol: Wright, 1981; pp. 5; 6.
5. Mayer O. Untersuchungen uber die Otosklerose. Wien: A. Holder, 1917.
6. Lindsay JR. Ann Otol Rhinol Laryngol 1974; 83: 33.
7. Paparella MM. Laryngoscope 1984; (in press).
8. Sercer A. Arch Ital Otol 1958; 69: Suppl. 34.
9. Gregoriadis S, Zervas J, Varletzidis E, Toubis M, Pantazoupoulos P, Fessas P. Arch Otolaryngol 1982; 108: 769.
10. Causse JB. Cahiers d'ORL 1980; 15:1, 49.

11. Yoo TJ, Stuart JM, Kang AH, Townes AS, Tomoda K. Ann Otol Rhinol Laryngol 1983; 92: 103.
12. Friedmann I. Acta Otorhinolaryngol Belg 1981; 35: 419.
13. Chevance LG, Causse J, Jorgensen MB, Bretlau P. Ann Otolaryngol Chir Cervicofac 1972; 89: 5.
14. Causse J, Chevance LG, Bel J, Michaux P, Tapon J. Ann Otolaryngol Chir Cervicofac 1972; 89: 563.
14a. Friedmann I, Galey FR, Odnert S. Am J Otol 1981; 3: 144.
14b. Friedmann I, Hodges GM, Graham MD. Ann Otol Rhinol Laryngol 1979; 89 (Suppl. 68): 241.
15. Katchburian E. J Anat 1973; 116: 285.
16. Wright IM. J Pathol 1977; 123: 5.
17. Shambaugh Jr GE. Adv Otorhinolaryngol 1977; 22: 35.
18. Kelemen G. Acta Otolaryngol (Stockh) 1934; 20: 211.
19. Ogilvie RF, Hall IS. J Laryngol Otol 1953; 67: 497.
20. Liston SL, Paparella MM, Mancini F, etal. Laryngoscope, 1984; 94: 1003.
21. Friedmann I. Pathology of the ear. Oxford: Blackwell, 1974; 128: 362.
22. Nager GT. Ann Otol Rhinol Laryngol 1973; 84 (Suppl. 22): 1.
23. Lindsay JR, Suga F. Arch Otolaryngol 1976; 102: 37.
24. Applebaum EL, Clemic JD. Laryngoscope 1977; 87: 1753.
25. McKenna RJ, Schwinn CP, Soong KY, Higinbotham NL. Cancer 1964; 17: 42.
26. Friedmann I, Osborn DA. Pathology of granulomas and neoplasms of the nose and paranasal sinuses. Edinburgh: Churchill Livingstone, 1982.
27. Bergstrom I, La Vonne. Laryngoscope 1977; 87 (Suppl. 6): 1.
28. Hamersma H. ORL 1973; 36: 21.
29. Nager GT, Kennedy DW, Kopstein E. Ann Otol Rhinol Laryngol 1982; 91: 5.
30. Goodhill V. Laryngoscope 1950; 60: 1.
31. McCaffrey TV, McDonald TJ. Laryngoscope 1979; 99: 1735.
32. Hirschl S, Katz A. Hum Pathol 1974; 5: 171.
33. Wolfowitz BL, Schmaman A. South Afr Med J 1973; 47: 1397.
34. Copeman WSC. Br Med J 1963; ii: 1526.
35. Goodwill CJ, Lord J, Knill-Jones RP. Ann Rheum Dis 1972; 31: 170.

Menière's disease

History

This disease derives its name from the Parisian physician, Prosper Menière,[1] who first described it in 1861 as a syndrome characterized by paroxysmal attacks of vertigo associated with unilateral deafness and tinnitus. Shakespeare mentions the association of deafness and 'falling sickness' in Julius Caesar.[2] There is no doubt that the syndrome was recognized before Menière's account, although attributed to a cerebral rather than to a labyrinthine disorder.

The obvious difficulty in studying the pathology of Menière's disease lies not only in obtaining suitable specimens for light and electron microscopy, but also in the variety of neuro-otological conditions that have been referred to by this term.[3] In the case described by Menière, the labyrinth was found to be filled with a blood-stained fluid, and for many years it was assumed that the disease was caused by haemorrhage into the inner ear.

Site and sex

Both ears may be affected from the onset; in many patients the second ear is not affected until many years after the first. There is a slight preponderance of male patients.

Histopathology

Hallpike & Cairns[4] described the histological findings in the labyrinth of two patients who died following severance of the auditory nerve to cure Menière's disease. The saccule and scala media were grossly distended and Corti's organ showed degeneration. In one case there was also degeneration of the vascular stria, the macula and the wall of the semicircular canals. These findings were later confirmed by other workers and

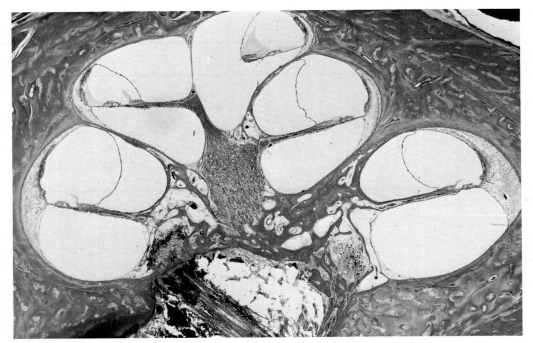

Fig. 15.1 The cochlea in Menière's disease. The cochlear duct is distended, with the result that the peripheral attachment of the vestibular membrane (Reissner's membrane) has been displaced toward the axis of the cochlea; the membrane, therefore, assumes an almost perpendicular position instead of its normal slope. The bulging of the membrane is due to the increased pressure of the endolymph within the duct (cochlear hydrops).

Haematoxylin–eosin   × 55

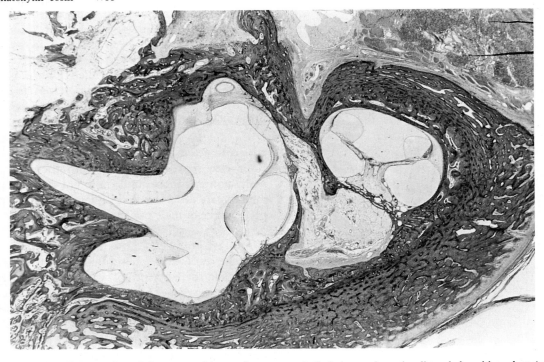

Fig. 15.2 Midmodiolar section of the temporal bone of an anencephalic baby to show the distended cochlear duct (on the right) and the ruptured saccular wall in the distended vestibule. Comparable with other types of idiopathic endolymphatic hydrops (e.g. in Fig. 15.1).

Haematoxylin–eosin   × 12.5

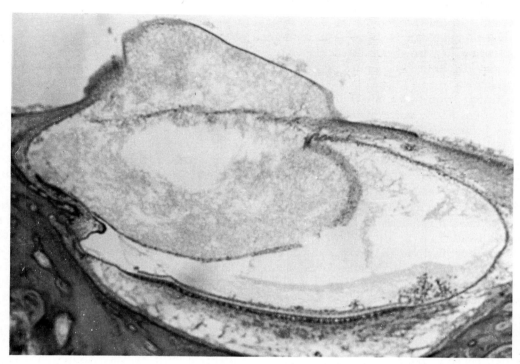

Fig. 15.3 Detail of ruptured saccular wall (as in Fig. 15.2) which appears to have been sealed off by coagulated perilymph. Such ruptures of the membranous labyrinth have been considered as the mechanism causing the attack of vertigo in patients suffering from idiopathic cochlear hydrops (e.g. in Menière's disease).   Haematoxylin–eosin   × 60

the term 'endolymphatic hydrops' came to be used synonymously with Menière's disease.[5-7] Nevertheless, while it is recognized that the most significant change in the inner ear is *endolymphatic hydrops*, the cause of this change has remained obscure.

Under some pathological conditions, as in Menière's disease, the transport of fluids across the inner ear neuroepithelium may be disrupted and the endolymphatic space may become distended and the function of the inner ear impaired. It has been suggested that the initial lesion is a change in the permeability of the intercellular junctions.

The vestibular membrane of Reissner—the vestibular wall of the cochlear duct which separates two fluids of different ionic composition—bulges into the scala vestibuli and may eventually rupture, allowing perilymph (with a low potassium content) to mix with endolymph (which has a high potassium content) (Fig. 15.1). After rupture, the pressures are equalized and the membrane may repair itself.

It is difficult to assess at necropsy the significance of endolymphatic hydrops and of the morphological changes in the inner ear, since these may represent only the particular phase that the disease was in at the time of the patient's death.[8] Reissner's membrane may be collapsed and may become fibrotic. Rupture of the membrane has been identified microscopically.[9, 10]

Pathogenesis

Rupture of the membranous labyrinth would most reasonably explain the episodic and paroxysmal nature of the clinical manifestations, for it is possible that, following such rupture, admixture of perilymph with endolymph might sufficiently alter the concentration of potassium in the former to interfere with neural excitation[11] (Figs 15.2, 15.3).

It has also been suggested that the disease may result from a primary disorder of the labyrinthine fluids. The condition might then be regarded as a failure of the mechanism that regulates the production and disposal of endolymph, recurrent attacks of endolymphatic hydrops resulting and in turn leading to permanent distension of the membranous labyrinth. The causes of such failure are unknown.

Labyrinthine hydrops leading to the partial or total dilatation of the entire membranous labyrinth may be associated not only with Menière's disease but, as 'Menière's syndrome', also with tuberculous meningitis,[12] amyotrophic lateral sclerosis,[13] congenital syphilis,[8] anencephaly[14] (Figs 15.2, 15.3) and otosclerosis.[15, 16] Some tumours may lead to increased labyrinthine tension and to clinical reactions not unlike those in Menière's disease.

Endolymphatic hydrops has been produced experimentally by obliterating the endolymphatic sac in the guinea pig and cat.[17, 18]

Developmental anomalies may contribute to the malfunction of the system (Figs 15.2, 15.3).[14] The crus commune was absent in both ears of a patient suffering from Menière's disease.[19] In view of the experimental finding that obliteration of the vestibular aqueduct produces endolymphatic hydrops in guinea pigs,[17] it is of interest that the vestibular aqueduct was found to be short and narrowed in a case of Menière's disease.[20]

Structures resembling inclusion bodies were found in the nuclei of the vestibular neurons of two patients with Menière's disease. Subsequent virological studies of Scarpa's vestibular ganglion in six cases of Menière's disease proved to be negative.[21]

Intracellular and extracellular laminated structures found in the basal lamina or in hair cells have attracted interest.[12, 22, 23] Such macromolecular structures may participate in the regeneration of the sensory epithelium leading to recovery after an attack of Menière's disease. The alternation of regenerative processes with the underlying degenerative process causing Menière's disease would explain the remissions after attacks.

More recently, interest has been stimulated in immunological mechanisms in the pathogenesis of some cases of Menière's disease. Raised circulating immune complex levels and a statistically significant increased incidence of autoantibodies was found in a study of 66 Menière's patients.[24] This strongly suggests an immunological disturbance and that circulating immune complexes may be an important aetiological factor in the pathogenesis of Menière's disease.

These observations are supported by the findings—experimental and human—that antibody titres to Type 2 collagen were higher in patients with Menière's disease than in control subjects, indicative of autoimmunity.[25] Our observations on some ultrastructural changes of the basal lamina, as mentioned, appear to point in the same direction. Similar studies by other authors have failed to confirm some of these findings.[26, 27]

Notwithstanding these observations, the aetiology and pathology of Menière's disease remain obscure. No real progress is to be expected until we have a more detailed knowledge of the vascular supply and innervation of the human labyrinth, the finer structure of the areas concerned with the production and resorption of the labyrinthine fluids, and the chemical composition of the latter under normal and pathological conditions.[28] Pathologists have ignored this important problem which requires the closest co-operation between pathologist and otologist.

REFERENCES

1. Menière P. Gaz Med Paris 1861; 16: 55, 88, 239, 379, 597.
2. Chalat NI. Amer J Otolaryngol 1979; 1: 52.
3. Cawthorne T. Ann Otol Rhinol Laryngol 1947; 56: 18.
4. Hallpike CS, Cairns H. J Laryngol Otol 1938; 53: 265.
5. Hallpike CS, Wright AJ. J Laryngol Otol 1940; 55: 59.
6. Rollin H. Z Hals Nas Ohrenheilk 1940; 31: 72.
7. Altmann F, Fowler EP. Ann Otol Rhinol Laryngol 1943; 52: 52.
8. Fraysse B. Maladie de Menière. Toulouse: Fournie, 1979: Thesis.
9. Koskas HJ, Linthicum FH Jr, House WF. Otolaryngol Head Neck Surg 1983; 91: 61.
10. Lawrence M. Acta Otolaryngol (Stockh) 1983; 95: 480.
11. Schuknecht HF. In: Pathology of the ear. Cambridge, Mass: Harvard University Press, 1974; 141: 241.
12. Friedmann I. In: Pathology of the ear. Oxford: Blackwell, 1974: 128, 362.
13. Kohut RI, Lindsay JR. Acta Otolaryngol (Stockh) 1972; 73: 402.
14. Friedmann I, Wright JLW, Phelps PD. J Laryngol Otol 1980; 94: 929.
15. Beales PH. Otosclerosis. Bristol: Wright, 1981: 5, 6.
16. Paparella MM. Ann Otol Rhinol Laryngol 1984; Suppl 112: 31.
17. Kimura RS. Ann Otol Rhinol Laryngol 1967; 76: 664.
18. Schuknecht HF, Northrop C, Igarashi M. Acta Otolaryngol (Stockh) 1968; 65: 479.

19. Gussen R. Ann Otol Rhinol Laryngol 1973; 82: 179.
20. Stahle J, Wilbrand HF. Acta Otolaryngol (Stockh) 1983; 95: 81.
21. Palva T, Hortling L, Ylikoski J, Collan Y. Acta Otolaryngol (Stockh) 1978; 86: 269.
22. Slepecky N, Hamernik R, Henderson D. Acta Otolaryngol (Stockh) 1981; 91: 189.
23. Engstrom H, Ades HW, Engstrom B, et al. Adv Otol Rhinol Laryngol 1977; 22: 93.
24. Brookes GB. Arch Otolaryngol 1985 (in press).
25. Yoo TY, Yazaway Y, Tomoda K, Floyd R. Science 1983; 222: 65.
26. Harris JP, Ryan AF. Am J Otolaryngol 1984; 5: 418.
27. Arnold W, Altermatt HJ, Gebbers JO, Pfaltz CR. Laryng Rhinol Otol 1985; 64: 1.
28. Altmann F. JAMA 1961; 176: 215.

16

The pathology of sensorineural hearing loss

ANATOMICAL CONSIDERATIONS

The term 'deafness' has been replaced by 'hearing loss' with the more hopeful implication that hearing can be improved by modern methods of audiology and microsurgery. This chapter deals with some of the causes of sensorineural deafness and describes various histopathological changes to be observed in the inner ear.

The inner ear is the site of the sensory apparatus of hearing and equilibrium. A knowledge of some of the anatomical and histological features of the normal inner ear is of assistance in considering the pathology of sensorineural hearing loss. The inner ear is located in the petrous portion of the temporal bone and is protected by the toughest part of the skull, the otic capsule.

The labyrinth, an essential part of the auditory organ, is a complex structure. It consists of a membranous tube lined by epithelium and is filled with endolymph (membranous labyrinth) contained within a bony tube, the osseous labyrinth, which is of corresponding complexity of shape and contains the perilymph. The membranous labyrinth is composed of the utricle, the three semicircular canals (each with an enlargement or ampulla which opens into it), the saccule, and the cochlea, which houses the organ of Corti. The membranous labyrinth is supplied by branches of the auditory nerve which pass to the maculae of the utricle and saccule, the cristae of the three ampullae and to the sensory cells of the organ of Corti.

The entrance of the nerve fibres is marked in the ampullae by a transverse inwardly projecting ridge (crista) and in the saccule and utricle by a thickening of the tunica propria (macula). At these places the epithelial lining is differentiated

Table 16.1 Histopathology of the organ of Corti

Site	Lesion	Aetiology of deafness
Sensory epithelium	Total absence or loss (abiotrophy)	Congenital; ageing
	Partial absence or degeneration of the sensory and supporting cells	Noise
		Drugs
Tectorial membrane	Shrinkage; retraction; adhesions	Congenital
		Viral (rubella and mumps)
		Anencephaly
Reissner's membrane	Distension	Menière's syndrome or disease
		Anencephaly
		Meningitis
		Trisomy 22
Vascular stria	Atrophy	Ageing, presbycusis
	Congestion and hyalinization	Diabetes mellitus
	PAS-positive deposits	Lange–Jervell syndrome
	Calcification (concretions)	Toxoplasmosis
		Budd–Chiari syndrome
		Alport's syndrome
	Vacuolation	Ototoxic agents
		Noise
	Granulations	Viral (rubella, measles)

to form a sensory epithelium or neuroepithelium; elsewhere it is a simple, undifferentiated epithelium.

The pathology of sensorineural hearing loss has been extensively studied and its causes are usually subdivided into congenital and acquired. Many difficulties stand in the way of an unambiguous biological classification of deafness, especially of congenital deafness. The auditory organ is liable to a number of adverse influences during growth, either causing failure to develop any of one or more parts of the auditory system or interrupting the process of development at any stage. Hearing loss may also be due to some processes which disturb or cause degeneration of the already wholly or partly developed apparatus of hearing.

Investigation of the pathology of deafness requires the application of a wide range of scientific methods. Histochemical studies as well as electron microscopy have provided an increasing amount of information on the morphology and function of the inner ear in health and disease. The pathological changes of the different constituents of the inner ear can be assessed in familiar general pathological terms (Table 16.1).

Changes of the sensory epithelium may be

complex. The neuroepithelium of the organ of Corti may be totally absent, as in various congenital syndromes, or there may be partial degeneration or absence of the hair cells and supporting cells. Basophilic deposits form in the vascular stria, the nature of which has remained obscure.[1] The tectorial membrane may be deformed and adherent to neuroepithelial remnants.

Together the varied microscopical lesions form the characteristic pathological features of cochleo-saccular dysplasia, first described in congenital deafness by Scheibe in 1892[2] and 1895.[3] It has been proposed that the term 'cochleosaccular dysplasia' should be applied to histopathological lesions of the pattern described by Scheibe (cochleosaccular pattern) and relating to developmental disorders causing congenital deafness; in contrast, the term 'cochleosaccular degeneration' should be applied to postnatal degeneration (abiotrophy) of a normally developed inner ear causing progressive sensorineural hearing loss.[4]

The principal histopathological findings include degeneration of the neuroepithelium both of the organ of Corti and of the macula of the saccule but not of the macula of the utricle. There is extensive atrophy of the vascular stria.

The *vascular stria*, forming the lateral wall of

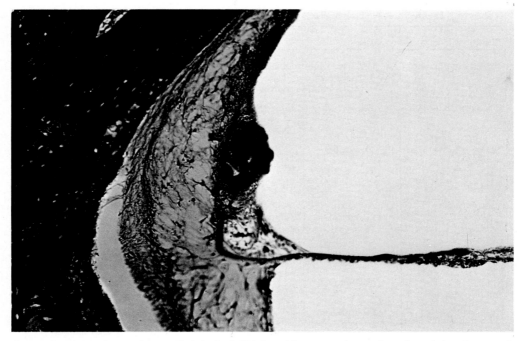

Fig. 16.1 Lange–Jervell syndrome of congenital deafness. PAS-positive matter is seen in a distended and ruptured capillary of the vascular stria. Periodic-acid/Schiff reaction × 120

the cochlear duct, is the site of various well-defined pathological lesions associated with various syndromes and diseases: atrophy in ageing and presbycusis; congestion and hyalinization in diabetes; periodic-acid/Schiff positive deposits in Lange–Jervell syndrome (Fig. 16.1); calcification and adhesions in Budd–Chiari syndrome, toxoplasmosis and Alport's syndrome; vacuolation caused by ototoxic substances and by noise; and inflammatory granulations in viral diseases (rubella and measles) (Fig. 16.2).

Reissner's membrane is distended when the endolymphatic pressure is increased, e.g. in Menière's disease or idiopathic endolymphatic hydrops (see page 297).

Ultrastructural changes of the sensory epithelium of the inner ear can be extensive. The cytoplasm of hair cells may show protrusions or ballooning followed by rupture of the outer cell membrane, distension of the rough endoplasmic reticulum with multiple Hensen bodies and marked reduction of the ribosomes. The outer hair cells contain various complexes of flattened membranous cisternae attached to the lateral walls of the outer hair cells. Some of the cisternae

form concentric whorls in the apical portion of the cytoplasm, the *Hensen bodies*, which are probably precursors of the lateral cisternae of the cell. Dense bodies and phagosomes may be present. The Golgi apparatus is affected by the concentration in it of toxic agents. The mitochondria may be damaged and contain ruptured cristae. Peripheral aggregations of chromatin and intranuclear viral inclusions may be present in the nuclei. Crystalline laminated or striated inclusions were observed in the hair cells.[5, 6]

CLASSIFICATION

The pathology of deafness may be conveniently classified according to the following scheme. No new categories are proposed, all having been selected from previous writings on the subject.[5, 7, 8]

1. Genetic

a) Pathology of deafnesss of genetic origin
    Lesions of the conductive apparatus
    (i) congenital abnormalities and malformations of the external and middle ear

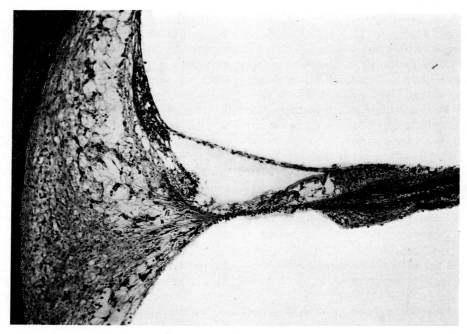

Fig. 16.2 Granulation tissue in the vascular stria of the cochlea of an aborted embryo. The mother had rubella during the first three months of her pregnancy.   Haematoxylin–eosin   × 130

(ii) complex congenital malformations (syndromes)

b) Lesions of the sensorineural apparatus of genetic origin

Aplasia

Abiotrophy (heredo-degenerative lesions)

Chromosomal aberrations

Syndromes—ectodermal
              mesenchymatous
              neuroectodermal

2. Embryopathies (antenatal)

Rubella, syphilis, toxoplasmosis, other infections—viral and bacterial; hormonal influences and metabolic disorders.

3. Perinatal

Infections, asphyxia, kernicterus, toxic, hormonal influences, metabolic disorders.

4. Postnatal

Infections—viral and bacterial, neoplasms, hormonal.

SYNDROMES OF DEAFNESS

There are a large number of syndromes in which deafness plays an important role. The classification of hearing loss has remained difficult and the simple division into conductive, sensorineural and mixed types contrasts sharply with the elaborate schemes developed by various authors. The labyrinthine structures may be completely absent or underdeveloped, or there may be partial defects of the bony or membranous structures or of both. There are many distinct types or syndromes: these may be classified as ectodermal, mesodermal and neuroectodermal, according to the combination of anomalies which are present: *essentially ectodermal*, e.g. Waardenburg's syndrome and Usher's syndrome; *essentially mesodermal*, e.g. Cogan's syndrome, Marfan's syndrome, Alport's syndrome, Pendred's syndrome, Lange–Jervell (cardio-auditory) syndrome and Hurler's syndrome; and *essentially neuroectodermal*, e.g. Recklinghausen's neurofibromatosis, Refsum's syndrome, the cerebellar degenerations and Jamaican neuropathy, mentioned only by title.

ECTODERMAL SYNDROMES

Waardenburg's syndrome

In 1951, P.J. Waardenburg,[9] a Dutch ophthalmologist, described a genetically-determined (autosomal dominant) syndrome of which unilateral deafness or deaf-mutism is a feature. The partial albinism of the hair of the scalp has given the condition one of its names 'white forelock syndrome'. Other components of the syndrome include white forelock or partial albinism in Black patients: lateral displacement of the medial canthus and other abnormal eye signs; partial or total heterochromia of the iris and joined eyebrows. These features may occur in different combinations and the commonest and most important one is sensorineural deafness with eyelid deformity and heterochromia or deep blue eyes.

Since its original description, over 1200 cases of the syndrome have been reported world-wide and in people of many races.[10] The syndrome accounts for about 2% of cases of deaf-mutism. The only report on the histopathology of the temporal bone in the world literature showed total absence of the organ of Corti.[11]

Usher's syndrome

Usher's syndrome consists of sensorineural deafness associated with retinitis pigmentosa. Microscopy includes malformed cochlea and degeneration of the spiral ganglion.

MESODERMAL SYNDROMES

Mesenchymatous tissues may be affected in various syndromes. The strict assessment of their role is difficult, whether or not they are associated with lesions of the ear, which may be localized in the mesenchymatous elements of the sensory organs and of the external and middle ear.

The following syndromes of obscure aetiology may be of interest.

Cogan's syndrome

Cogan's syndrome consists of perceptive deafness and non-syphilitic interstitial keratitis associated with vestibulo-auditory symptoms (vertigo, tinnitus and profound deafness).

Microscopically, new bone may be present in the cochlea and the organ of Corti is degenerated.

Marfan's syndrome

Marfan's syndrome is an ill-defined defect of connective tissue, usually hereditary, manifested by multiple abnormalities involving, in particular, the skeleton, the eyes (ectopia lentis), the external ears and the cardiovascular system (aneurysms). It is due to a generalized defect of the connective tissue in which collagen and bone formation are almost equally affected. This syndrome is usually recognized by the orthopaedic surgeon, and the otologist is rarely confronted with it.[11]

Alport's syndrome

This combines deafness and familial nephropathy. There may be a significant loss of neurones in the basal coils of the cochlea and basophilic deposits in the vascular stria.

The renal changes in hereditary nephritis with nerve deafness combine features of chronic glomerulonephritis, pyelonephritis, and interstitial nephritis, but lack some characteristics of each. Lipid-laden foam cells are present in the great majority of cases, often in long rows and nests in the lower renal cortex.[11]

Lange-Jervell syndrome

(Cardio-auditory syndrome of congenital deafness with an abnormal electrocardiogram.)

Histopathology (Fig. 16.1)

The most constant finding is a widespread degeneration of the sensory end organs of the cochlea and of the vestibular apparatus.

Reissner's membrane is collapsed and adheres to the vascular stria, to the tectorial membrane and/or to the remnants of the organ of Corti. The vascular stria contains unusual spherical inclusions of eosinophilic hyaline substance in every coil; these are most abundant in the apical coils. The deposits often protrude into the cochlear duct, and the ragged surface of the vascular stria appears to have been ruptured by the underlying hyaline or fibrillar material forming the deposit or inclusion. The deposited material is PAS-positive, a fact which suggests that it contains

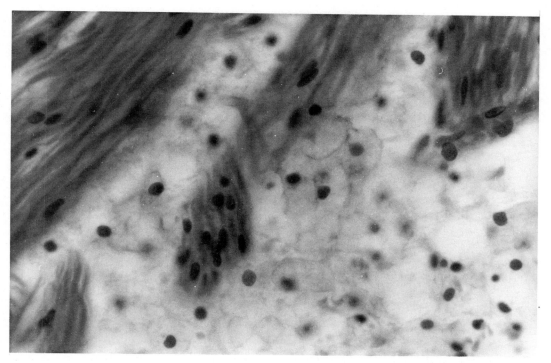

Fig. 16.3a Hurler's syndrome. The presence of vacuolated 'Hurler cells' have disrupted the vestibulocochlear nerve. Haematoxylin–eosin   × 250

mucopolysaccharides or allied substances.[11]

The most distressing aspect of this syndrome are fainting attacks and that some children have failed to recover from a fainting attack and died.

Special investigation of the conducting system of the heart revealed considerable narrowing of the sinu-atrial artery with intimal hyperplasia. The gradual narrowing of this artery and its intraneural branches may result in arrhythmia; should this become uncontrollable, death may ensue during a fainting attack.

Pendred's syndrome

Pendred's syndrome was described in 1890 by Vaughan Pendred, a British general practitioner, in two sisters who were deaf-mute and had goitre. It occurred in about 1 in 13 000 of the population. The syndrome consists of profound childhood deafness from birth, usually bilateral, and the development in childhood of a diffuse or nodular colloid goitre. The mental and physical development of the child is otherwise normal. Microscopy of the ear shows malformed cochlea and degenerative changes of the inner ear.[11]

OTHER CAUSES OF DEAFNESS

Mucopolysaccharidoses

The mucopolysaccharidoses form a group of lysosomal storage diseases due to an inherited deficiency of an enzyme capable of degrading glycosaminoglycans. Glycosaminoglycan is a term used 'generically' for hyaluronic acid, chondroitin and its 4- and 6-sulphates, dermatan and heparan sulphates, keratan sulphate and heparin.[12]

Figures 16.3a,b illustrate the characteristic vacuolated Hurler or gargoyle cells, disrupting the fascicles of the vestibulocochlear nerve within the temporal bone, in two cases of Hurler's disease.[13] The perivascular spaces of the mastoid process contain many vacuolated cells, and large areas of the mastoid are replaced by accumulation of Hurler cells. Light microscopy gave findings consistent with the diagnosis comparing well with those in other publications.[13a] It has been recognized by Hurler that the ear and hearing may be affected and Kittel[13b] notes that 28% of infants with this syndrome were hard of hear-

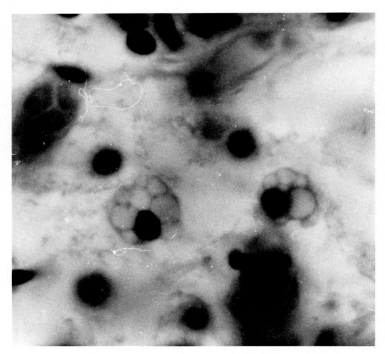

Fig. 16.3b Typical vacuolated 'Hurler cells'. The cell is distended by multiple vacuoles (lysosomes) surrounding the nucleus. Haematoxylin–eosin   × 500

ing or totally deaf. The hearing loss may be sensorineural or conductive, usually due to otitis media.

Deafness associated with chromosomal aberrations

Chromosomal aberrations are responsible for a number of severe anomalies. The presence of an extra chromosome (trisomy) may lead to anomalies associated with deafness. Cochlear anomalies associated with presence of the additional chromosome in trisomy 13–15 include *Patau's syndrome*, characterized by deafness, ocular defects and absence of the olfactory bulbs and tracts. Deafness is common in *Down's syndrome* (trisomy 21 and trisomy 22). Multiple malformations of the ear were described in a prematurely born infant with trisomy 22.[14]

Viral infections

Viral infections of the inner ear have been produced experimentally.[16] Microscopy of natural infections often shows inflammatory granulation tissue in the vascular stria of the organ of Corti or elsewhere.[11] Herpes zoster may cause facial palsy and affect the inner ear (*herpes zoster oticus*) (Fig. 16.4a,b).

The histopathological findings in the temporal bones of two infants—a 5-day-old male infant whose mother had rubella in the fifth week of pregnancy and a 3-day-old infant with maternal rubella in the eighth week of pregnancy—included large inflammatory granulations in the vascular stria, protruding far into the scala media and causing adhesions between Reissner's membrane and the vascular stria (Fig. 16.2).[11] Among other changes there was neuroepithelial degeneration of the organ of Corti. Similar findings have been reported by others:[15, 17] the changes appear to have occurred at a time when the organ of Corti had reached morphological maturation. This could be interpreted as reflecting continued interaction between virus and cell as is indicated by other stigmata of the rubella syndrome. It can therefore be suggested that the rubella virus acts not only by arresting the de-

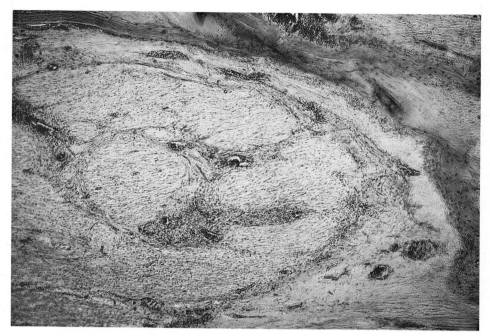

Fig. 16.4a Herpes zoster oticus. Facial nerve with perivascular lymphocytic infiltration.
Haematoxylin–eosin   × 65

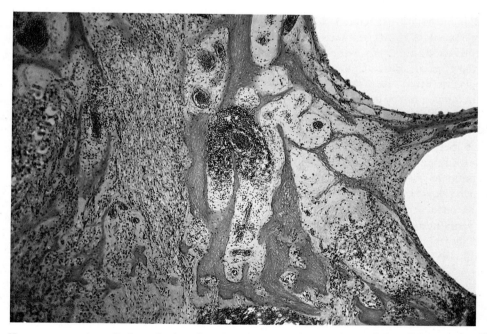

Fig. 16.4b Herpes zoster oticus. Perivascular lymphocytic infiltrate (cuffing) in the modiolus of the cochlea. There are no neurones of the spiral ganglion present.
Haematoxylin–eosin   × 70

velopment of the auditory apparatus, but that it continues to be active in the cells of the developing or fully developed auditory organ.[18]

Idiopathic facial palsy (Bell's palsy)

Bell's palsy is a fairly common disorder of unknown aetiology. Its cause may be of vascular, viral or allergic nature. Relatively common among diabetics, Bell's palsy may be the first manifestation of diabetes mellitus, resulting from ischaemia of the facial nerve that may be caused by diabetic angiopathy.[19] Facial palsy is fairly common in severe hypertension; sometimes it is bilateral in these patients. Although the mechanism is uncertain, a blood clot was found in the facial canal in the only two reported cases in which there was a necropsy.

The development of facial palsy, it is interesting to note, has led to the detection of severe hypertension caused by a renal tumour.[20]

There is evidence that viral infection is sometimes a cause of acute peripheral facial palsy.[21] Whether or not activation of a latent virus is responsible has not been proven. Axonal degeneration is the main microscopical finding in these cases.

Facial palsy can be associated with various viral infections such as herpes zoster,[11] mumps and infectious mononucleosis associated with infection by the Epstein–Barr virus.

Facial palsy is often the presenting sign of a malignant neoplasm of the ear.

Idiopathic sudden deafness

Interest has been attracted by the challenging problems of idiopathic sudden deafness which can be defined as spontaneous sudden sensorineural hearing loss in patients with no known previous ear or hearing problems. Its pathogenesis has remained obscure despite some improvement in its clinical management,[22, 23] but may be viral or vascular. Mumps virus has been isolated from the perilymph of a patient with mumps who suffered sudden deafness.[24] Cytomegalovirus has been isolated from the ear in at least one case.[25] Autoimmune inner-ear disease may be responsible in some cases.[26] Immunological mechanisms may play an aetiological role in ear diseases, many of which have been con-

sidered to be of idiopathic nature. Various cellular constituents of the immune system, as well as immunoglobulins, have been identified within the inner ear, suggesting that it may possess an active immune system. While it is possible that many of the idiopathic diseases will eventually prove not to be immunologically mediated, the result of the intensive investigations carried out will assist in a better understanding of some of the basic mechanisms of host immunity involved in ear disease.[26a, 26b] The usual clinical picture consists of bilateral progressive sensorineural deafness, often with tinnitus and reduced vestibular responses. The diagnosis is based mainly on a characteristic clinical course and response to treatment with steroid and immunosuppressive drugs. Eight temporal bones, six of them from individuals with unilateral sudden deafness and two from a person with bilateral sequential sudden deafness, showed pathological changes not unlike those seen in labyrinthitis of known viral aetiology.[27, 28, 29]

Acquired deafness

In young children, as in adults, deafness can be acquired. It can be a complication of measles and mumps. It can also accompany or follow meningitis (notably tuberculous meningitis), otitis media, trauma to the head, certain neoplasms (notably tumours of the vestibulocochlear nerve) and diabetes mellitus. Post-inflammatory ossifying labyrinthitis may ensue (see below) (Fig. 13.23).[30] Unusual causes include hearing loss due to typhoid:[31] this was known to earlier authors, such as Manassé,[32] who attributed the lesion to 'toxic neuritis'.

Labyrinthitis ossificans

Partial or total bony obliteration mainly of the cochlea may result from various causes: meningococcal or pneumococcal meningitis, Pendred's syndrome, Cogan's syndrome (page 306), chronic otitis, syphilis (Fig. 13.21), systemic bone disease, vascular obstruction (as experimentally produced in animals), otosclerosis and leukaemia (see Fig. 17.37).

Ototoxic drugs (iatrogenic deafness)

There is a wide range of drugs which are capable

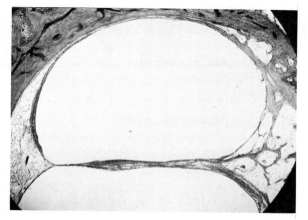

Fig. 16.5 Neomycin ototoxicity. There is complete degeneration of the organ of Corti following the use of a neomycin spray in the treatment of a child with cystic fibrosis of the pancreas.

Haematoxylin–eosin   × 30

of causing deafness or dizziness by causing toxic degeneration either of the inner ear or of the higher centres of hearing and equilibrium (Fig. 16.5).[33] The peculiar sensitivity of the eighth nerve has not yet been satisfactorily explained. Many of the drugs that are ototoxic, have no apparent chemical similarity—for example thalidomide (the teratogenic glutarimide hypnotic), ethacrynic acid (a carboxylic acid diuretic) and sodium aminoarsenate (Atoxyl, an early trypanocidal aminoarsenate). However, most ototoxic antibiotics belong to the aminoglycoside group of antibiotics derived from streptomycetes.

Sensorineural deafness may be caused by the carboxylic acid diuretics (the so-called 'loop diuretics' or 'high-ceiling diuretics', including bumetanide, frusemide and ethacrynic acid), powerful diuretics which inhibit cellular metabolism and the enzymes participating in electrolyte transport.[34] Ethacrynic acid causes oedema and cystic degeneration of the vascular stria.[35] Studies of the combined effect of kanamycin and ethacrynic acid show that the concurrent administration of two or more ototoxic drugs has an enhanced toxic effect on the inner ear.[36] The selective ototoxicity of atoxyl can be employed as a model system for comparative studies of ototoxic agents.[37, 38]

The earliest ultrastructural signs of degeneration, regardless of the drug administered, occur in the outer hair cells and in the vestibular epithelium. Abnormal otoconia may be formed.

Hearing loss due to noise and other physical agents

Repeated exposure to high levels of noise is a potent cause of deafness, particularly in certain industrial occupations and in places of public or private entertainment where there is over-amplification of sound. Proximity to explosions or to gunfire is also liable to result in deafness. In some cases of industrial deafness, the hearing loss involves only a limited range of sound-wave frequencies.

There are considerable difficulties in the study of noise-induced hearing loss. The term 'acoustic trauma' is used for those permanent losses of hearing that follow immediately after brief exposure to a very intense noise and 'occupational noise-induced hearing loss' to those that result from long exposure to noise in industry.[39]

The pathological changes in the vascular stria following acoustic trauma have been noted to be similar to those observed following large intravenous doses of ethacrynic acid (see above).[40]

Hair cells and cochlear nerve endings can degenerate within days following excessive exposure to sound; the outer hair cells are more susceptible than the inner hair cells. In the cochlear nucleus the small cochlear nerve endings are especially susceptible to acoustic trauma.[41]

The effects of ageing and of noise on the hearing level appear to be additive.[42] Sound occurring in nature seldom exceeds 100 decibels (dB). Industrial noise pollution often produces noises above this level and for long periods. Noise-induced degenerative patterns in the human ear exhibit a characteristic 'knife-sharp' demarcation line between the damaged and undamaged areas.[43] Even lower levels of noise may damage the outer hair cells. High intensity sound (noise) produces considerable changes in the cilia, which may be converted into large complex 'giant' structures affecting the function of the sensory cells.

Ageing and hearing loss

Hearing loss and loss of balance control in the aged is of gradual onset and forms part of the progressive deterioration of the physiological functions associated with the ageing process. These are of a general nature, affecting any cell of any tissue and organ, although different cell systems may become vulnerable in particular ways. There are some changes in the mitochondria of some cells of aged animals which may be selectively affected, leading to alterations in their matrix.[44]

There are other cellular and subcellular processes participating in various degenerative syndromes which find expression in extreme old age. The pathological changes of hearing loss of the aged (presbycusis) include atrophy of the vascular stria, of the basilar membrane and of the spiral liagament.[45]

The hair-cell population decreases with age in parallel with atrophy of the spiral nerves. The vestibular end organs may also be affected and there is an age-related progressive reduction of the number of vestibular sensory cells and nerve fibres over the age of 40 years.[46] The cells contain a great deal of lipofuscin yet the physiological ability of such persons may not be substantially impaired, probably as a result of compensation by the surviving cells.

Vascular diseases causing hearing loss

Progressive or sudden hearing loss can be caused by localized or systemic vascular disease. In the first category the vessels of the vascular stria and the internal auditory artery and its branches— which are terminal arteries—play a significant role, e.g. in diabetes mellitus[47, 48] and in various congenital syndromes associated with deafness. The vestibular end organs appear to be more resistant than the organ of Corti to the effects of surgical severance of the labyrinthine artery.[49]

The cause of so-called idiopathic sudden deafness varies (page 302). A vascular disorder such as spasm, oedema or arteritis, or combinations of several vascular factors have been incriminated.[50]

Polyarteritis causing deafness has been reported.[51] *Wegener's granulomatosis* involving the ear may cause deafness.[52–54]

Cogan's syndrome (non-syphilitic interstitial keratitis with hearing loss and vestibular disorder) may be associated with aortic valvular disease and systemic vasculitis. Atypical cilia have been demonstrated in the nasal mucosa of deaf-blind children with Cogan's syndrome.[55]

Relapsing perichondritis (see p. 257)

Sensorineural hearing loss has been reported in some cases.

Meningeal carcinomatosis

Saenger,[56] in 1900, may have been the first to report deafness caused by meningeal carcinomatosis with infiltration of the vestibulocochlear nerve as it crosses the subarachnoid space. In a series of 5 cases in which hearing loss was the first manifestation of proven leptomeningeal carcinomatosis, the primary growths were in the lungs in 2 cases but were unknown in the other 3 cases.[57]

REFERENCES

1. Hiraide F, Paparella MM. In: Hearing loss and dizziness. Tokyo: Igaku-Shoin, 1985.
2. Scheibe A. Arch Otolaryngol 1892; 21: 12.
3. Scheibe A. Z Ohrenheilk 1895; 27: 95.
4. Nadol JB. In press.
5. Friedmann I. Pathol Annual 1978; 13: 373.
6. Slepecky N, Hamernik R, Henderson D. Acta Otolaryngol (Stockh) 1981; 91: 189.
7. Friedmann I. Bull Int Pathol 1975; 16: 9.
8. Friedmann I. In: Principles and practice of surgical pathology. Vol. 2. New York: Wiley & Son, 1983; 1541.
9. Waardenburg PJ. J Hum Genet 1951; 3: 195.
10. Wang L, Karmody CS, Pashyan H. Otolaryngol Head Neck Surg 1981; 89: 666.
11. Friedmann I. Pathology of the ear. Oxford: Blackwell, 1974: pp. 128; 362, 369–380, 385, 396.
12. Gerlings PG, Dekleyn A. Proc R Neth Acad 1946; 49: 28.
13. Friedmann I, Spellacy E, Crow J, Watts RWE. J Laryngol 1985; 99: 29.
13a. Kelemen G. J Laryngol 1966; 80: 791.
13b. Kittel G. Z Laryngol etc. 1963; 42: 206.
14. Arnold W, Schnuknecht HF, von Voss H. Laryng Rhinol 1981; 60: 545.
15. Brockhouser PE, Bordley JE. Arch Otolaryngol 1973; 98: 252.
16. Davis LE, Johnson RT. Lab Invest 1976; 34: 349.
17. Lindsay JR, Carruthers DG, Hemmenway WG et al. Ann Otol 1953; 62: 1201.
18. Lindsay JR. Arch Otolaryngol 1973; 98: 258.
19. Korczyn AD. Lancet 1971; i: 108.
20. Kumar S, Winearls CG, Owen DL. Br Med J 1982; 285: 1266.
21. Djupesland G, Berdal P, Johanessen TA. Arch Otolaryngol 1976; 102: 403.
22. Shaia FT, Sheehy JL. Laryngoscope 1976; 86: 389.
23. Morrison AW. Br J Hosp Med 1978; 19: 237.

24. Westmore GA, Pickard BH, Stern H. Br Med J 1979; i: 14.
25. Davis LE, Nager GT, Johnson RT. Ann Otol Rhinol Laryngol 1979; 88: 198.
26. McCabe B. Ann Otol Rhinol Laryngol 1979; 88: 585.
26a. Veldman JE, Roord JJ, O'Connor AF et al. Laryngoscope 1984; 94: 501.
26b. Harris JP, Ryan AF. Am J Otolaryngol 1984; 5: 418.
27. Schuknecht HF, Kimura RS, Naufal PM. Acta Otolaryngol (Stockh) 1973; 76: 75.
28. Smith GA, Gussen R. Arch Otolaryngol 1976; 102: 108.
29. Karmody CS. Laryngoscope 1983; 93: 1527.
30. Suga F, Lindsay JR. Ann Otol Rhinol Laryngol 1977; 86: 17.
31. Debaine JJ, Peytral C, Basset JM, Lefebure B. Ann Otolaryngol Chir Cervicofac 1977; 94: 943.
32. Manasse P. Handbuch der pathologische Anatomie des menschlichen Ohres. Wiesbaden: JF Bermann, 1917.
33. Hawkins Jr JE. Ann Otol Rhinol Laryngol 1959; 68: 698.
34. Horn KL, Langley LR, Gates GA. Arch Otolaryngol 1977; 103: 539.
35. Quick C, Duvall AJ. Laryngoscope 1970; 80: 954.
36. Nakai Y. Laryngoscope 1977; 87: 1548.
37. Anniko M, Wersall J. Acta Otolaryngol (Stockh) 1975; 80: 167.
38. Anniko M. Thesis. Stockholm: Balder AB, 1977.
39. Hinchcliffe R. Br J Hosp Med 1970; 4: 303.
40. Duval 3rd AJ, Warde WD, Lauhala KE. Ann Otol Rhinol Laryngol 1974; 83: 498.
41. Morest DK, Bohne BA. Hearing Res 1983; 9: 145.
42. Burns W, Robinson DW. Ciba Found Symp 1970; 177.
43. Johnson LG, Hawkins Jr JE. Ann Otol Rhinol Laryngol 1976; 85: 725.
44. Rowlatt C. In: Cristofallo LVJ, Holěcková E, eds. Cell impairment in ageing and development. New York and London: Plenum Press, 1975: 215.
45. Schuknecht HF. Arch Otolaryngol 1964; 80: 369.
46. Bredberg G. J Laryngol Otol 1967; 81: 739.
47. Engstrom H, Bergstrom B, Rosenhall U. Arch Otolaryngol 1974; 100: 411.
48. Kovar M. ORL 1973; 35: 42.
49. Sando I, Ogawa A, Jafek BW. Ann Otol Rhinol Laryngol 1982; 91: 136.
50. Coyas A. Ann Otolaryngol Chir Cervicofac 1977; 94: 387.
51. Gussen P. Arch Otorhinolaryngol 1977; 217: 263.
52. McGill TJL. Arch Otolaryngol 1978; 104: 140.
53. Friedmann I, Bauer F. J Laryngol Otol 1973; 87: 449.
54. McCaffrey TV, McDonald TJ, Pacer GW, De Remee RA. Otolaryngol Head Neck Surg 1980; 88: 586.
55. Fox B, Bull TB, Arden GB. J Clin Path 1980; 33: 327.
56. Saenger A. Munch Med Wschr 1900; 47: 341.
57. Alberts MC, Terence CF. J Laryngol Otol 1978; 92: 233.

Neoplasms of the ear

Tumours of the ear are commoner than has generally been assumed: they are liable to be overlooked if the patient's symptoms, as often happens, are those of a chronic aural infection. Chronic otorrhoea may be an accompaniment of benign or malignant tumours of the ear, and by the time severe pain, haemorrhage, facial palsy, sudden deafness and other alarming symptoms ensue, the tumour may have spread too widely into the surrounding bone or soft tissues for eradication to be practicable. The importance of adequate sectioning, as a regular practice, of all tissue removed surgically from the ear has repeatedly proved its reality. This practice enables the diagnosis of many aural tumours to be made earlier than would otherwise have been the case: coupled with a general clinical awareness of the occurrence of cancer of the ear, it has led to a considerable improvement in diagnostic standards. It must be stressed that the only hope of successful treatment lies in the establishment of the diagnosis at as early a stage as possible in the course of the disease. The application of the methods of exfoliative cytology to the investigation of aural disease may offer further advances in early diagnosis. There is no doubt, however, that the most important factor in diagnosis is appreciation of the possible grave significance of chronic otorrhoea, particularly in older people; any change in the quality or severity of the symptoms in patients with chronic otorrhoea should be regarded as a danger signal and its causes must be fully investigated.

In the following account benign and malignant tumours arising in the ear will be dealt with in that order (see Tables 17.1 and 17.2). The ear may also be invaded by tumours in adjacent structures. It may be noted at the outset that by

Table 17.1 Benign neoplasms of the ear

Surface epithelial	Squamous cell papilloma Keratoacanthoma Epidermoid cyst Pigmented naevi
Glandular	Adenoma Ceruminous adenoma Choristoma
Neurogenic	Schwannoma Neurofibroma Neuroma (facial nerve) Meningioma
Vascular	Hamartoma (angiolipoma) Capillary haemangioma Cavernous haemangioma Paraganglioma
Lymphoreticular system	Plasmacytoma
Connective tissue	Fibroma Lipoma Chondroma Osteoma (exostosis)

Tumour-like conditions	Aural polyp or granulation
	Cholesterol granuloma
	Epidermoid cholesteatoma
	Tympanosclerosis
	Angiolymphoid hyperplasia
	  (Kimura's disease)
	Chondrodermatitis nodularis
	  helicis
	Specific granulomas
	Wegener's granuloma
	Fibrous dysplasia
	Eosinophilic granuloma

far the commonest and most important of all aural tumours are the squamous carcinomas, and that the most dangerous are those that arise in the middle ear, for they are the ones that may not attract the attention of the patient or his doctor until the disease is too far advanced to be eradicated.

Haemorrhagic discharge coupled with severe pain and facial palsy are the symptoms of a deeply placed aural tumour, usually a carcinoma of the middle ear that has already spread beyond the confines of the latter and so presents an often insuperable therapeutic problem. Complete excision of the temporal bone has been practised, occasionally with success. Radiotherapy and cytotoxic drugs may improve the outlook in cases of some varieties of tumours, such as the uncommon rhabdomyosarcoma of the ear.

Incidence

Neoplasms of the ear are comparatively rare, with an estimated incidence of 6 in 1 000 000 people[1] or in 1 in 16 312 new out-patients at a teaching hospital.[2]

Classification

The classification of tumours of the ear may be based on topographical considerations. Alternatively, the classification may be based on the tissue of origin. The two approaches can be combined.

TUMOUR-LIKE LESIONS OF THE EAR

There are various tumour-like lesions of the ear listed in Table 17.1. Some of these have been

Table 17.2 Malignant neoplasms of the ear

Surface epithelial	Squamous cell carcinoma Basal cell carcinoma Malignant melanoma
Glandular	Ceruminous adenocarcinoma Adenocarcinoma of mucous glands Carcinoid
Neurogenic	Malignant Schwannoma Glioma, gliosarcoma
Vascular	Haemangiopericytoma Haemangiosarcoma (Kaposi) Malignant paraganglioma
Lymphorecticular system	Malignant lymphoma Leukaemia Mycosis fungoides
Connective tissue	Fibrosarcoma Chondrosarcoma Osteosarcoma Rhabdomyosarcoma

**Secondary tumours
   from**
	Parotid, breast, lungs, kidney,
	   prostate, rectum,
	   nasopharynx

described in previous sections, for instance aural polyps and granulations, epidermoid cholesteatomas and some bone diseases. Two unusual tumour-like lesions, chondrodermatitis nodularis helicis and angiolymphoid hyperplasia with eosinophils (Kimura's disease), will be discussed here.

Chondrodermatitis nodularis helicis

Nodular chondrodermatitis of the auricle is an inflammatory lesion of traumatic origin. There are foci of non-specific inflammatory granulation tissue in the subcutaneous tissue forming small nodules that give the condition its name. The skin may be ulcerated over the nodules and the cartilage in their vicinity may show degenerative changes (Fig. 17.1).

Angiolymphoid hyperplasia with eosinophils (Kimura's disease)[3–5]

This benign condition is characterized by the development of single or multiple subcutaneous nodules occurring mainly in the auricular region of young persons. It is probably inflammatory, but the cause of the inflammation is unknown. In

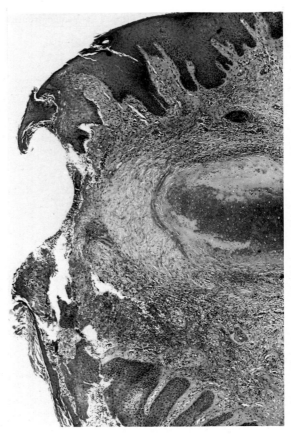

Fig. 17.1 Chondrodermatitis nodularis helicis. The ulcerated auricle is infiltrated by non-specific inflammatory granulation tissue surrounding degenerated elastic cartilage.

Haematoxylin–eosin   × 30

some cases the bite or sting of an arthropod may have been its origin. The condition is mentioned here because it commonly presents as a swelling in the scalp behind one ear.

The histological picture in the active phase has been misinterpreted as angiosarcomatous in a number of cases.[6] The lesions are formed in the dermis or subcutaneous tissue of any part of the body, although most frequently of the head. They are characterized by intensive angioblastic activity, with the formation of many fine branching channels of capillary calibre, lined by large hyperchromatic endothelial cells. There is an abundant infiltrate of lymphocytes; follicle formation is usual and germinal centres may be conspicuous. Numerous eosinophils are present in the tissues and there may be a substantial rise in

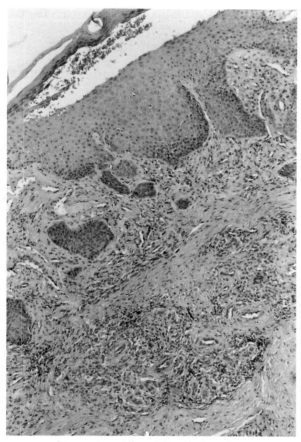

Fig. 17.2 Angiolymphoid hyperplasia (Kimura's disease). There is perivascular aggregation of lymphocytes with interspersed histiocytes and eosinophils.

Haematoxylin–eosin   × 70

the number of eosinophils in the blood. The lesions heal with fibrosis (Figs. 17.2, 17.3).

A histologically identical condition, confined to the subcutaneous tissue behind the lobule of the auricle, is thought to result from the rupture of an epidermoid cyst (see page 318).

TUMOURS OF SQUAMOUS EPITHELIAL ORIGIN

BENIGN

Squamous cell papillomas of the skin of the auricle or in the external acoustic meatus occur mainly in the older age groups. Their chief importance is their liability to become malignant.

Keratosis obturans, an obscure condition affecting the external meatus, may be mentioned in this context. It is a form of hyperkeratosis of the epidermis lining the meatus; it may cause the patient a great deal of local irritation and discomfort, and occasionally it leads to the development of squamous carcinoma (Fig. 17.4).

Basal cell papilloma (also called sebaceous naevus or seborrhoeic dermatitis so that it is not confused with basal cell carcinoma) is composed of uniform darkly-stained basal cells. There are

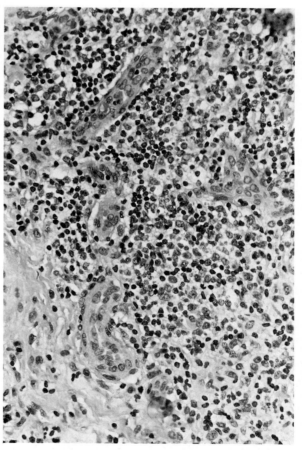

Fig. 17.3 Angiolymphoid hyperplasia (Kimura's disease). There is perivascular aggregation of lymphocytes with interspersed histiocytes and eosinophils.

Haematoxylin–eosin   × 370

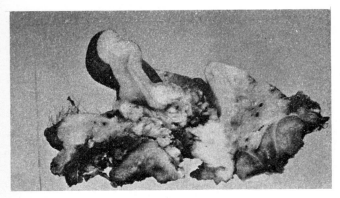

Fig. 17.4 Completely excised temporal bone and external ear for invasive squamous cell carcinoma. The patient had suffered from chronic keratosis obturans and developed, after many years, a squamous cell carcinoma. The picture shows the tumour obstructing the external auditory meatus invading and destroying the deeper structures of the middle and inner ear. There is a large necrotic tumour invading the petrous portion of the temporal bone (bottom right).

Haematoxylin–eosin   × 2

usually several keratotic cysts within the epithelial layer filled with closely-laminated keratin. The basal lamina is well defined and intact.

Keratoacanthoma may develop on the auricle. As in other situations it must be distinguished particularly carefully from squamous carcinoma.

Cysts

Epidermoid cysts ('sebaceous cysts') often occur on the auricle. Clusters of small epidermoid cysts are commonly found in the angle between the auricle and the mastoid region: they are prone to infection. Rupture of a cyst into the adjoining connective tissue results in the formation of a lipogranuloma. In some cases a lesion indistinguishable from angiolymphoid hyperplasia may be a sequel of the rupture of a cyst (see page 316). The occurrence of squamous carcinoma in this area may be a complication of these cystic lesions, which originate from the follicles.

Pseudocysts of the auricles may occur, mainly in young and middle-aged men. Bilateral pseudocysts in an old man were described.[6a] Microscopy showed the cyst wall composed of partly degenerated auricular cartilage and lined by some

amorphous eosinophilic material filling the cyst cavity. A traumatic origin has been suggested but the pathogenesis is obscure.

Pilomatrixoma. The so-called 'benign calcifying epithelioma' of Malherbe may be found behind the auricle, which is one of its commonest sites.[7] This lesion is sometimes said to result from desiccation and calcification of the contents of an epidermoid cyst, with residual proliferation of foci of the cells of the lining of the latter.

MALIGNANT

Squamous carcinoma

Squamous carcinoma is the commonest neoplastic disease of the ear, any part of which may be its site of origin. Although the auricle is the most frequent site of these growths, those that arise in the external acoustic meatus and in the middle ear are particularly important because their presence may long escape detection, while their early symptoms are likely to be obscured by otorrhoea or other evidence of a long-standing pre-existing disease.

The majority of cancers of the ear present in the auricle (Fig. 17.5). The auricle was the site of 69% of a series of 273 malignant neoplasms of the ear: 22.9% of these auricular tumours were squamous carcinomas.[8, 9] In another series of 92 neoplasms of the ear, 41 were squamous carcinomas: of these, 17 (42%) arose on the auricle and 24 (58%) in the external auditory meatus.[10, 11] The overall histological appearance and differentiation were similar at both sites but there were some differences between the two in terms of age, sex and prognosis. 6% (1 patient out of 17) of the patients with auricular cancer died of causes related to the tumour, in contrast to 52% (11 out of 21 of those who could be followed up) with carcinomas of the external auditory canal.

A squamous carcinoma of the auricle or external meatus may present as an ulcer that soon shows all the features typical of primary squamous cancer of the skin. It may invade and destroy the auricular cartilage (Fig. 17.6). Alternatively, the lesion may be a proliferative, polypoid growth. The tumours that arise in the middle ear or invade it progressively excavate the surround-

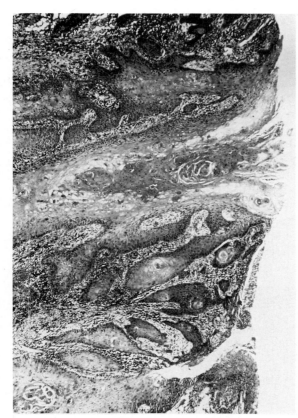

Fig. 17.5 Well-differentiated invasive squamous cell carcinoma of the pinna arising from the hyperkeratotic epidermis. There is some reactive lymphocytic infiltrate surrounding the neoplastic tissue which is completely excised.

Haematoxylin-eosin   × 35

Aetiology

There is, normally, no squamous epithelium in the middle ear, and the squamous carcinomas that arise there must develop either from squamous epithelium that is present as a result of disease or from the respiratory type of epithelium by a process of metaplasia. It is possible that chronic otitis media—occasionally, in ears treated by tympanoplasty[12] and its complications such as 'epidermoid cholesteatoma' (page 270) may be predisposing factors.

It has been said that more than half the patients who have squamous carcinoma of the

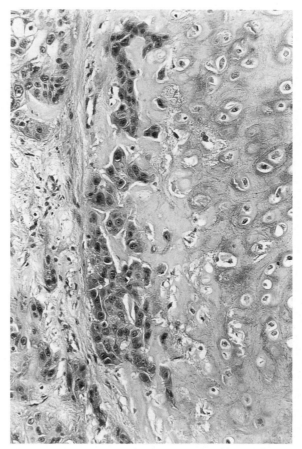

Fig. 17.6 Squamous carcinoma infiltrating the cartilage of the pinna of an old woman suffering from carcinoma of the external auditory meatus.

Haematoxylin–eosin   × 146

ing bone, extend into the mastoid, auditory tube or external meatus and invade any of the adjacent structures (Fig. 17.4). Secondary infection, necrosis and bleeding are the rule. Death may result from haemorrhage, or from meningitis or brain abscess following invasion of the cranial cavity. The histological appearances are characteristic and, as in other situations, the tumours may differ markedly in their degree of differentiation: most are well-differentiated, keratinizing growths (Fig. 17.7). Metastatic involvement of the regional lymph nodes may be present by the time the initial lesion is diagnosed: the upper deep cervical and retro-auricular nodes are those most liable to be affected. Perivascular spread is uncommon (Fig. 17.8).

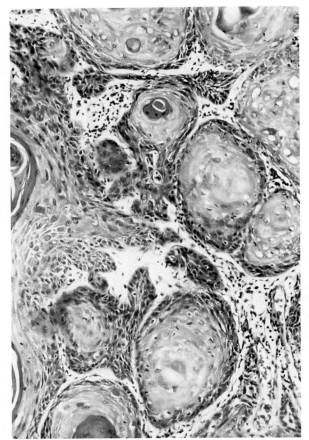

Fig. 17.7 Well-differentiated primary squamous carcinoma of the ear. The disease in this case presented with the clinical picture of chronic otitis media.

Haematoxylin–eosin   × 140

middle ear have had chronic infection of the ear:[8, 9, 9a] the relationship between the chronic infection and the development of the cancer is thought to be significant.[13, 14] If this is the case, the greater efficacy of modern methods of treatment of otitis media by antibiotics and surgery may well bring about an important decrease in the incidence of cancer of the middle ear and, possibly, also of cancer of the external auditory meatus.

The factors that lead to the development of squamous cancer of the auricle are not related to middle-ear disease. They are the usual factors concerned in the development of squamous carcinoma of the skin generally. Damage to the epidermis of the auricle by exposure to sunlight may be one of these factors.[10, 11]

It is pertinent to note that there is often considerable difficulty in telling whether a given tumour has arisen in the external acoustic meatus or in the middle ear or its extensions (Fig. 17.4). This is due to the fact that in many instances the growth has spread to involve both regions before its presence is recognized (Fig. 17.9).

Basal cell carcinoma

Basal cell carcinoma is common on the external ear. In the series of 273 cases of cancer of the ear referred to above (page 318) there were 61 instances (41%) of basal cell carcinoma.[8] Although they grow slowly, basal cell carcinomas may invade deeply into the underlying bone and are therefore liable to recur after surgical excision. Most of them are pure basal cell growths but

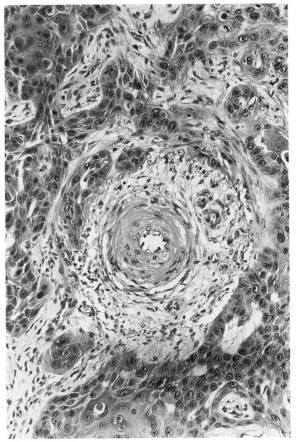

Fig. 17.8 Perivascular lymphatic spread of squamous carcinoma of the middle ear.

Haematoxylin–eosin   × 240

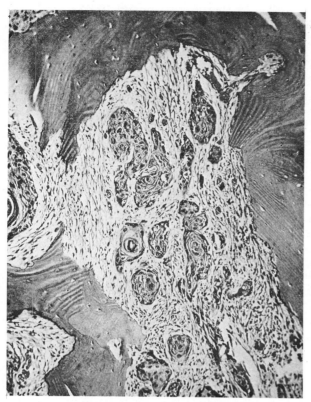

Fig. 17.9 Mastoid bone invaded by well-differentiated squamous carcinoma. There is much fibrosis and bone destruction. There was a 40-year history of otitis media.

Haematoxylin–eosin   × 140

basisquamous carcinomas also occur. As elsewhere, it is exceptionally rare for pure basal cell carcinomas of the auricle to metastasize; in contrast, the basisquamous tumours are commonly said to be liable to do so, although this view is now often regarded as doubtful.[12]

GLANDULAR TUMOURS

Choristoma

Choristoma is a congenital tumour formed by histologically normal tissue displaced during embryonic development. The developmental error in cases of choristoma of the ear occurs around the proximal part of the second branchial arch. The displaced epithelial rests form salivary gland tissue and may extend into the middle ear. Alternatively, the epithelial cell rests may be trapped during development in the temporal bone and proliferate so as to form a tumour of the middle ear.[15]

First described in 1961,[16] only 10 cases of choristoma of the middle ear had been reported by 1978.[17] Some of these were attached to the facial nerve. The tumours have also been reported in the auditory tube and the external auditory meatus. Associated ossicular and other malformations have been described.[18] This benign lesion is composed of salivary gland tissue and is non-neoplastic. In the case of a published example of adenoid cystic carcinoma of the middle-ear cleft, this tumour may have arisen from a choristoma of the middle ear.[19]

Benign adenoma of the middle ear

The benign adenomas of the middle ear, as a distinctive group, are of recent recognition[20] and constitute a rare type of tumour of the ears.[20a] A review in 1982 referred to only 37 cases in all.[21] Such tumours have been usually included with the cerumen gland tumours, although the middle-ear mucosa does not possess any apocrine glands. Choristomas have been mentioned as the tissue of origin. Both may develop from displaced or trapped embryonic cell rests of glandular type.

Whether or not these are truly benign tumours, their bland uniform morphology does not reflect a potential for malignant behaviour.[21] Adjoining soft tissues and bone may, however, be invaded by the more aggressive tumours of this kind and the clinical signs have to be taken into account to determine the nature of primary middle-ear adenomas.[22, 23]

Microscopy shows the tumours to be composed of relatively uniform cuboidal to low columnar cells forming acini (Fig. 17.10a). Some may display a papillary pattern. Tissue removed from the deeper parts of the mastoid process was invaded by the well differentiated adenomatous tumour illustrated in Figure 17.10b. This underlines the difficulty in distinguishing benign from malignant type adenomas noted also by other authors.[22, 24]

In a published case[21] argyrophile granules were demonstrated by light microscopy corresponding ultrastructurally to membrane-bound secretory granules of mucinous character which were

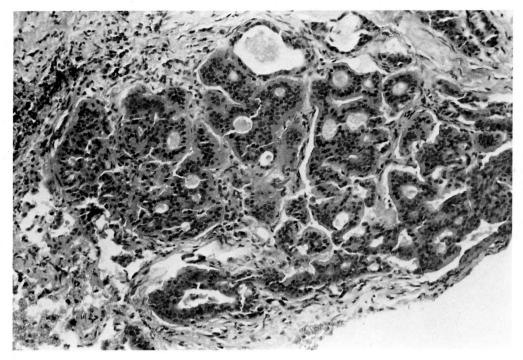

Fig. 17.10a Well-differentiated adenocarcinoma of the middle ear considered to be an adenoma. The neoplastic tissue consists both of acini and of solid areas.

Haematoxylin–eosin × 225

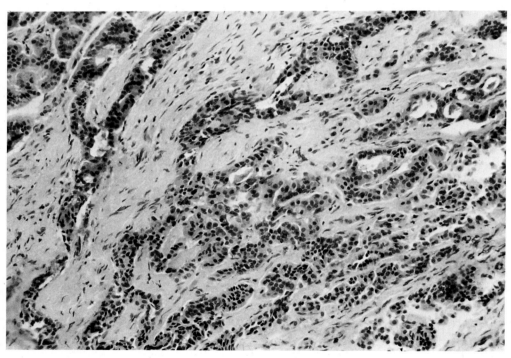

Fig. 17.10b Tissue from the mastoid process infiltrated by the adenocarcinoma as in Fig. 17.10a.

Haematoxylin–eosin × 225

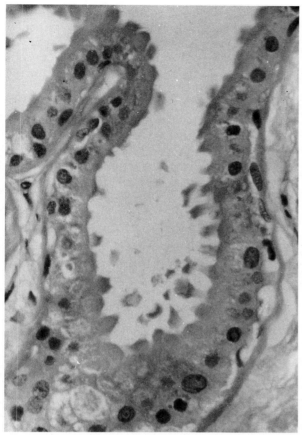

Fig. 17.11 Normal apocrine ceruminous glands. The superficial part of the cytoplasm is 'budding' into the lumen. The myoepithelial layer can be made out peripheral to the epithelium.

Haematoxylin–eosin × 450

located in the apical portion of the cells in contrast to the more dispersed distribution of the usually smaller neurosecretory granules in glomus tumours. The nature of these granules is not known but I have seen similar granules in the apical part of the cells of ceruminous glands and tumours.

Adenocarcinoma of the middle ear

This is very rare: only 17 cases have been reported in the literature.[25] The neoplasm may arise from the mucosa of the middle ear, the Eustachian tube or the mastoid air cells.

Patients treated by extensive surgical resection and radiation therapy have remained free of disease for 10 years after treatment.[25]

TUMOURS OF THE CERUMINOUS GLANDS[26]

These are important tumours in the region, not so much on the grounds of their frequency but because of their unpredictable natural course and difficult terminology.

The true frequency of these comparatively rare tumours is difficult to assess but it is certainly higher than the number of published cases would suggest. On the other hand, as suggested by a recent critical review of the literature,[27] several of the reported cases ought to be excluded because of diagnostic inaccuracies.

The use of the term 'ceruminoma' should only be used for those tumours arising from the modified apocrine sweat glands (ceruminous glands) of the external auditory meatus.[28] It has been pointed out[27] that to 'label them all under one term such as ceruminoma, hidradenoma or otherwise is erroneous'. In the survey of 273 aural cancers already mentioned (page 318), 20% were listed as 'ceruminomas'.[9] Clinically, tumours that arise from the ceruminous glands of the external auditory meatus (Fig. 17.11) grow slowly, may remain unnoticed for years, or present as trivial polyps and occasionally with the symptoms of and signs of mastoiditis.[29]

Histopathology

Various aspects of these tumours and of their histological classification require some detailed consideration.

Their structure is characterized by two types of cells: columnar cells forming the internal layer and myoepithelial cells that rest on a well-defined basal lamina. The columnar cells contain large granular apocrine secretion (Fig. 17.11). These appearances are similar to those of the sweat gland tumours and also to the salivary and mucous gland tumours.

The *classification* of the tumours of ceruminous glands is difficult. Different workers have given different names to what are clearly identical tumours and have arrived at various histogenic interpretations. Some writers include in their proposed classification growths that others do not even consider to arise from the ceruminous glands of the external auditory meatus.

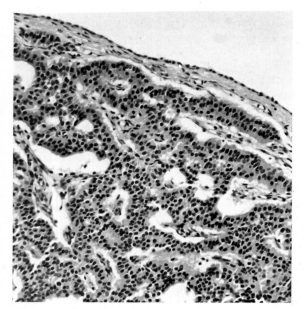

Fig. 17.12 Well-differentiated ceruminous adenocarcinoma consists of acini lined by a twin-layered epithelium.

Haematoxylin-eosin   × 126

The most generally acceptable classification that has been proposed up to now is that of Wetli and his associates[30] based on light and electron microscopic features, in particular on the predominant pattern and on their biological behaviour with particular reference to the presence or absence of invasion. It recognizes that there may be an overlap but four more or less distinct types may be recognized.

1. Ceruminous adenoma
The ceruminous adenoma is a well-differentiated localized proliferation of the glands (Fig. 17.12). Microscopy shows acini formed by two layers of the epithelium as in normal cerumen glands, and marked proliferation of the myoepithelial cells. The adenomas are considered to be benign and local excision is the treatment of choice. The clinical behaviour of some of these tumours may, however, contradict their apparently 'benign' morphological features.

2. Adenoid cystic or cribriform ceruminous
adenocarcinoma
This is the commonest type of the rare ceruminous-gland tumours and its clinical behaviour is characterized by extensive local infil-

tration, invasion of the middle-ear cleft and perineural invasion. Adenoid cystic carcinomas arise from the ceruminous glands of the external auditory meatus; but similar neoplasms of the adjacent parotid salivary gland may spread to the meatus.

The cribriform pattern is the characteristic and pathgnomonic feature of the tumour. The tumour cells form small duct-like structures or larger masses with interspersed cystic spaces to give a cribriform or lace-like pattern. Adenoid cystic carcinomas may show other cellular patterns in addition to the cribriform appearance. Tubulo-glandular structures and solid cellular areas are variable in extent (Fig. 17.13a,b). A higher proportion of solid areas has been con-

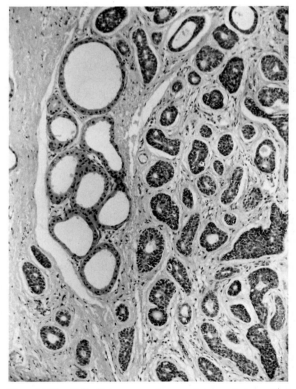

Fig. 17.13a Cribriform ceruminous adenocarcinoma. Both normal (above) and neoplastic ceruminous glands are shown. The structure of tumours of the ceruminous glands may reproduce that of almost any variety of sweat gland tumour arising in the skin of other parts of the body.

Haematoxylin-eosin   × 70

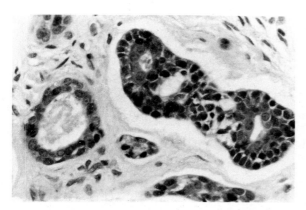

Fig. 17.13b Higher magnification shows acini lined by two layers of epithelial cells.

Haematoxylin–eosin   × 234

sidered by some authors to indicate a worse prognosis but that has not been confirmed.[31, 32] A cylindromatous pattern may be seen in some tumours.

Outlook. The outlook of all types of ceruminoma is variable.[33] This is exemplified by my experience of four cases of the cribriform type.[14] One patient died 2 years after the disease presented; local recurrence had followed radical surgery and radiotherapy. Two patients were alive and their disease had not recurred 5 years and 22 years respectively after its presentation. The fourth patient was alive 24 years after the tumour was recognized; there was repeated local recurrence in this case. It is important to note that the cribriform type of tumour of the ceruminous glands has a particular tendency to metastasize to the lungs and to the kidneys.[26] This must be considered regularly when the patient comes for follow-up examination.

3. Ceruminous gland adenocarcinoma

This tumour is difficult to differentiate from primary adenocarcinoma of the middle ear. But their site in the external auditory meatus and the eosinophilic cytoplasm of the cells may assist in their correct identification.[32]

4. Pleomorphic ceruminous gland tumours ('mixed' tumours)

Pleomorphic ceruminous gland tumours are not common and may have to be distinguished from similar tumours arising in the parotid gland which having spread into the external auditory meatus and may present as primary tumours of the ear. For this reason en bloc surgical excision with removal of the parotid gland is advised for these tumours of the ear. The microscopical picture does not differ from that of the salivary gland tumours of this type.[33]

Ultrastructure

Only single examples of ceruminoma have been examined under the electron microscope.[30, 34] No specific ultrastructural features have been reported. The epithelial cells have prominent apical caps containing much glycogen and protrude into the lumen of the glands. The cytoplasm is rich in glycogen and contains some lipid droplets, a small number of mitochondria and scanty cisternae of the rough endoplasmic reticulum. There are well-defined desmosomes and the epithelial cells are connected by junctional complexes at the apex. There is a distinct basal lamina but no myoepithelial cells were seen in the examined cases. I have examined the ultrastructure of three ceruminous adenocarcinomas which displayed similar features but contained myoepithelial cells.

Extramammary Paget's disease[35] affecting the external auditory meatus has been observed in association with a ceruminous gland carcinoma.

Behaviour

The behaviour of the neoplasms arising from the ceruminous glands of the auditory meatus cannot be predicted from their microscopical features. I have classified them as 'intermediate neoplasms' meaning that they form a group between the benign and malignant neoplasms. Invasiveness appears to be the only definite evidence of their malignancy (Fig. 17.14a,b). Contemporary opinion tends to be in favour of regarding all ceruminomas as potentially malignant, irrespective of whether or not invasive growth has been identified in the biopsy specimen.

Tyrosine crystals in ceruminoma

The presence of tyrosine crystals in salivary gland tumours has been reported. Similar tyrosine deposits have been recognized in a ce-

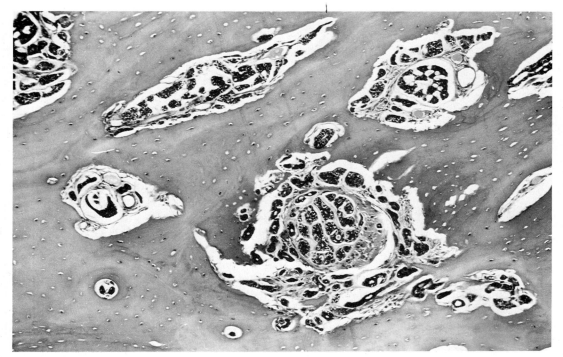

Fig. 17.14a Cribriform adenocarcinoma of ceruminous glands invading temporal bone.
Haematoxylin–eosin   × 100

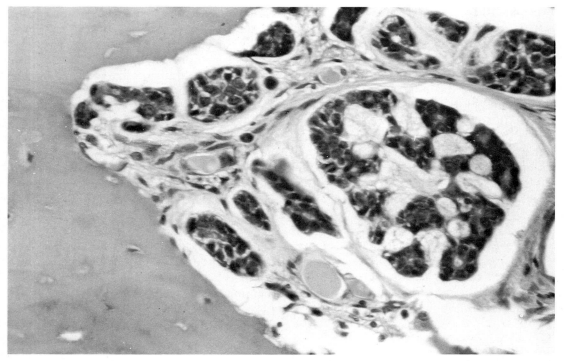

Fig. 17.14b Cribriform ceruminous adenocarcinoma invading mastoid air cells (same specimen as Figure 17.14a).
Haematoxylin–eosin   × 300

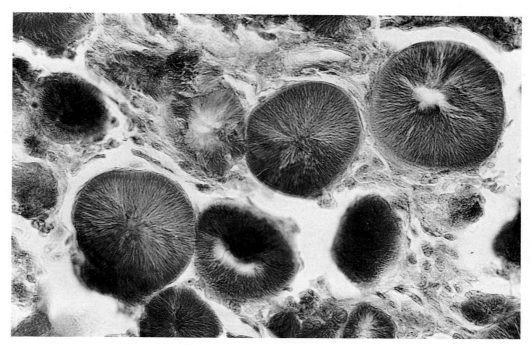

Fig. 17.15 Tyrosine crystals of flowery pattern occupying the tumour acini.
Van Gieson   × 400

ruminous gland tumour in a 42-year-old man, removed from the right external auditory meatus.[36]

Microscopy showed randomly distributed crystalline deposits surrounded by myo-epithelial cells and occluding the neoplastic acini. The needle-shaped crystals formed sheaves and petal-like clusters and were best demonstrated in sections stained by Van Gieson's stain (Fig. 17.15). Under polarized light the crystals were birefringent and displayed Maltese-cross figures. The surface of the tumour was covered by squamous epithelium and there were normal ceruminous glands in the subepithelial stroma.

Similar crystalline deposits have been described in pleomorphic adenomas of the parotid gland in a series of 5 cases; 4 of the patients were black and 1 was white.[32] 6 further examples, all in Black patients, were included in a series of 121 pleomorphic salivary gland tumours seen at the University of Cape Town in a period of 20 years.[37] Other workers too have confirmed the greater frequency of this peculiarity in Black patients.[38]

NEUROENDOCRINE TUMOURS

CARCINOID TUMOURS OF THE EAR

The term 'carcinoid tumour' has been coined by Oberndorfer in 1907[39] to describe a distinctive neoplasm of the intestinal tract. Recent histochemical and ultrastructural investigations have shown that these tumours may present in various organs and that they belonged to the group of the so-called apudomas. The APUD cell system consists of cells with a high content of amines, the capacity for endocrine activity and the production of a variety of vasoactive polypeptide hormones.[40] They are characterized microscopically by the formation of cords, ribbons and festoons of sheet-like cellular areas. The cytoplasm contains argyrophil granules and under the electron microscope neurosecretory granules are seen. Multiple immuno-reactive peptides can be identified in the cells by the immunoperoxidase methol; e.g. calcitonin, VIP, somatostatin, ACTH.

Carcinoid tumours may display four main his-

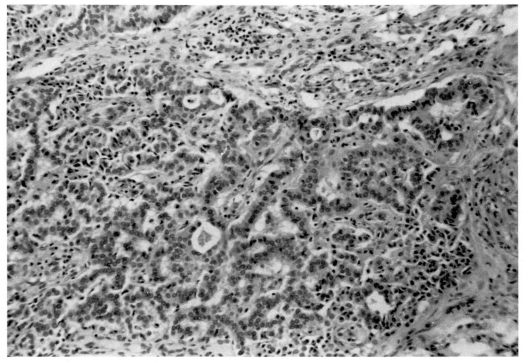

Fig. 17.16 Mixed carcinoid tumour of the ear. This field is from an area formed of columnar cells, arranged partly in strands partly forming acinus-like structures. Small numbers of paraganglionic cells are scattered among the columnar cells.
Haematoxylin–eosin   × 200

tological patterns:[41] 1) comprising solid lobules or masses; 2) in which the cells show a trabecular or cord-like arrangement; 3) with tubular or rosette-like features; and 4) of mixed structure.

Incidence

Carcinoid tumours of the middle ear are very rare. A carcinoid tumour of the middle ear displaying adenomatous features was described.[42] Another carcinoid tumour of the middle ear, apparently arising in a glomus jugulare tumour, was associated with a long history of diarrhoea, flushing and severe headaches consistent with the so-called carcinoid syndrome and cured by the removal of the tumour.[43] A mixed type of carcinoid tumour arising in the middle ear of a middle-aged man showed a somewhat varied histological pattern.[44] It was partly glandular and on frozen sections was interpreted as a low-grade adenocarcinoma (Fig. 17.16). Elsewhere the tumour had a more solid appearance resembling a paraganglioma composed of nests of ovoid or

spheroidal cells separated by a vascular fibrous stroma (Fig. 17.17). Stained with the Grimelius method, the cells of both the glandular and paraganglionic tissue contained argyrophil granules (Fig. 17.18a). Under the electron microscope there were large numbers of neurosecretory granules in both types of cell and this confirmed the diagnosis of carcinoid tumour of mixed pattern (Fig. 17.18b).

The Grimelius stain and electron microscopy are essential methods in the differential diagnosis of adenomatous tumours of the ear showing trabecular arrangement.[45, 45a]

Typical carcinoid tumours and undifferentiated small cell neuroendocrine carcinoma form the two ends of a spectrum of neoplasms with neuroendocrine differentiation. Tumours with intermediate histological and biological characteristics occur but are poorly understood.

Endocrine cells sharing some properties with neurones such as the presence of neurosecretory granules have been called paraneurones.[45b]

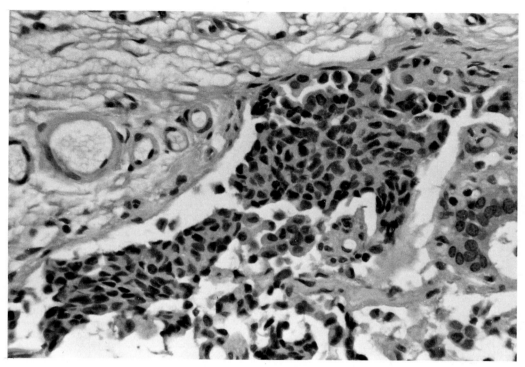

Fig. 17.17 Carcinoid tumour arising in the middle ear of a middle-aged man (same case as in Figure 17.16). Shows the paraganglionic cells forming large masses in fibrous tissue. Part of a glandular acinus is seen (right margin). Following partial resection of the temporal bone the patient has remained free of the tumour for several years.

Haematoxylin–eosin   × 500

PARAGANGLIOMA OF THE JUGULO-TYMPANIC BODIES

Anatomy
The extra adrenal non-chromaffin paraganglionic system is known to be widely distributed in the body, subserving the same function as the carotid

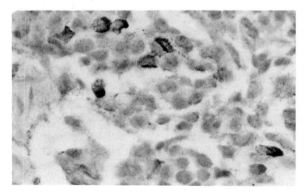

Fig. 17.18a Specimen as in Figure 17.16 and 17.17. Grimelius stain shows argyrophilic cells.

× 465

body by responding to chemical changes in the blood.[46, 47] There are two non-chromaffin paraganglia in the temporal bone of great otological importance: the glomus tympanicum and the glomus jugulare. It is of some interest that a tympanic paraganglion appears to have been the first of the paraganglia to have been described. Valentin, in 1840,[40] found it in the tympanic canaliculus and gave it the name 'gangliolum tympanicum'. But our present knowledge of the morphology, sites and structure of the non-chromaffin paraganglia of this anatomical region is in a large part due to the work of Guild, who in 1941,[49] described the 'glomus jugulare' or jugular body and in 1953[50] their incidence in the temporal bone and their anatomy.

More than half of the glomus formations found are in the adventitia of the dome of the jugular bulb, along the jugular fossa—part of the course of Jacobson's nerve (tympanic branch of the glossopharyngeal nerve); and an-

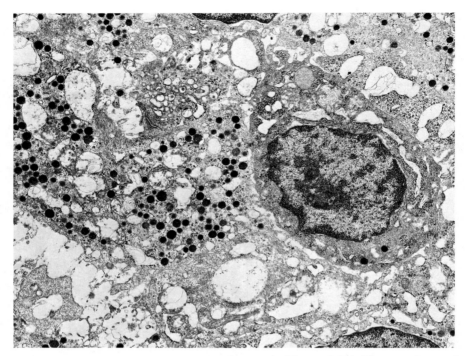

Fig. 17.18b Mixed carcinoid tumour of the ear (same specimen as in Figure 17.18a). Electron micrograph showing large numbers of dense neurosecretory granules in both paraganglionic cells and columnar cells.   × 15 000

other fifth are in the osseous canal (tympanic canalicus) through which the nerve of Jacobson enters the middle ear from the jugular fossa (glomus jugulare): In about one-fourth of the ears, there might occur glomus formations in the mucosa of the cochlear promontory, along the tympanic plexus portion of the course of the nerve of Jacobson (glomus tympanicum).

Histology
Paraganglionic cells are derived from the neural crest and migrate in close association with autonomic ganglion cells—hence the name *paraganglion*. The epithelioid principal cells (chief cells) form groups or strands with smaller sustenacular cells and pericytes in a vascular stroma. The principal cells have a granular cytoplasm; electron microscopy shows that they contain large numbers of neurosecretory granules. The neuroendocrine nature of these cells has been confirmed.[51] The jugulotympanic paraganglia, in common with others, synthesize and store catecholamines which are sequestered in dense-core cytoplasmic granules.

Tumours of the jugulotympanic bodies
The relationship of certain unusual, vascular tumours of the ears with the jugular glomera was first recognized by the pathologist Otani and reported by Rosenwasser in 1945.[52, 53] This led to a fresh evaluation of a number of tumours that had been published, under various names, by earlier authors and to their retrospective correct identification.

Nomenclature
The nomenclature of these tumours is still confused. Among the names that are in use are 'non-chromaffin paraganglioma' (used here), 'chemodectoma' and 'tympanic tumour of carotid body type'. It is noteworthy that it is exceptional for even the slight degree of chromaffinity of the average carotid body tumour to be found in the tumours of the jugulotympanic bodies.

Incidence
Paragangliomas represented about 15% of 92 neoplasms of the ear studied at the University of Minnesota in the period 1964–1975.[54] This incid-

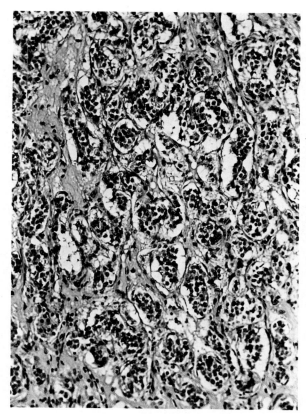

Fig. 17.19 Paraganglioma of a glomus jugulare showing the characteristic alveolar pattern. It presented as an aural polyp as shown in Figure 17.24.

Haematoxylin–eosin   × 160

ence was higher than the 9% in my experience of 295 tumours of the ear at the Institute of Laryngology and Otology, London.[55] Paragangliomas of the jugulotympanic bodies are commoner in women. Most of the patients are aged between 40 and 60 years when the condition presents. There are several records of more than one case occurring in a family,[56] but most patients have no known family predisposition.

Histopathology
The microscopical picture displays the features of a paraganglioma arising in any location. Compact groups of polyhedral epithelioid cells, also called 'chief cells', are often delineated by a well-defined reticulum network and lie in intimate relationship to capillary blood vessels (Figs 17.19, 17.20). The alveolar pattern is particularly

well-demonstrated in preparations stained to show the reticulin fibres. The epithelioid or chief cells usually have a moderately abundant, finely granular cytoplasm. The tumour cells contain a moderate number of mitochondria, a prominent Golgi apparatus and occasional profiles of dilated smooth endoplasmic cisternae.

The nuclei of the chief cells are generally rounded, but may sometimes exhibit irregularity though conclusion regarding behaviour cannot be drawn from the histological pattern alone. A common feature of all these tumours is their ability to produce catecholamines, a property which they share with the adrenal medulla and tumours derived therefrom though the concentration in the cells of chemodectomas is rarely sufficient to exhibit the chromaffin reaction. Nevertheless, the characteristic secretory granules can be visualized under the electron microscope (Fig. 17.21a,b) and can also be demonstrated by the formaldehyde-induced-fluorescence technique.[57] There are also sustentacular cells, which do not contain granules but have a close relation to nerves as well as to the chief cells, and thus are regarded as chemoreceptor cells. It is noteworthy that there was enhanced secretion of catecholamines in a malignant paraganglioma of the carotid body.[58]

Electron microscopy has confirmed that pericytes and nerve fibres are present in the walls of the capillaries of the tumours as they are in those of normal paraganglia.

Histological types. Some authors have distinguished three main types:[59] 1) *the classical type*, described above, in which the structure closely reproduces that of the normal paraganglion; 2) *adenomatous type*, consisting predominantly of epithelial aggregates, with minimal stroma; and 3) *angiomatous type*, in which the vascular component of the tumour is usually conspicuous. However, most examples of the tumours include areas that correspond to all three of these types, and there is little advantage in trying to differentiate them in this way. The adenomatous type may have to be distinguished from a carcinoid tumour.

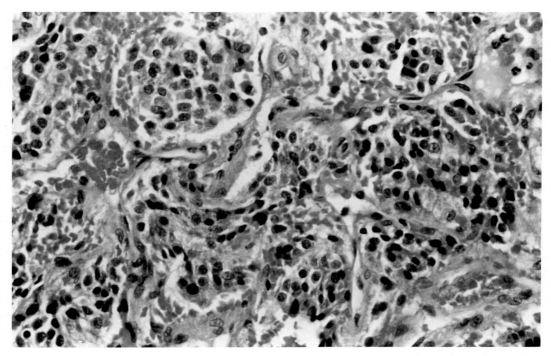

Fig. 17.20 Paraganglioma of the glomus tympanicum. Note characteristic cell-balls formed by spheroidal paraganglionic cells around narrow capillaries.   Haematoxylin–eosin   × 490

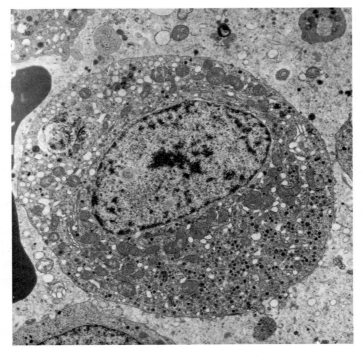

Fig. 17.21a Paraganglioma of a glomus jugulare. Electron micrograph showing a rounded tumour cell containing large numbers of electron-dense membrane-bound neurosecretory granules.   × 7000

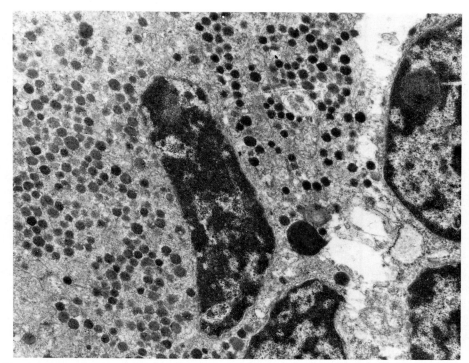

Fig. 17.21b Paraganglioma of a glomus jugulare. Electron micrograph showing a large number of electron-dense neurosecretory granules in the cytoplasm of a paraganglionic cell.   × 14 000

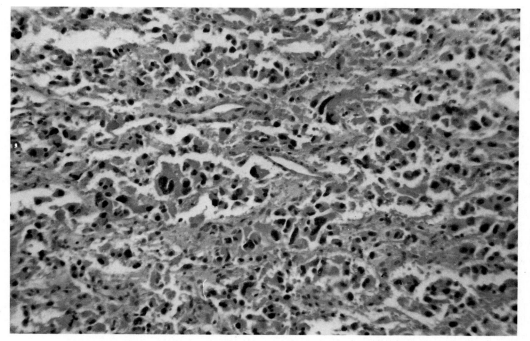

Fig. 17.22 Malignant paraganglioma of the middle ear. The nuclei are irregular and often bizarre. The cells are in groups separated by fibrous septa forming some glomerular structures.

Haematoxylin–eosin   × 160

Provided by Dr P. Gruskin, St Vincent's Medical Center, Los Angeles, Cal, USA.

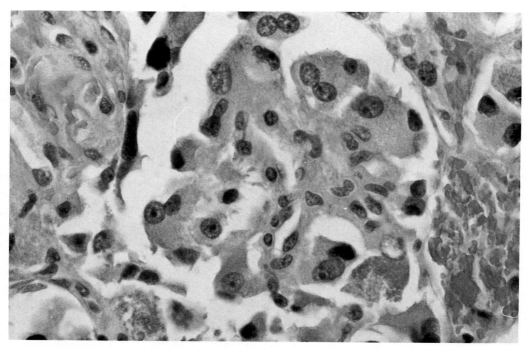

Fig. 17.23 Detail of glomerular formation of tumour cells (as specimen in Fig. 17.22).
Haematoxylin–eosin   × 48

Course and behaviour
Paragangliomas grow slowly, and it is common for symptoms to be present over several years before the diagnosis is made. Invasion of the roof of the jugular fossa is followed by extension into the tympanic cavity, destruction of the ossicles, and perforation of the tympanic membrane.

Malignant paraganglioma of the ear is very rare. Microscopy shows considerable nuclear irregularity of size and shape (Fig. 17.22). The alveolar pattern is less prominent than in a benign tumour of this kind. Occasionally, glomerular-like structures may be formed (Fig. 17.23). Metastatic subcutaneous deposits can develop in the course of the disease.

Presentation in the external acoustic meatus in the form of a vascular mass is liable to be mistaken clinically and microscopically for a simple aural polyp, the protuberant mass of oedematous, vascular granulation tissue that may develop in association with chronic otitis media (Fig. 17.24). Once again, the necessity for microscopical examination of all polyps and other surgical speci-

mens from the ears is stressed, and at the same time it must be observed that the presence of tissue that is in every way characteristic of these tumours may still be overlooked. A tendency to bleeding, which may even take the form of a sudden sharp haemorrhage from the meatus, is characteristic.

The tumour may extend into the mastoid process or into the petrous part of the temporal bone. Some authors regard these growths as 'cranial-base tumours'. Occasionally, tumour that has invaded the mastoid may penetrate the bone to infiltrate the subcutaneous tissue and skin. It can resemble a cerebello-pontine angle tumour.

Presenting as a tumour of the base of the skull with distension of the foramen jugulare, the tumour occasionally extends into the internal jugular vein to appear in the neck and even extend as far as to the heart.[60] Invasion of the jugular vein may be followed by metastasis, particularly to the lungs and liver. The regional lymph nodes may also be infiltrated. Usually the metastasizing tumours are as well-differentiated

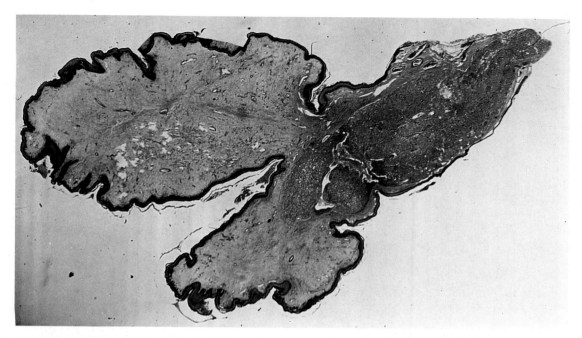

Fig. 17.24 Paraganglioma of the middle ear. This example presented as an aural polyp projecting into the external acoustic meatus. The picture shows that the 'polyp' is formed of inflamed and oedematous connective tissue covered by epidermis: tumour tissue is confined to the stalk of the polyp (right), where it accounts for the rather darker appearance, contrasting with the paler, oedematous connective tissue of the rest of the lesion.

Haematoxylin–eosin   × 9

as those that are only locally invasive, but in rare instances they are anaplastic, showing pleomorphism and many mitotic figures (Figs 17.23, 17.24).

There can be no doubt that all paragangliomas of the jugulotympanic glomera must be regarded as malignant.[61] Schwartz & Israel[62] described a young woman who had a paraganglioma of the right glomus jugulare and developed extensive secondary deposits in the lungs 3 years after surgical removal of the primary tumour. It is relevant that 20 cases of carotid body tumours with distant metastasis have been collected.[63] Recurrent bilateral tumours of the tympanic bodies have been reported in association with a family history of paragangliomas.[64, 65]

In the present context, there are no indications as to the cause of this tumour, although there have been reports of enlarged carotid bodies in relation to chronic hypoxaemia[66] and an increase in the incidence of carotid-body tumours at high altitudes.[67]

The relationship with hypoxia is of interest. In Peru there is a comparatively high incidence of paragangliomas of the head and neck in people born and living at altitudes of 2100–4350 m.[67] All the carotid-body tumours among the patients in one series were benign; one glomus jugulare tumour, in the same group, was malignant. A quantitative histological study on the carotid bodies of 10 normal rats and 10 rats living in a hypobaric chamber at a pressure of 460 mmHg (61.3 kPa) from 25 to 96 days showed a fourfold increase in the mean combined volume of the carotid bodies; there was an increase in vascularity which may be a mechanism to increase blood flow and thus oxygen transport to a hypoxic organ.[68]

Hyperplasia of the carotid bodies occurred in association with right ventricular cardiac hypertrophy complicating hypoxaemia and with left ventricular hypertrophy secondary to systemic hypertension.[69] Proliferation of the sustentacular cells was found.[70] It would be interesting to study the structure of the jugulotympanic bodies under similar conditions.

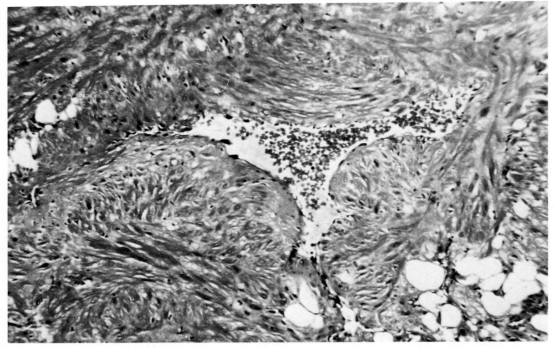

Fig. 17.25 Vascular hamartoma (angiofibrolipoma). Incidental finding in the tympanic cavity. Cushion-like endothelial formations protrude into the lumen. There are fibromatoid areas and also some fatty tissue.

Haematoxylin–eosin   × 200

TUMOURS AND TUMOUR-LIKE LESIONS OF THE CONNECTIVE TISSUE

Some tumours have been included in Tables 17.1 and 17.2 for the sake of completeness and will not be described.

Hamartoma (Fig. 17.25)

Clinically the rare angiolipomatous hamartomas, which by definition are benign, may resemble more sinister neoplasms such as Schwannomas of the vestibulocochlear nerve and cancer. Hamartomatous cerebral tissue in the middle ear is shown in Figure 17.26.

FIBROUS AND VASCULAR TUMOURS

The commonest benign connective tissue tumours of the auricle and external auditory meatus are *fibromas* and *haemangiomas* (Fig. 17.4). Occasionally these extend into the tympanic membrane. An *aggressive fibrous histiocytoma* was described in the external auditory meatus.[71]

A comprehensive review of the literature up to 1973 has traced 211 sarcomas of the ear, among them 64 rhabdomyosarcomas.[75]

Fibrosarcoma

Fibrosarcoma of the auricle is a rare tumour. Fibrosarcoma involving temporal bone and temporalis muscle 5 years after radiation therapy and nitrosourea therapy for cerebral glioma was reported recently.[72] Radiation-induced fibrosarcoma is rare but may follow 3–38 years after radiotherapy.[73]

Angiosarcoma

The auricle may also be involved in *Kaposi's angiosarcomatosis*. It is essential that the possibility of angiolymphoid hyperplasia be considered in any case in which the diagnosis of angiosarcoma is suggested by the appearances of the biopsy tissue.

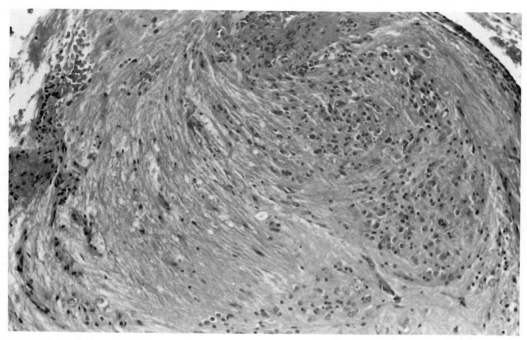

Fig. 17.26 Hamartomatous cerebral tissue found in the tympanic cavity. Normal brain tissue covered by squamous epithelium. Clinically a tumour was suspected.

Haematoxylin–eosin   × 180   *Provided by Dr P.H. Gruskin, St Vincent's Medical Center, Los Angeles, Cal, USA.*

CARTILAGINOUS AND BONY TUMOURS

Chondroma

Chondromas of the auricle have been reported. They may be bilateral. Malignant change has been observed.

Osteoma

The commonest of the osseous tumours of the temporal bone that come to the attention of the otologist are undoubtedly the osteomas (or exostoses—see below) of the acoustic meatus. Most of these growths arise from the tympanic ring and so adjoin the tympanic membrane; they present as single or multiple, often bilateral, nodules. Microscopically, they range in structure from dense sclerotic bone (ivory or eburnated osteoma) to soft spongy bone (cancellous osteoma) (Fig. 17.27). Some of the cancellous lesions are probably attributable to a reactive hyperplasia of bone caused by chronic inflammation or other factors. Osteomas of the external acoustic meatus occur relatively frequently in swimmers; the signific-

ance of this association is obscure.[74] There is no uniformity in the literature with regard to a distinction between 'exostosis' and 'osteoma'. For practical purposes it is permissible to refer to all bony lesions of the auditory apparatus as osteomas, without attempting to distinguish specifically between hyperplastic inflammatory lesions, hamartomas and true neoplasms.

Chondrosarcoma and osteosarcoma

These may arise in the bony wall of the meatus or elsewhere in the temporal bone.

MUSCLE TISSUE TUMOURS

Leiomyoma

A patient with a benign leiomyoma of the auricle was reported.[76]

Rhabdomyosarcoma

Rhabdomyosarcoma is the commonest sarcoma of the ear and occurs almost exclusively in children. In a review of literature prior to 1973, 64 cases of rhabdomyosarcoma were accepted.[75] The

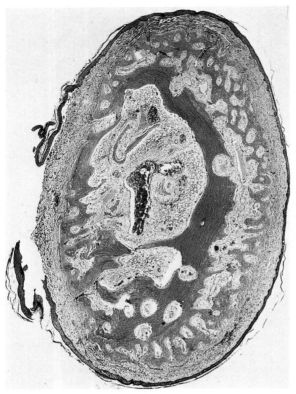

Fig. 17.27 Osteoma ('exostosis') of the external auditory meatus. The bone is covered by condensed dermal connective tissue and thinned epidermis.

Haematoxylin–eosin   × 19

more recent literature contains several additional case-reports.[77, 78]

The clinical manifestations as in cases of other malignant neoplasms of the ear may be misinterpreted as otitis media, usually of long duration. Histologically, most aural rhabdomyosarcomas are of the differentiated pleomorphic striated type. The demonstration of cross-striation is not an essential feature of diagnosis (Figs 17.28, 17.29, 17.30). Histochemical methods demonstrating the presence of dermin and electron microscopy are of diagnostic importance. Electron microscopy reveals the presence of malignant rhabdomyoblasts in various stages of differentiation containing immature sarcomeres and myofilaments.[79, 80]

Rhabdomyosarcoma of the ear may extend into the mastoid process (Fig. 17.30) and may penetrate into the parapharyngeal tissues, compressing the walls of the nasopharynx and oropharynx.[81] It may invade the posterior cerebral fossa. The prognosis is poor, but has been considerably improved by the introduction of extended therapy with cytotoxic drugs. 11 out of 24 patients with rhabdomyosarcoma of the ear were alive 2–7 years after multimodal chemotherapy.[82]

MALIGNANT MELANOMA

Primary malignant melanomas are rare and may occur at any age. At least three cases in early childhood are on record.[83] The tumour arises on the auricle or, occasionally, in the external auditory meatus.[84] Malignant melanoma in the middle ear and inner ear is probably always metastatic from a primary growth elsewhere in the body; peripheral facial palsy may be the first clinical manifestation (Fig. 17.31a, b).[85] In a series of 82 patients with malignant melanoma arising on the external ear, there were local recurrences in 23.5% of the patients after treatment, and 45.5% of the patients developed metastases to other parts of the body.[86] Early diagnosis is the key to effective treatment.[87]

NEUROGENIC TUMOURS

Schwannoma

Terminology
The terminology of the neurogenic tumours is confused, in large part because clinical usage of pathological nomenclature does not conform to the histopathological features. Tumours of the vestibulocochlear nerve are often referred to as 'acoustic neuromas', a term that, I believe, should be reserved for the histologically-featureless tumour-like lesions of traumatic origin that form, for example, on the chorda tympani.

The neurilemma or endoneurium is identical with the basal lamina material that plays an important role in the ultrastructural pattern of eighth nerve tumours (see page 342) but the term derived from it, *neurilemmoma*, has been spelt in so many ways that, in my opinion, it might with advantage be replaced by *Schwannoma* (the

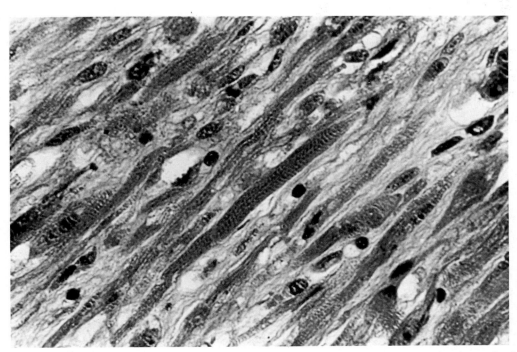

Fig. 17.28 Rhabdomyosarcoma of the ear. Striated rhabdomyoblasts are seen forming the main tumour in the internal auditory meatus (specimen as in Figure 17.29).   PTAH   × 600

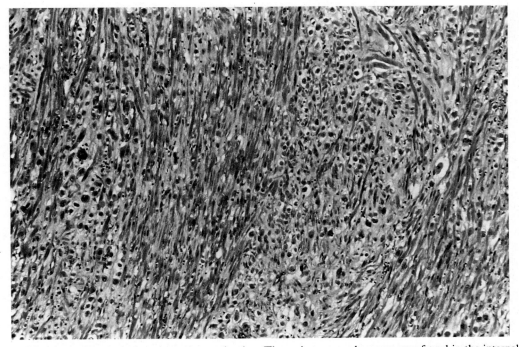

Fig. 17.29 Rhabdomyosarcoma presenting as an aural polyp. The main tumour, however, was found in the internal auditory meatus and had spread through the temporal bone. Bundles of spindle-shaped cells formed the greater part of the growth. In many places they are separated by large round rhabdomyoblasts. The latter appeared to predominate in the polypoid structures removed in the first instance.

Haematoxylin–eosin   × 225

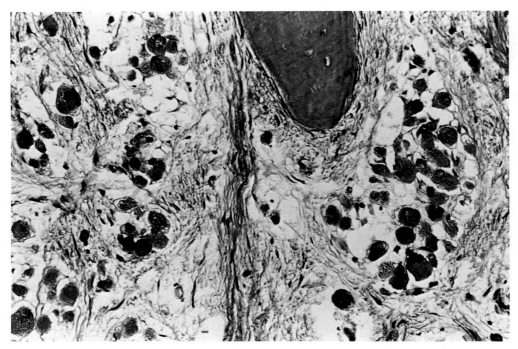

Fig. 17.30 Rhabdomyosarcoma of the ear. Bulky rhabdomyoblasts have invaded parts of the temporal bone.
Haematoxylin–eosin   × 320

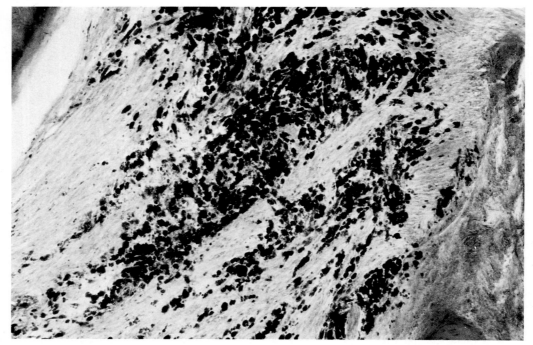

Fig. 17.31a Metastatic malignant melanoma invading the vestibulocochlear nerve and Scarpa's ganglion.
Haematoxylin–eosin   × 100

Provided by Dr J. Farkashidy, General Hospital, Toronto, Ont, Canada.

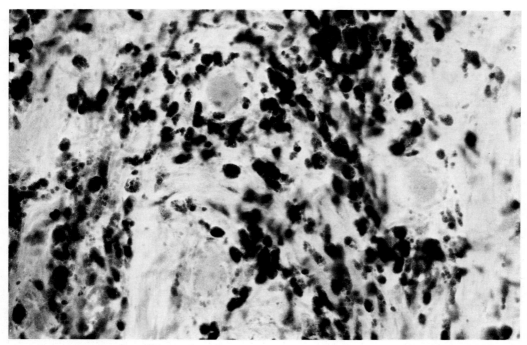

Fig. 17.31⟨i⟩ Metastatic malignant melanoma invading the vestibular nerve. Neurons surrounded by melanoblasts are seen (same specimen as in Fig. 17.31a).

Haematoxylin–eosin   × 400

Schwann cells are, of course, the cells forming the myelin sheaths of nerves).

The *Schwannoma of the vestibulocochlear* nerve is the most common neurogenic tumour of the aural region. Occasionally, such tumours may occur on the external ear,[88] along the facial nerve and in the region of the foramen jugulare.[89]

Usually the Schwannoma of the vestibulocochlear nerve presents clinically in the third or fourth decade. Women are affected more often than men. In spite of a history of loss of hearing of long duration, the tumour may remain undiagnosed (Fig. 17.32) and the symptoms may be misinterpreted for a cerebello-pontine angle tumour.

Origin and incidence
The majority of the tumours arise from the vestibular branch of the vestibulocochlear nerve. However, the cochlear branch was found on examination of a series of temporal bones to be the primary site in 3 out of 4 previously undiagnosed cases.[90] The true incidence of the tumour is unknown. The tumour may only be detected when

temporal bones are regularly examined histopathologically. The finding of occult Schwannomas in 0.9% of routinely-examined temporal bones[91] indicates greater incidence in the general population. Schwannomas of the eighth nerve account for about 8% of intracranial neoplasms. The tumour is usually unilateral, but bilateral instances are not rare. Some regard the bilateral tumours as a *forme fruste* of Recklinghausen's disease.

Histopathology
The features of peripheral-nerve tumours under the light microscope are variable, and the tendency has been to classify them in a single group as Schwannoma. This is not justifiable. Schwannomas and neurofibromas can be distinguished.

Schwannomas are generally encapsulated. They are composed of two readily-distinguishable types of tissue, a compact spindle-cell pattern with nuclear palisading forming Verocay bodies (the so-called Antoni type A) (Fig. 17.33), admixed in variable proportions with a looser and

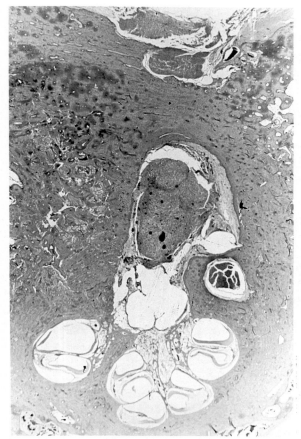

Fig. 17.32 Schwannoma of the vestibulocochlear nerve in the dilated internal auditory meatus. The tumour was a post-mortem finding. The patient, a man of 70, had been admitted to hospital critically ill in a comatous condition. The correct diagnosis was not made during life. Midmodiolar section of the temporal bone.

Haematoxylin-eosin   × 8

often more pleomorphic spindle-cell tissue with foam cells (Antoni type B).[92, 93, 94]

Neurofibromas, which may be diffuse or plexi-form, are tumours derived from the fibroblasts of the perineural tissue, are unencapsulated and do not contain Verocay bodies. They may be solitary or multiple. When multiple they constitute the condition of neurofibromatosis (Recklinghausen's disease). It is noteworthy that Schwannomas may also be present in neurofibromatosis. Neurofibromas of the vestibulocochlear nerve may form large bulky masses and may be confused with a myxoma. The cells of neurofibromas have comma-shaped or 'tear-drop' nuclei with a fine chromatin pattern. Myxomas are composed of stellate cells with elongated cytoplasmic tails and their nuclei tend to be more hyperchromatic than those of the cells of neurofibromas.

Ultrastructure

The ultrastructure of Schwannomas has many characteristic features. The convoluted densely packed processes of the Schwann cells form a network in which there are some widely scattered nuclei or nuclei forming small groups.

The processes of the Schwann cells are enveloped by dense layers of homogeneous basal lamina material, another dominant feature of these tumours. There are some characteristic

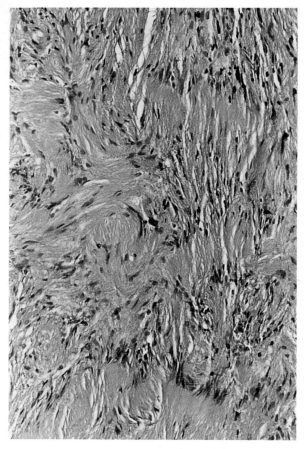

Fig. 17.33 Schwannoma of the vestibulocochlear nerve. The interwoven bundles of fibres and the palisading of the nuclei of the tumour Schwann cells are seen (case as Figure 17.32).

Haematoxylin–eosin   × 150

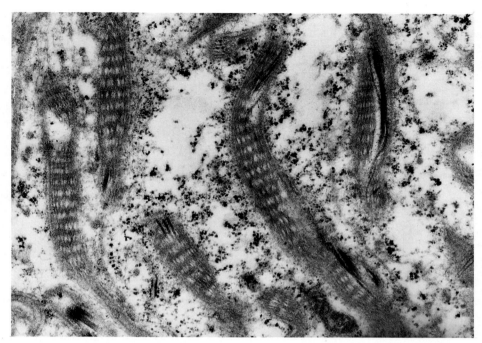

Fig. 17.34 Schwannoma of the vestibulocochlear nerve. Electron micrograph showing multiple bands of long-spacing collagen. A characteristic ultrastructural feature of Schwannomas.   × 10 650

banded structures in the basal lamina. Although not entirely specific, they are almost always present in Schwannomas of the vestibulocochlear nerve and offer a valuable clue to the diagnosis (Fig. 17.34).[95-98] Intercellular and intracellular examples of these structures formed by long-spacing collagen have been interpreted as stages of an enzymatically-induced degradation of collagen in which lysis of the collagen leads to splitting of the degenerating or decomposing fibres, thus revealing their subfibrillar structure.

Differences can be demonstrated in the collagen in Schwannomas, neurofibromas and fibromas.[99] Collagen in Schwannomas is composed mainly of thin, argyrophile, weakly birefringent fibres formed by thin collagen fibrils (type 3 collagen). Fibromas contain only thick, non-argyrophile strongly birefringent fibres composed of thick collagen fibrils (type 1 collagen). In neurofibromas collagen of both these types is found in different areas.

Surgical consideration

Microsurgical methods for the removal of Schwannomas of the vestibulocochlear nerves allow total removal of the tumour in a large proportion of cases while preserving the facial nerve. For surgical purposes it is helpful to class the tumour into these groups: those confined to the internal auditory meatus; those projecting into the cerebellopontine angle but not causing pressure on the brain stem or cerebellum and those large enough to press on the brain stem and cerebellum.

Malignant Schwannoma

Malignant neurogenic tumours are rare and malignant Schwannomas of the vestibulocochlear nerve have rarely been reported.[94] Some irregularity of nuclear shape and size is fairly common but cannot be regarded as a morphological index of malignant change in a Schwannoma of the vestibulocochlear nerve.

Neuroma of the chorda tympani

This tumour-like lesion is rare and may present, in some cases of chronic otitis media, behind the tympanic membrane embedded in inflammatory granulation tissue. It is analogous with the post-traumatic neuroma which may result after trans-

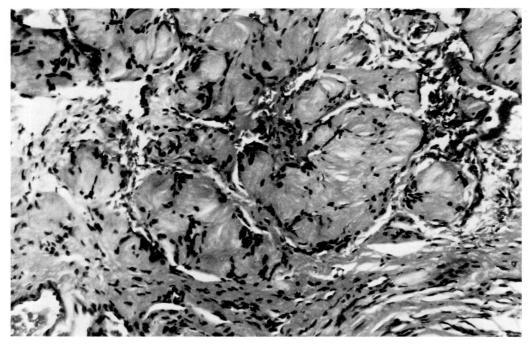

Fig. 17.35a Tactile (Pacinian) neurofibroma of the stapedius tendon. Microscopy shows the tumour to be composed of lobular structures resembling the Pacinian corpuscles (normal pressure receptors). Higher magnifications showed the individual structures to consist of balls of elongated cells arranged in lamellae and separated by delicate collagen fibres. Some seemed to have a central core of spindle-shaped cells, others of some homogenous myelin-like material.

Provided by Drs H. van Goethem and J. Marquet, University of Antwerp, Belgium.   Haematoxylin–eosin   × 190

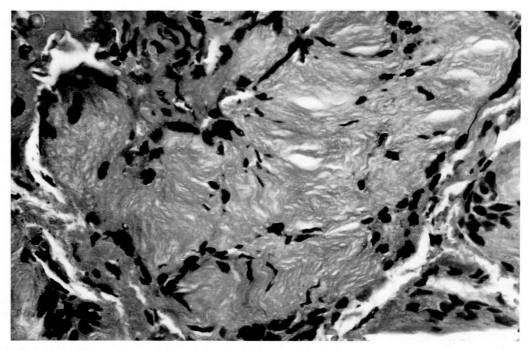

Fig. 17.35b A tactile-like structure composed of elongated cells. probably Schwann cells, with scattered nuclei.
Haematoxylin–eosin   × 480

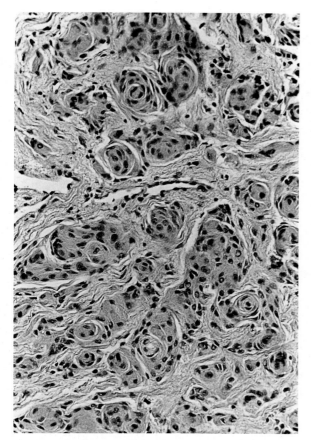

Fig. 17.36 Meningioma of the temporal bone. The tumour consists of meningiothelia and fibroblast-like cells forming characteristic 'whorls'.

Haematoxylin–eosin   × 150

labyrinthe section of the vestibular nerve for the treatment of dizziness.[100]

Tactile (Pacinian) neurofibroma

Tactile neurofibromas have been described in the skin.[101] A similar tumour removed from the stapedius muscle or tendon is the first to have been found in the middle ear.[102] Microscopy shows the tumour to be composed of lobular structures resembling the Pacinian corpuscles—the normal pressure receptors (Fig. 17.35a). Higher magnification showed the individual structures to consist of balls of elongated cells arranged in lamellae and separated by delicate collagen fibres (Fig. 17.35b). Some contained a central core of spindle-shaped cells or of some homogenous myelin-like material.

Meningioma involving the temporal bone[103]

Meningioma of the temporal bone may present in two forms: 1) as an extension of an intracranial meningioma; 2) unaccompanied by an intracranial meningioma. It may invade the internal auditory meatus and present as a cerebellopontine-angle tumour (Fig. 17.36). Occasionally aggressive meningiomas may spread within the lumen of the internal jugular vein, presenting as a swelling of the neck. I have seen such a case misdiagnosed as a carotid body tumour.

Tumours of the cerebellopontine angle

The commonest tumours of this site are in order of occurrence: acoustic Schwannoma of the vestibulocochlear nerve, meningioma, epidermoid cholesteatoma, and Schwannoma of the facial or of other cranial nerves in the posterior cerebral fossa. In a series of 1354 cerebellopontine-angle tumours studied by the Otologic Medical Group, Los Angeles,[104] there were 91.3% Schwannomas of the vestibulocochlear nerve; 3.1% meningiomas; 2.4% epidermoid cholesteatomas and the remainder Schwannomas of various nerves.

There were a further 25 rare tumours occurring as cerebellopontine-angle lesions. 7 patients had arachnoid cysts in the cerebellopontine angle. 5 patients had tumours of blood-vessel origin in the cerebellopontine angle: 4 haemangiomas and 1 haemangioblastoma. In 2 cases the tumour was an astrocytoma, and in 2 cases, a medulloblastoma. 6 other tumours were located in the cerebellopontine angle: 2 dermoids, 2 lipomas, 1 chondrosarcoma and 1 malignant teratoma. Paragangliomas may present as cerebellopontine-angle tumours and may invade the cerebellum.

The benign lesions occurring in the cerebellopontine angle can sometimes be removed by an approach that maintains hearing. Particularly in the case of arachnoid cysts, a retrolabyrinthine approach can establish the diagnosis and treat the disease while preserving hearing. Prognosis for malignant lesions in this location is poor because total removal is difficult, if not impossible, without injuring adjacent vital brain-stem structures.

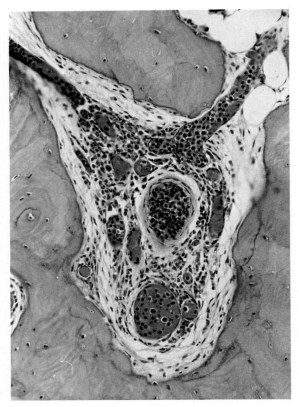

Fig. 17.37 Myeloid leukaemia. A fibrovascular space in the mastoid process is infiltrated by leukaemic cells.

Haematoxylin-eosin   × 160

MISCELLANEOUS LESIONS

Leukaemia

Leukaemic infiltration of the temporal bone and of the inner ear is common but its true incidence is not known (Fig. 17.37). Occasionally an apparently purulent discharge suggestive of otitis media may be a presenting sign.[14] I have observed this in chloroma, confirmed by autopsy which revealed green-coloured deposits of leukaemic cells in the temporal bone and orbit together with similar infiltrates in the dura and elsewhere in the body.

Burkitt's lymphoma

Involvement of the mastoid process by Burkitt's lymphoma has been reported.[105]

Mycosis fungoides

An instance of this disease presenting with pulsating tinnitus and facial palsy has been described. It involved the middle-ear cleft and the central nervous system. Sézary cells were found in the cerebrospinal fluid.[106] This cell, also called the 'mycosis fungoides cell', has a characteristic markedly convoluted nucleus confirmed by electron microscopy.[107]

SECONDARY TUMOURS

Secondary tumours of the ear are more common than the number of published cases would suggest, because of the apparent lack of interest by pathologists in the barren regions of the temporal bone.

The temporal bone and the ear may be the site of lymph-borne or blood-borne metastatic deposits and it may be directly invaded by a growth arising in the Eustachian tube or spreading along it from the postnasal region. The external ear may be invaded by neoplasms of the parotid gland and these may be difficult to distinguish from tumours of the ceruminous glands.

In a series of 145 temporal bones removed routinely at necropsy, I found 6 instances of secondary cancer, various parts of the ear being involved, including the mastoid process, the facial or vestibulocochlear nerve and the major veins. The primary growth was situated in a parotid gland in one case, in the larynx in three cases (Fig. 17.38a,b) in the rectum once and in a breast once.

In a review of 103 published cases, in 17.7% the primary tumour was carcinoma of the breast, in 11.8% a bronchial carcinoma and in 9.8% a renal carcinoma.[108] In an examination of 19 temporal bones from 11 patients who had metastatic deposits in the bone, the distant primary growths included one adenocarcinoma of the breast, 2 adenocarcinomas of the prostate, one squamous cell carcinoma of the tonsil, 3 cases of malignant melanoma, and 2 adenocarcinomas the primary site of which could not be determined. The remaining 2 cases were malignant lymphomas.[85] Such findings lend strong support to the value of systematic investigation at necropsy of the tem-

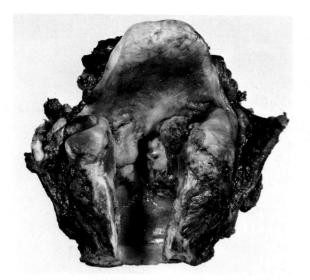

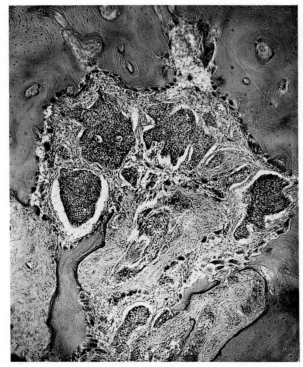

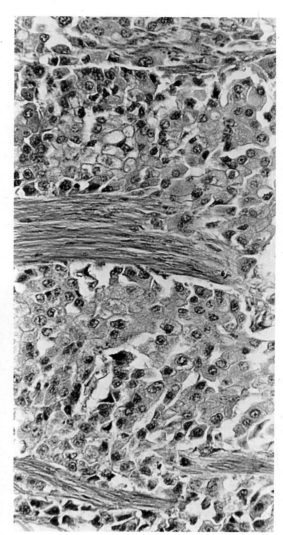

Fig. 17.39 Vestibulocochlear nerve and Scarpa's ganglion infiltrated by metastatic carcinoma of bronchial origin disrupting the nerve fibres.

Haematoxylin–eosin   × 200

Fig. 17.38a and b Primary squamous cell carcinoma of the larynx. The tumour spread along the internal jugular vein and invaded the mastoid process as shown in (**b**).

Haematoxylin–eosin   × 75

poral bones in confirming that they are not uncommon sites of secondary deposits. Mammary, bronchial, renal (Fig. 17.39), prostatic[109, 110] and rectal[111] rendered neoplasms (Fig. 17.40) are the most frequent sources of metastatic tumour in the temporal bone. The latency of both primary and secondary neoplasms of the ear and temporal bone has been recognized; although the secondary tumour in the ear may be, in fact, the first and even the only clinical manifestation of a distant primary tumour. Metastatic malignant melanoma to both eighth nerves developed 6 years after the excision of a melanoma from the right shoulder.[112]

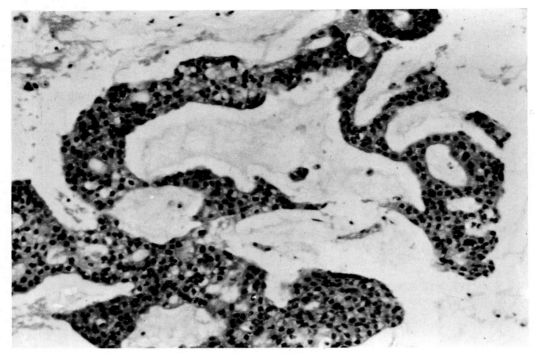

Fig. 17.40 Metastatic mucoid adenocarcinoma in the temporal bone. The primary growth was in a breast.
Haematoxylin-eosin   × 340

REFERENCES

1. Lodge WO, Jones HM. Smith MEN. Arch Otolaryngol 1955; 61: 535.
2. Fairman HD. In: Ballantyne J, Groves J, eds. Scott Brown's Diseases of the ear, nose and throat. 4th ed. London: Butterworths, 1979; 321.
3. Kimura T, Yoshimura S, Ishikawa E. Trans Soc Pathol Jpn 1948; 37: 179.
4. Wells GC, Whimster I. Br J Dermatol 1969; 81: 1.
5. Nelson SM, Meyers SD. Trans Am Acad Opthalmol Otolaryngol 1977; 86: 680.
6. Reed RJ, Terazakis N. Cancer 1972; 29: 489.
6a. Fukamizu H, Imaizumi SH. Arch Dermatol 1984; 120: 1238.
7. Yadav YC. J Laryngol 1969; 83: 935.
8. Saenger A. Munch Med Wschr 1900; 47: 341.
9. Conley J, Schuller DE. Laryngoscope 1976; 86: 1147.
9a. Wagenfield DJH, Kean ET, Nostrand AWP, et al. Laryngoscope 1980; 90: 912.
10. Alberts MC, Terence CF. J Laryngol Otol 1978; 92: 233.
11. Chen KTK, Dehner LP. Arch Otolaryngol 1978; 104: 247.
12. Kleinsasser O, Schulze W, Glanz H. HNO 1984; 32: 61.
13. Diamant M. Acta Otolaryngol (Stockh) 1954; (Suppl. 118): 54.
14. Friedmann I. Pathology of the ear. Oxford: Blackwell, 1974; 128: 362.
15. Peron DL, Schuknecht HF. Arch Otolaryngol 1975; 101: 498.
16. Taylor GD, Martin HF. Arch Otolaryngol 1961; 73: 651.
17. Abadir WF, Pease WS. J Laryngol Otol; 92: 247.
18. Caplinger CB, Hora JF. Arch Otolaryngol 1967; 85: 365.
19. Cannon RC, McLean WC. Otolaryngol Head Neck Surg 1983; 91: 96.
20. Hyams VJ, Michaels L. Clin Otolaryngol 1976; 1: 17.
20a. Mills SE, Fechner RE. Am J Surg Pathol 1984; 8: 677.
21. Riches WG, Johnson WH. Am J Clin Path 1982; 77: 153.
22. Jahrsdoerfer RA, Fechner RE, Selman JW, Moon CN, Powell JB. Laryngoscope 1983; 93: 1041.
23. Eden AR, Pincus RL, Parisier SC, Som PM. Laryngoscope 1984; 94: 63.
24. Pallanch JF, McDonald TJ, Weiland LH et al. Laryngoscope 1982; 92: 47.
25. Schuller DE, Conley JJ, Goodman JH, Clausen KP, Miller WJ. Otolaryngol Head Neck Surg 1983; 91: 280.
26. Pulec JL. Laryngoscope 1977; 87: 1601.
27. Hicks GW. Laryngoscope 1983; 93: 326.
28. Goodhill V. Ear diseases, deafness and dizziness. Hagerstown, MD: Harper and Row, 1979.
29. Jahnke V, Bender Gotze C. Laryngol Rhinol Otol (Stuttg) 1975; 54: 692.
30. Wetli CV, Pardo V, Millard M, Gerston K. Cancer 1972; 29: 1169.

31. Friedmann I, Osborn DA. The pathology of granulomas and neoplasms of the nose and paranasal sinuses. Oxford: Blackwell, 1982.
32. Thackray AC, Lucas RB. Tumours of the major salivary glands. Washington: AFIP, 1974: Fasc 32.
33. Perzin KH, Gullane P, Conley J. Cancer 1982; 50: 2873.
34. Michel RC, Woodard BH, Shelburne JD, Bossen EH. Cancer 1978; 41: 545.
35. Fliegel Z, Kaneko M. Cancer 1975; 36: 1072.
36. Friedmann I. J Clin Pathol 1983; 97: 465.
37. Nochomovitz LE, Kahn LB. Arch Pathol 1974; 97: 141.
38. Thomas K, Hutt MRS. J Clin Path 1981; 34: 1003.
39. Oberndorfer S. Frankfurt Z Pathol 1907; 1: 426.
40. Pearse AGE, Polak JM. Gut 1971; 12: 783.
41. Riddle PJ, Font RL, Zimmerman LE. Hum Pathol 1982; 13: 459.
42. Murphy GF, Pilch BZ, Dickerstein GR, Goodman GI, Nadol GB. Am J Clin Path 1980; 73: 816.
43. Farrior JB, Hyams VJ, Bemke RH, Brown FJ. Laryngoscope 1980; 90: 110.
44. Friedmann I, Galey FR, House WF, Carberry JN, Ward PP. J Laryngol 1983; 97: 465.
45. Inoue S, Tanaka K, Kannae S. Virchows Arch (Pathol Anat) 1982; 396: 357.
45a. Manni JJ, van Haelst UJGM, Kubat K, Marres EHMA. HNO 1984; 32: 419.
45b. Fujita T. Arch Histol (Jpn) 1977; Suppl. 40.
46. Glenner GG, Crimley PM. Atlas of tumour pathology. Washington DC: AFIP, 1974: Second Series, Fasc 9.
47. Kleinsasser O. Arch Ohrenheilk 1970; 184: 214.
48. Valentin G. Arch Anat Phys Wiss Med 1940; 287.
49. Guild SR. Anat Rec 1941; 79 (Suppl. 2): 28.
50. Guild SR. Ann Otol Rhinol Laryngol 1953; 62: 1045.
51. Lawson W. Laryngoscope 1980; 90: 120.
52. Rosenwasser H, Otani S. Proc Roy Soc Med 1974; 67: 259.
53. Rosenwasser H. Arch Otolaryngol 1945; 41: 64.
54. Chen KTK, Dehner LF. Arch Otolaryngol 1978; 104: 253.
55. Friedmann I. Pathology of the ear. Oxford: Blackwell, 1974; 175.
56. Veldman JE, Mulder PHM, Sjef HJ, et al. Arch Otolaryngol 1980; 106: 547.
57. Falck B, et al. J Histochem Cytochem 1962; 10: 348.
58. Strauss M, Nicholas GG, Abt AB, Harrison TS, Seaton JF. Otolaryngol Head Neck Surg 1983; 91: 315.
59. Schade R. Brit J Cancer 1953; 7: 449.
60. Chretien PB, Engelman K, Hoye RC, et al. Am J Surg 1971; 122: 7400.
61. Gerlings PG. Pract Otorhinolaryngol 1970; 32: 164.
62. Schwartz ML, Israel HL. Arch Otolaryngol 1983; 109: 269.
63. Rangwala AF, Sylvia LC, Becker SM. Cancer 1978; 42: 2865.
64. House WF, Graham MD. Arch Otolaryngol 1973; 98: 58.
65. Kowatsch K, Carson M, Ramel MP, Bourdiniere G. Rev Laryngol Rhinol Otol (Bord) 1978; 99: 747.
66. Arias-Stella J, Valcarel J. Hum Pathol 1976; 7: 361.
67. Saldana MJ, Salem LE, Travenzan R. Hum Pathol 1973; 4: 251.
68. Laidler P, Kay JM. J Pathol 1975; 124: 27.
69. Smith P, Jago R, Heath D. J Pathol 1982; 137: 287.
70. Heath D, Smith P, Jago R. J Pathol 1982; 138: 115.
71. Cremer H, Totouk V, Sutter S. Laryng Rhinol Otol 1983; 62: 77.
72. Case Record 40-1983. N Eng J Med, 1983; 309: 843.
73. Gane NFC, Lindup R, Strickland P, Bennett MH. Brit J Cancer 1970; 24: 705.
74. Harrison DFN. Ann Roy Coll Surg Engl 1962; 31: 187.
75. Naufal PM. Arch Otolaryngol 1973; 98: 44.
76. Inoue F, Marsumoto K. Arch Dermatol 1983; 119: 445.
77. Deutsch M, Felder H. Laryngoscope 1974; 84: 586.
78. Dehner LP, Chen KT. Arch Otolaryngol 1978; 104: 399.
79. Friedmann I, Harrison DFN, Tucker WN, Bird ES. J Clin Pathol 1965; 18: 63.
80. Hosoda S, Suzumi H, Kawabe Y, et al. Cancer 1971; 27: 29.
81. Jaffe BF, Fox JE, Batsakis JG. Cancer 1971; 27: 29.
82. Schuller DA. Arch Otolaryngol 1979; 105: 689.
83. Shanon E, Samuel Y, Adler A, Rapoport Y, Redianu C. Arch Otolaryngol 1976; 102: 244.
84. Friedmann I, Radcliffe A. J Laryngol Otol 1954; 68: 114.
85. Jahn AF, Farkshidy J, Berman JM. J Otolaryngol 1979; 8: 85.
86. Conley J. Pack Medical Foundation 1979; p. 106.
87. Balch CM, Soong SJ, Milton GW, et al. Cancer 1983; 52: 1748.
88. Fodor RI, Pastore PN, Frable MA. Laryngoscope 1977; 87: 1760.
89. Clemic JD, Noffsinger D, Derlacki EL. Trans Am Acad Opthalmol Otolaryngol 1977; 84: 687.
90. Thomsen J, Jorgensen MB. Arch Klin Exp Ohren Nas Kehlheilk 1973; 204: 175.
91. Stewart TJ, Liland J, Schuknecht HF. Arch Otolaryngol 1975; 101: 91.
92. Abell MR, Hart WR, Olsen JR. Hum Pathol 1970; 1: 503.
93. Asbury AK, Johnson PC. Major Probl Pathol 1978; 9:
94. Grushkin P, Carberry JN. In: House WF, Luetje CM, eds. Acoustic tumours. Vol. 1: Diagnosis. Baltimore: University Park Press, 1980: Ch. 6.
95. Luse SA. Neurology 1960; 10: 881.
96. Friedmann I, Cawthorne T, Bird ES. J Ultrastruc Res 1965; 12: 92.
97. Conley FK, Rubinstein IJ, Spence AM. Acta Neuropathol 1976; 34: 293.
98. Nemetchek-Gansler H, Meinel A, Nemetscek T. Virchows Arch (Pathol Anat) 1977; 375: 185.
99. Junqueira LCU, Moates GS, Kaupert D, Shigihara KM, Bolonhani TM, Krisztan RM. J Neuropathol Exp Neurol 1981; 40: 123.
100. Linthicum FH, Alonso A, Denia A. Arch Otolaryngol 1979; 105: 654.
101. Macdonald DM, Wilson-Jones E. Histopathol 1977; 1: 247.
102. Goethem van H, Friedmann I, Marquet J. J Laryngol 1985; 99: 187.
103. Nager GT. Ir J Med Sc 1966; Series 6, 483: 69.
104. Brackmann DE, Bartels LJ. Otolaryngol Head Neck Surg 1980; 88: 555.
105. Oyetunji NMA, Lapado AA. J Laryngol 1981; 95: 1063.

106. Zackheim HS, Lebo CF, Wasserstein P, et al. Arch Dermatol 1983; 119: 311.

107. Haber H, Milne JA. In: Systemic pathology 1980, 2nd ed. Vol. 6. Edinburgh: Churchill Livingstone; 2783.

108. Hill BA, Kohut RI. Arch Otolaryngol 1976; 102: 568.

109. Applebaum EL, Dolsky RL. Trans Am Acad Opthalmol Otolaryngol 1977; 84: 154.

110. Franks LM. Lance 1956; ii: 1037.

111. Sadek SAA, Dixon NW, Hardcastle PF. J Laryngol Otol 1983; 97: 459.

112. Harbert F, Liu J-Ch, Berry RG. J Laryngol Otol 1969; 83: 889.

Index